British Poultry Standards

Seventh Edition

British Poultry Standards

Complete specifications and judging points of all standardised breeds and varieties of poultry as compiled by the specialist affiliated Breed Clubs and recognised by the Poultry Club of Great Britain

Seventh Edition

Co-edited by
J. Ian H. Allonby
Trustee, Standards Lead
Poultry Club of Great Britain

Philippe B. Wilson
MChem(Hons) PhD MRSC MRSB FLS FHEA
Trustee, Chairman Poultry & Eggs Committee
Poultry Club of Great Britain

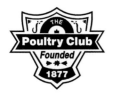

The Poultry Club
OF GREAT BRITAIN

WILEY Blackwell

This edition first published 2019
© 2019 Poultry Club of Great Britain
Edition History [John Wiley and Sons 6e, 2009]

The right of J. Ian H. Allonby and Philippe B. Wilson to be identified as the authors of this work has been asserted in accordance with law.

Registered Office(s)
John Wiley & Sons, Inc., 111 River Street, Hoboken, NJ 07030, USA
John Wiley & Sons Ltd., The Atrium, Southern Gate, Chichester, West Sussex, PO19 8SQ, UK.

Editorial Office
9600 Garsington Road, Oxford, OX4 2DQ, UK

For details of our global editorial offices, customer services, and more information about Wiley products visit us at www.wiley.com.

Wiley also publishes its books in a variety of electronic formats and by print-on-demand. Some content that appears in standard print versions of this book may not be available in other formats.

Limit of Liability/Disclaimer of Warranty

The contents of this work are intended to further general scientific research, understanding, and discussion only and are not intended and should not be relied upon as recommending or promoting scientific method, diagnosis, or treatment by physicians for any particular patient. In view of ongoing research, equipment modifications, changes in governmental regulations, and the constant flow of information relating to the use of medicines, equipment, and devices, the reader is urged to review and evaluate the information provided in the package insert or instructions for each medicine, equipment, or device for, among other things, any changes in the instructions or indication of usage and for added warnings and precautions. While the publisher and authors have used their best efforts in preparing this work, they make no representations or warranties with respect to the accuracy or completeness of the contents of this work and specifically disclaim all warranties, including without limitation any implied warranties of merchantability or fitness for a particular purpose. No warranty may be created or extended by sales representatives, written sales materials or promotional statements for this work. The fact that an organization, website, or product is referred to in this work as a citation and/or potential source of further information does not mean that the publisher and authors endorse the information or services the organization, website, or product may provide or recommendations it may make. This work is sold with the understanding that the publisher is not engaged in rendering professional services. The advice and strategies contained herein may not be suitable for your situation. You should consult with a specialist where appropriate. Further, readers should be aware that websites listed in this work may have changed or disappeared between when this work was written and when it is read. Neither the publisher nor authors shall be liable for any loss of profit or any other commercial damages, including but not limited to special, incidental, consequential, or other damages.

Library of Congress Cataloging-in-Publication Data

Names: Allonby, J. Ian H., editor. | Wilson, Philippe B., editor.
Title: British poultry standards : complete specifications and judging points of all standardized breeds and varieties of poultry as compiled by the specialist affiliated breed clubs and recognized by the Poultry Club of Great Britain / co-edited by J. Ian H. Allonby, Philippe B. Wilson.
Description: Seventh edition. | Chichester, UK ; Hoboken, NJ : John Wiley & Sons, 2018. |
Identifiers: LCCN 2018023892 (print) | LCCN 2018035716 (ebook) | ISBN 9781119509172 (Adobe PDF) | ISBN 9781119509196 (ePub) | ISBN 9781119509141 (hardcover)
Subjects: LCSH: Poultry–Judging. | Poultry breeds. | Poultry–Standards.
Classification: LCC SF485 (ebook) | LCC SF485 .B75 2018 (print) | DDC 636.5/1–dc23
LC record available at https://lccn.loc.gov/2018023892

Cover image: © The Poultry Club of Great Britain
Cover design by Wiley

Set in 9.5/11 pt SabonLTStd-Roman by Thomson Digital, Noida, India

10 9 8 7 6 5 4 3 2 1

Contents

Turkeys 345

Waterfowl 363
Geese 363

Acknowledgements

The Editors and the Poultry Club of Great Britain (PCGB) wish to acknowledge the Breed Clubs for their cooperation in compiling this new edition. Additionally, the PCGB thanks Jed Dwight, Rupert Stephenson, Tim Daniels, Joshua Kittle, Christopher Parker, Victoria Roberts, Michael Corrigan, Graham Hicks, John Tarren, David Scrivener, Alan Davies, Malcom Thompson, Geoff Parker, the Breed Clubs and Arnaud Asselin for providing illustrations and photographs. Illustrations of Dominique are from the American Standard of Perfection 1974.

Introduction

Standards for pure breeds of poultry owe their origin to the popularity of exhibition and the need for a benchmark by which they could be judged fairly; individual exhibits of a breed needed to be judged against each other. There was a call, therefore, for uniformity of type (encompassing body, shape, and carriage) together with a breed's colouration while taking into account egg production and table values in those classified as Utility. Apart from these attributes, Standards needed to embody the ideal characteristics which defined not only each individual breed to make them distinctive from others but also the specific colours and markings of particular varieties within a breed. Standards needed to be formulated to serve as a guide for breeders, exhibitors, and judges alike.

It was as long ago as 1865 that the Poultry Club authorised the publication of the first *Standard of Excellence in Exhibition Poultry*, edited by W.B. Tegetmeier and published by Groombridge & Sons. This was the first book of its kind in the world. Two years later, in 1867, it was adopted by the American Poultry Society and published in the United States by A.M. Halsted, complete with alterations and additions to suit the fancy in America.

The original Poultry Club lasted just three years before being disbanded with the second, and current, Poultry Club of Great Britain being founded in 1877. During the intervening period, W.B. Tegetmeier's *The Poultry Book* was published in 1867, followed by a new edition in 1873. This book contained not only the original British 'Standards of Excellence' but outlined comparisons with those of America – notably that the original 'Scale of Points' for each exhibit was 15 in Britain while being 100 across the Atlantic.

It was Lewis Wright who next published Standards for exhibition poultry in his 1873 work *The Illustrated Book of Poultry*, making every attempt to achieve uniformity in the way the Standards were set out. Each bird was considered perfect to begin with and allocated 100 'Points of Merit', from which various points for 'Defects to be Deducted' were to be subtracted. The defects and points varied from breed to breed. Clearly, after this, it must have been realised that 15 points were inadequate when grading exhibits and, in Britain too, the 'Scale of Points' in each breed Standard was to total 100 from then on.

A Scale of Points for each breed is important. While judges in Britain may not necessarily award a percentage mark when awarding prizes, it is a breed's 'Scale of Points' which highlights, at a glance, the features which are regarded as significantly important for that particular breed. This may or may not be so apparent in the actual wording of the Standards as the following examples reveal: 'Colour' in Andalusians accounting for 50 points, 60 in a Hamburgh, but just 9 in Old English Game Bantams, while a Norfolk Black Turkey's 'Head' is considered to be worth 20 points in comparison with a lowly 5 for this feature in a Sebastopol Goose where 'Conditioning & Feathering' attract 40 points. Scales of Points can be useful, too, when comparisons between different breeds and species are made to arrive at the award of Show Champion.

After the second Poultry Club was founded in 1877, its initial series of Standards Books for Poultry was initiated. The first edition of *Poultry Club Standards*, edited by Alexander Comyns, was published by the Poultry Club in 1886 with subsequent editions of 1901

British Poultry Standards, Seventh Edition. Edited by J. Ian H. Allonby and Philippe B. Wilson.
© 2019 Poultry Club of Great Britain. Published 2019 by John Wiley & Sons Ltd.

edited by T. Threlford, published by Casell & Company; 1905 edited by Lewis Wright, also published by Casell & Company; 1910, 1922, and the sixth in 1923, all edited by William W. Broomhead; then the seventh in 1926, with the last of the first series, the eighth, published in 1930. Following the Second World War, *Poultry World* took over as publisher and here the modern-day series of editions began. The first edition was published in 1954; the second in 1960; the third in 1971, edited by C.G. May; the fourth in 1982, edited by David Hawksworth; and then the fifth in 1997 and sixth in 2008 were both edited by Victoria Roberts. Publishers changed during the series to Butterworths, to Blackwell, and to John Wiley & Sons, which acquired Blackwell Publishing in 2007 to become Wiley Blackwell.

Right from the very beginning, therefore, the Poultry Club has remained guardian of the Standards without necessarily being the body responsible for framing them. This task is normally undertaken by the specialist Breed Club or by the originator of a new breed or variety. So seriously, however, is this guardianship imposed, and accepted by the clubs, that until a new variety is admitted to Standard it remains unrecognised by show authorities whose events are staged under the rules of the Poultry Club of Great Britain.

Current procedures for the admittance of a new breed or variety of an existing breed to Standard are comprehensive. A Provisional Standard must first be submitted to the relevant Breed Club not only for its recommendation but also for postal ballot approval by its members. Once this is received, the proposed Standard with particulars of origin and breeding together with a list of breeders and the ballot papers must then be submitted for full standardisation by the Poultry Club. This is when further criteria, including a signed declaration, have to be met – the breed or variety has to satisfy Council as to its purity and whether it breeds true to type and colour; specimens of the proposed breed or variety need to have been exhibited in non-Standard classes; three rung generations of the new breed or colour should be available for inspection by the Poultry Club; a new breed has to possess distinctive characteristics and a new colour variety has to conform to the character of the breed concerned. The only exception to these procedures is when a recognised breed is imported from another country in which it has already been accepted to Standard.

Since the middle of the last century the introduction of hybrid strains of layers and broilers has meant that, commercially, pure breeds of poultry have been kept less and less. However, the fact that these hybrids owe their origin to Standard pure bred poultry is appreciated. The Poultry Club not only represents our hobby with the Department for Environment, Food, and Rural Affairs (DEFRA) but as custodian of British Poultry Standards is involved with the preservation of these traditional breeds, especially those that have originated in Britain. The significance of the pool of genetic resources retained in the pure breeds is recognised as important should hybrid strains need to be remade due to disease.

To safeguard publication interests the Poultry Club has agreed not to accept or authorise publication of any alterations to existing Standards for a period of two years from the issue of this edition. The Poultry Club, through its affiliated Breed Clubs, maintains the strictest watch on these Standards of Excellence. It will not allow alterations or amendments until its governing Council has made a thorough examination of all the circumstances. Once established, whole-scale alterations to existing Standards due to fashion should not happen. They should not stray too far from the original. In this way the Poultry Club can be truly said to be the guardian of the Standards and so plays its part in ensuring that our pure breeds of poultry will be part of the heritage we pass on to future generations.

Indeed, with recent advances in the science of agricultural feeds, some breeds may be increasing in size. This is less an issue for large fowl examples; however, in order to maintain the dichotomy between the two sizes of most breeds, it is important for breeders and ourselves as the guardians of the Standards to maintain a watchful eye on size deterioration. Furthermore, greater numbers of breeds are seeing decreases in the size differences between their bantam and large fowl equivalents – a worrying factor when assessing Standards with strictly stipulated weights. The Standards established within this and earlier editions provide distinct judging points to guide and inform the judge, exhibitor, and breeder. Although strictly defined, each Standard can be used as a guide to establish the viability of stock and provides the blueprint for judges to carry out their duties at shows.

This edition has been thoroughly revised and edited, with numerous changes to breed pictures and profiles providing a well-defined update for contemporary breeding, judging, and exhibiting. It is also intended for use as a manual to aid in the instruction and identification of breeds for the novice through to the veterinary surgeon.

J. Ian H. Allonby and Philippe B. Wilson

Standard feather markings

Plate 1

1 Hackle feather conforming to Standard as applying to brown Leghorn and other males of black-red colouring. Note the absence of shaftiness, black fringing, and tipping. The actual colour of the outer border varies in different breeds between dark orange and pale lemon. In such breeds the saddle hackle should conform closely to the neck hackle.

1A Faulty hackle in the same breeds. There is considerable shaftiness, the striping runs through, and the feather is tipped with black. Striping is also indefinite and fouled with red.

2 Hackle feather conforming to Standard from the partridge Wyandotte male. There is no shaftiness and the striping is very solid and distinct. In partridge Wyandottes lemon-coloured hackles are a desirable exhibition point.

2A Faulty neck hackle in the same breed. Note that the black striping runs through to the tip and is irregular in shape. There is also a distinct black outer fringing to the gold border.

3 Standard hackle feather from a male of the gold-laced Wyandotte and similar breeds with a rich bay ground colour. Note the intensity of the centre stripe, absence of shaftiness, and freedom from blemish in the outer border. Note also the soundness of colour in the underfluff.

3A Faulty hackle feather from similar breeds, showing indistinct striping, with foul colour, shaftiness, and black running through to the tip. Underfluff is a mixture of red and dark grey.

4 Standard hackle feather from a male of the light Sussex and similar breeds of ermine markings, such as light Brahma, Columbian Wyandotte, and ermine Faverolles. The demand is for a solid black centre with a clear white border extending to the underfluff. Green sheen is an important feature.

4A Faulty hackle from similar breeds, showing black fringing to the border, black tipping, and shaftiness in the quill. Underfluff also lacks distinction.

5 Perfect tri-coloured hackle feather from a speckled Sussex male. The black striping is solid, with green sheen, and the border is the desired rich mahogany colour, finishing with a clean white tip. Note clarity of the undercolour.

5A Faulty speckled Sussex hackle feather showing almost complete lack of black striping, varying ground colour in the border, and indistinct white tipping.

6 Neck hackle conforming to a Standard Andalusian male. The so-called Andalusian blue is a diffusion of black and white, and in male hackles a dark border or lacing surrounds the slate-blue feather. Undercolour is sound and even.

6A Faulty hackle from same breed. The colour generally is blotchy and lacing is indefinite.

7 Standard neck hackle of a Rhode Island Red male. No attempt has been made to show the ultra-dark red usually seen in show specimens, but the colour seen here conforms with Standard and should be agreeable for exhibition. Note the purity of the undercolour – a very important point in this breed.

7A Faulty hackle feather from the same breed, showing uneven ground colour, black tipping, and smutty undercolour, which is a very severe defect in a Rhode Island Red.

8 Hackle from an Ancona male, conforming closely to Standard. Note the clear V-shaped white tipping, complete absence of shaftiness, rich green sheen, and solidity of the dark underfluff, a particularly strong point in the breed.

8A Faulty hackle feather from the same breed, showing indistinct tipping of greyish-white and faulty undercolour not dark to skin.

9 Hackle feather conforming to Standard from a buff Orpington male, very similar, except for the exact shade, to feathers from other buff breeds, such as Cochins and Rocks. Note the even colour throughout, absence of shaftiness, and sound colour in the underfluff, with a quill buff to the skin.

9A Faulty hackle feather from a similar breed, showing severe shaftiness, uneven ground colour with a darker fringe, and an impure undercolour.

British Poultry Standards, Seventh Edition. Edited by J. Ian H. Allonby and Philippe B. Wilson.
© 2019 Poultry Club of Great Britain. Published 2019 by John Wiley & Sons Ltd.

Plate 1

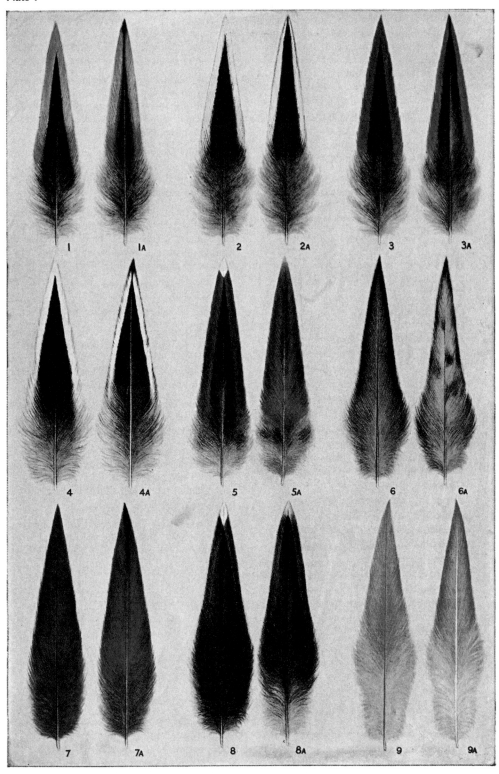

Plate 2

1 Standard hackle from a barred Plymouth Rock male and similar breeds. Note the points of excellence – barring practically straight across the feather, sound contrast in black and blue-white, barring and ground colour in equal widths, and barring carried down the underfluff to the skin. The tip of the feather must be black.

1A Faulty saddle or neck hackle from a similar variety. There is a lack of contrast in the barring, with a dull grey ground colour and V-shaped bars.

2 Hackle as the Standard description from a silver Campine, in which males are inclined to hen feathering. Note that the black bar is three times the width of the ground colour and the tip of the feather is silver.

2A In this faulty hackle (also from a silver Campine male) the ground colour is too wide and the barring narrow. The feather is without a silver tip.

3 Standard hackle from a Marans male. In this and some similar breeds evenness of the banding is not essential, but it is expected to show reasonable contrast. It should, however, carry through to the underfluff.

3A From the same group of breeds this feather is far too open in the banding and lacks uniformity of marking. It is also light in the undercolour.

4 Standard markings of a female body feather in Plymouth Rocks and similar barred breeds where barring and ground colour are required to be of equal width. Note that barring runs from end to end of the feather and that the tip is black.

4A Faulty feather from same group. Note the absence of barring to the underfluff and the V-shaped markings; also blurred and indistinct ground colour.

5 Sound body feather from a silver Campine female showing a Standard silver tip and barring three times as wide as the ground colour, as in the male. Gold Campine feathers are similar but different in the ground colour.

5A Faulty female feather, again from a silver Campine. Here again, as in 2A, barring is too narrow in relation to the silver ground colour and the tip of the feather is black.

6 Body feather from a Marans female, conforming to Standard requirements. Note that the markings are less definite than in Rocks and Campines, and the black is lacking in sheen, while the ground colour is smoky white.

6A Faulty Marans female feather. Lacks definition and contrast in the banding, which is indefinite in shape, the blotchy ground colour making an indistinct pattern.

7 Excellent body feather from a partridge Wyandotte female, showing correct ground colour and fine concentric markings. Note the complete absence of fringing, shaftiness, and similar faults. Fineness of pencilling is a Standard requirement.

7A From the same breed this faulty female feather shows a rusty red ground colour and indistinct pencilling, with faulty underfluff.

8 Body feather of Standard quality from an Indian or Cornish Game female. The illustration shows clearly two distinct lacings with a third inner marking. Lacing should have a green sheen on a rich bay or mahogany ground.

8A Faulty feather from the same breed. Missing are evenness of lacing and central marking. The outer lacing runs off into a spangle tip.

9 Standard feather from a laced Barnevelder female. In this breed the ground colour should be rich with two even and distinct concentric lacings. Quill of the feather should be a mahogany colour to the skin.

9A Faulty Barnevelder female feather, showing a spangle tip to outer lacing and irregular inner markings on the ground colour that is too pale.

Plate 2

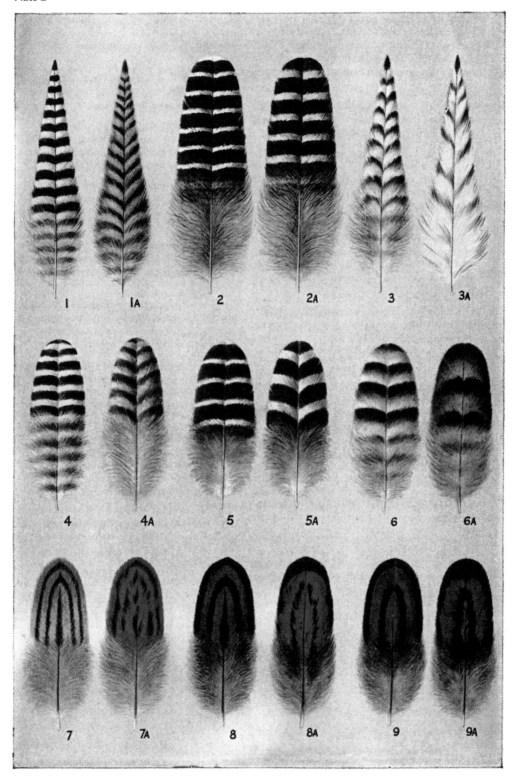

Plate 3

1 Standard markings on a silver-laced Wyandotte female feather, showing very even lacing on a clear silver ground colour and rich colour in the underfluff. In this breed clarity of lacing is of greater importance than fineness of width.

1A Faulty female feather from the same breed. In this there is a fringing of silver outside the black lacing, which is irregular in width and runs narrow at the sides. Undercolour is also defective.

2 Excellent feather from a gold-laced Wyandotte. In this the ground colour is a clear rich golden bay and there is a complete absence of pale shaft. Undercolour is sound and lacing is just about the widest advisable.

2A This shows a very faulty feather from the same breed. It portrays a mossy ground colour with blotchy markings and an uneven width of lacing at the sides of the feather. Undercolour is not rich enough.

3 Standard markings on an Andalusian female feather showing well-defined lacing on a clear slate-blue ground and good depth of colour in the underfluff. The dark shaft is desirable and is not classed as a fault.

3A Faulty feather from a female of the same breed. In this the ground colour is blurred and indistinct, and the lacing is not crisp, while the undercolour lacks depth.

4 This shows a feather from an Ancona female, almost perfect in Standard requirements. The white tipping is clear and V-shaped and the undercolour is dark to the skin.

4A Faulty feather from a female of the same breed. Here the tip of the feather is greyish-white and lacks the necessary V-shape, while the undercolour is not rich enough.

5 An almost perfectly marked feather from a speckled Sussex female – though the white tip might be criticised by some breeders as rather too large. The black dividing bar shows a good green sheen and the ground colour is rich and even.

5A As a contrast this faulty feather shows a blotchy white tip and lack of colour in the underfluff. The ground colour is also uneven.

6 An excellent example of 'mooning' on the feather of a silver spangled Hamburgh female. Note the round spangle and the clear silver ground with sound undercover.

6A In this feather from the same breed the spangling at the tip is not moon-shaped and there is too much underfluff and insufficient silver ground colour to the body of the feather.

7 A good example of the desired colour in Rhode Island Red female plumage. Note the great depth of rich colour and the sound dark undercolour.

7A Faulty colour in a feather from the same breed. Here the middle of the feather is paler and inclined to shaftiness, and the colour generally is uneven.

8 Standard plumage in females of Australorp and similar breeds of soft feather with a rich green sheen. Note the brilliance of colour and the general soundness of the underfluff.

8A This shows a common fault in similar breeds, a sooty or dead black colour without sheen and lacking lustre. This sootiness is, however, usually accompanied by a dark undercolour.

9 Standard colour and feather in the buff Rock female and similar breeds which perhaps vary in exact shade and in quantity and softness of the underfluff. Note the clear even buff and lack of shaftiness or lacing, also the sound rich undercolour.

9A This feather from a similar buff breed shows very bad faults – mealiness and bad undercolour with a certain amount of pale colour in the shaft.

Plate 3

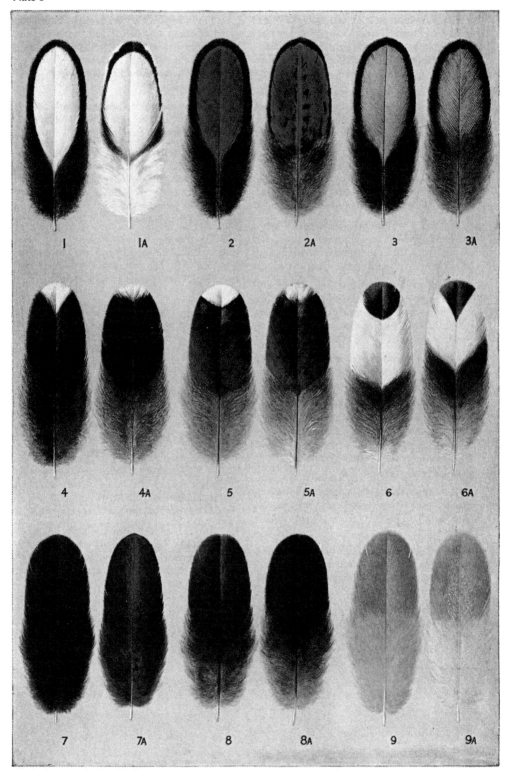

Plate 4

1 This shows a typical Standard bred feather from a Derbyshire Redcap female. Note the rich ground colour and the crescentic black markings, which are really midway between spangling and lacing.

1A In this faulty feather from a female of the same breed the ground colour is uneven and lacks richness, while the black tip is too small and indefinite and too closely resembles moon-shaped spangling.

2 This is a Standard example of the webless type of plumage associated with Silkies in which the feather vane has no strength and the barbs no cohesion. This plumage is common in all colours.

2A Faulty feather from the same breed. In this the middle of the feather is too solid and lacks silkiness, while the fluff has insufficient length.

3 A delicately pencilled body feather from a silver grey Dorking female. Note the silvery colour and absence of ruddy or yellow tinge in the ground colour. This type of feather is also usual in duckwing females of various breeds.

3A Faulty colour in a female feather from the same breed. Here there is a distinctly incorrect ground colour and pronounced shaftiness.

4 A good example of a Standard bred colour and markings in the body feather of a brown Leghorn female, where the ground colour is a soft brown shade and the markings finely pencilled. This type of feather is common to many varieties of partridge or grouse colouring.

4A This shows a body feather from the same breed, in which the ground colour is ruddy and the shaftiness is pronounced – both severe exhibition faults.

5 A well-chosen example of the irregularity in markings of an exchequer Leghorn female. In this breed the black and white should be well distributed but not regularly placed, and the underfluff should be parti-coloured black and white.

5A This faulty feather from the same breed shows a too regular disposition of markings, the body of the feather being almost entirely black and the white markings almost resembling lacing.

6 This is a Standard feather from the breast of a silver Dorking, and with slight variations of shade from pale to rich salmon applies to a number of varieties with black-red or duckwing colouring. Colour should be even with as little pale shaft as possible.

6A A faulty sample of a breast feather from the same group. Here the ground colour is washy and disfigured by pale markings known as mealiness.

7 Standard markings in a North Holland Blue female. Note the defined but somewhat irregular banding on a distinctly bluish ground. No banding or other requirements in the underfluff are called for in the Standard.

7A This shows a faulty female feather in the same breed, which is not closely standardised for markings. The ground colour is smoke-grey instead of blue, and is blotchy, with uneven markings.

8 A good example of clear colour in an unlaced or self-blue female feather, where no lacing is permissible, such as in blue Leghorns, blue Wyandottes, etc. Note the even pale blue shade and absence of any form of markings. This is an example of the true-breeding blue colour found in Belgian bantams.

8A This faulty female feather is a dull dirty grey instead of clear blue, and has blotchy markings as well as a suggestion of irregular lacing.

9 A good sample of exquisitely patterned thigh fluff in Rouen drakes. The ground colour is a clear silver and the markings a delicate but clear black or dark brown. These markings are sometimes known as chain mail.

9A Another good Rouen feather – this time from the duck. Ground colour is very rich and markings intensely black, though seldom so regular and even as in domestic fowl.

Plate 4

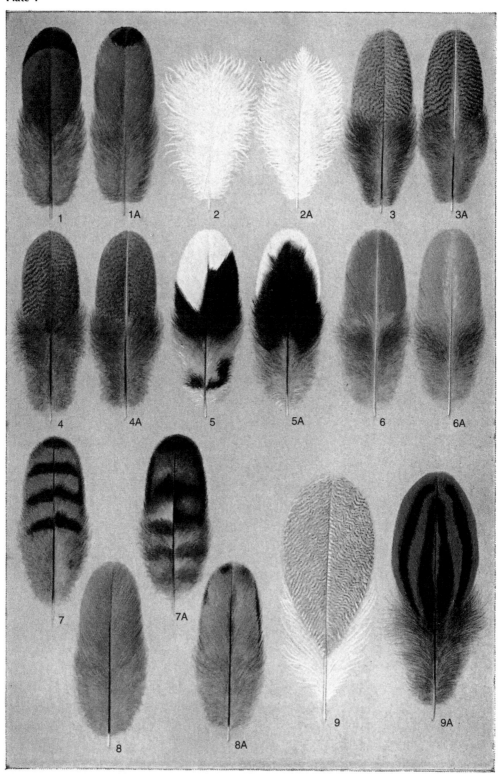

Chief points of the fowl

(Figures 1–6)

Figures 1 and 2 illustrate the chief points of the various breeds of fowl.

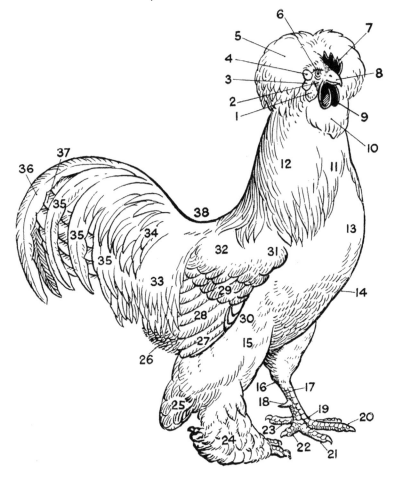

1	Muffling	14	Keel	27	Primary flights
2	Face	15	Thigh	28	Wing bay
3	Ear-lobe	16	Hock joint	29	Wing bar
4	Ear	17	Shank	30	Wing covert
5	Crest	18	Spur	31	Shoulder
6	Eye	19	Foot	32	Wing bow
7	Comb	20	Middle toe	33	Saddle hackle
8	Beak	21	Third toe	34	Tail coverts
9	Wattles	22	Fourth toe	35	Side hangers
10	Beard	23	Fifth toe	36	Tail sickle
11	Neck	24	Footings	37	Main tail
12	Neck hackle	25	Vulture hock	38	Back
13	Breast	26	Abdomen		

Figure 1

British Poultry Standards, Seventh Edition. Edited by J. Ian H. Allonby and Philippe B. Wilson.
© 2019 Poultry Club of Great Britain. Published 2019 by John Wiley & Sons Ltd.

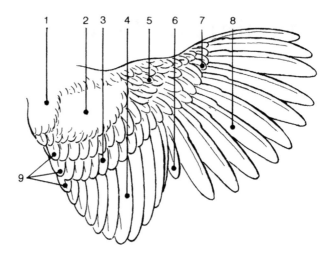

Figure 2

1 Shoulder butt or scapulars
2 Wing bow coverts
3 Wing bar or speculum (lower wing coverts)
4 Secondaries
5 Wing bow coverts
6 Axial feather (not waterfowl)
7 Flight coverts
8 Primaries
9 Tertiaries (mainly waterfowl)

Figure 3 Types of comb

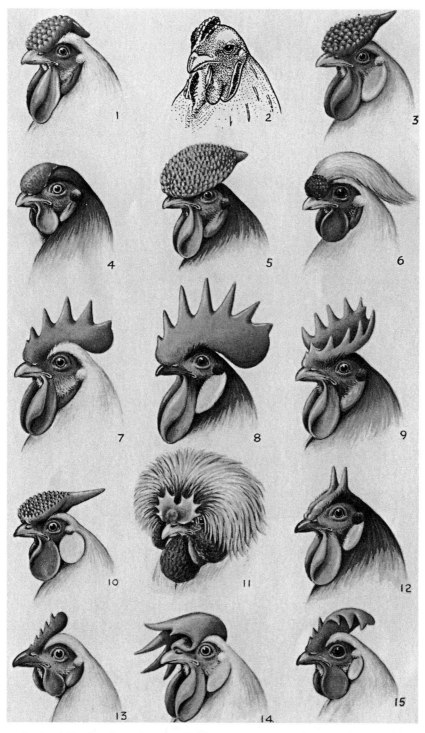

1 Rose, leader following line of neck 2 Triple or pea 3 Rose, short leader 4 Walnut 5 Cap
6 Mulberry 7 Medium single 8 Large single 9 Cup 10 Rose with long leader 11 Leaf 12 Horn
13 Small single 14 Folded single 15 Semi-erect single

Figure 4 Leg types

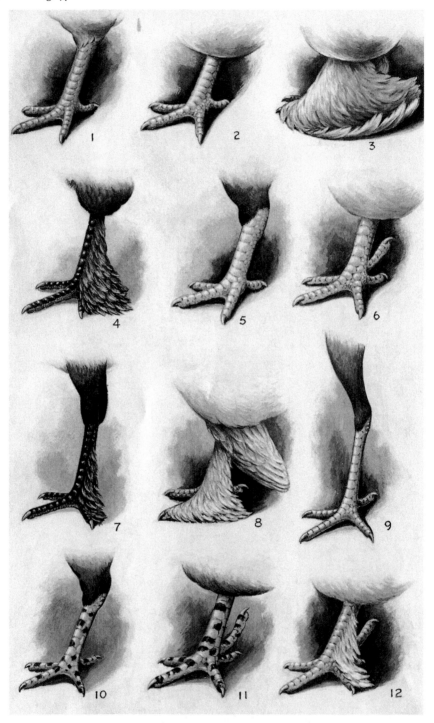

1 Clean legged, flat side (Leghorns) **2** Clean legged, round shanks (Game) **3** Heavy feather legged, and feathered toes, i.e. foot feather **4** Feather legged, no feathers middle toe (Croad Langshan) **5** Short round shanks (Indian Game) **6** Five toed (Dorking) **7** Slightly feathered shanks (Modern Langshan) **8** Feather legged and vulture hocked (Sultan) **9** Thin round shanks (Modern Game) **10** Mottled shanks (Ancona) **11** Mottled and five toed (Houdan) **12** Feather legged and five toed (Faverolles)

Figure 5   Types of tail

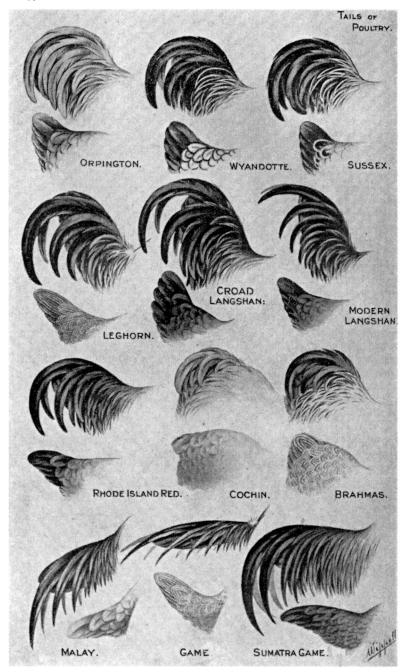

Figure 6

 1 Neck hackle, male (striped)
 2 Neck hackle, female (laced)
 3 Saddle hackle, male (striped)
 4 Pencilled hackle (female)
 5 Ticked hackle
 6 Tipped neck hackle, male, as in spangled Hamburgh
 7 Striped hackle, male, showing outer fringing of colour – a fault
 8 Striped saddle hackle, male, showing open centre (desired only in pullet-breeder)
 9 Pencilled feather, cushion, female, as in silver grey Dorking and brown Leghorns
10 Barred neck hackle (male)
11 Triple pencilled back (female)
12 Laced
13 Faulty laced (i.e. horseshoed)
14 Spangled (moon-shaped)
15 Speckled. White tick and two other colours on feather
16 Shoulder feather in spangled varieties
17 Poland laced crest (pullet)
18 Poland crest, female
19 Crescent marked
20 Barred or finely pencilled as in Hamburgh. Bars and spaces same width
21 Double laced
22 Tipped, showing V-shaped tip, as in Ancona
23 Barred as in barred Rock, shows barring in undercolour. To finish with black bar
24 Laced and ticked, as in dark Dorking
25 Elongated spangle, as in Buttercup
26 Finely pencilled, as in dark Brahma female
27 Barred, as in Campine. Finishes with white end. Light bars a quarter to a third of the width of dark bars
28 'Silkie' (no webbing)
29 Fine in pencilling, as in black marks of black-red, and duckwing Game
30 Barred Rock sickle
31 Buff laced
32 Wing marking on flight feather
33 Laced sickle
34 Saddle hackle mackerel marked (Campine cockerel)

Figure 6   Feather markings

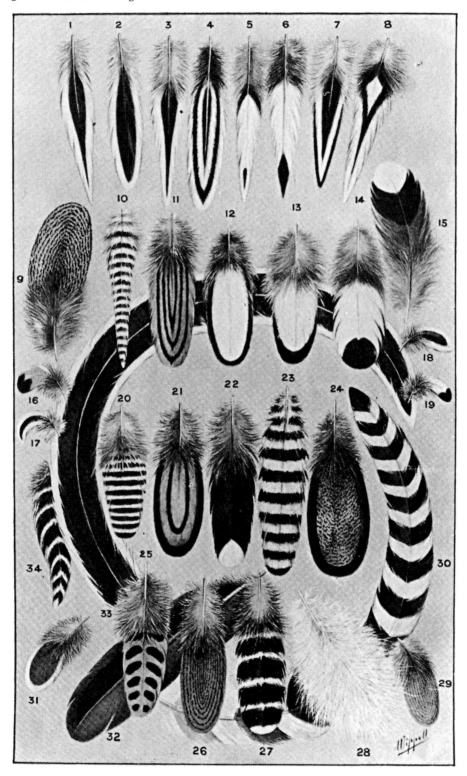

Complete classification of pure breed poultry

British Poultry Standards, 7th edition

CHICKENS

Hard Feather

Carlisle Old English Game
Indian Game
Modern Game
Old English Game Bantam
Oxford Old English Game

Soft Feather: Heavy

Australorp
Autosexing breeds:
   Brussbar, Dorbar,
   Rhodebar, Wybar
Barnevelder
Brahma
Cochin
Croad Langshan
Dorking
Faverolles
Frizzle
German Langshan
Marans
New Hampshire Red
Orloff
Orpington
Plymouth Rock
Rhode Island Red
Sussex
Wyandotte

Soft Feather: Light

Ancona
Appenzeller Spitzhauben
Araucana
Rumpless Araucana
Autosexing breeds:
   Legbar, Cream Legbar,
   Welbar
Derbyshire Redcap
Hamburgh
Leghorn
Minorca
Poland
Scots Dumpy
Scots Grey
Silkie
Welsummer

Asian Hard Feather

Asil
Ko Shamo
Kulang
Malay
Nankin Shamo
Satsumadori
Shamo

True Bantam

Belgian Bearded Bantams:
   Barbu d'Anvers, Barbu
   de Boitsfort, Barbu
   d'Everberg, Barbu de
   Grubbe, Barbu d'Uccle,
   Barbu de Watermael
Booted

British Poultry Standards, Seventh Edition. Edited by J. Ian H. Allonby and Philippe B. Wilson.
© 2019 Poultry Club of Great Britain. Published 2019 by John Wiley & Sons Ltd.

Taiwan
Thai Game
Tuzo
Yakido
Yamato-Gunkei

Dutch
Japanese
Pekin
Rosecomb
Sebright
Serama
Suffolk Chequer

Rare True Bantam

Burmese
Nankin
Ohiki

Rare Soft Feather: Heavy

Crèvecoeur
Dominique
Houdan
Ixworth
Jersey Giant
La Flèche
Modern Langshan
Norfolk Grey
North Holland Blue
Sulmtaler
Transylvanian Naked Neck

Rare Soft Feather: Light

Andalusian
Appenzeller Barthüner
Augsburger
Ayam Cemani
Brabanter
Brakel
Breda
Bresse-Gauloise
Campine
Dandarawi
Fayoumi
Friesian
Groninger
Kraienköppe
Lakenvelder
Marsh Daisy
Old English Pheasant Fowl
Sicilian Buttercup
Spanish
Sultan
Sumatra
Thüringian
Vorwerk
Yokohama

TURKEYS

Heavy

Bourbon Red
Bronze
Crimson Dawn/Black-
   winged Bronze
Narragansett
Nebraskan

Light

Blue
Buff
Crollwitzer (Pied)
Harvey Speckled
Norfolk Black
Slate
White

DUCKS

Heavy	Light	Bantam
Aylesbury	Abacot Ranger	Black East Indian
Blue Swedish	Bali	Call
Cayuga	Campbell	Crested
Muscovy	Crested	Silver Appleyard Miniature
Pekin	Hook Bill	Silver Bantam
Rouen	Indian Runner	
Rouen Clair	Magpie	
Saxony	Buff Orpington	
Silver Appleyard	Welsh Harlequin	

GEESE

Heavy	Medium	Light
African	Brecon Buff	Chinese
American Buff	Buff Back	Czech
Embden	Grey Back	Franconian
Skåne	Pomeranian	Pilgrim
Toulouse	West of England	Roman
		Sebastopol
		Shetland
		Steinbacher

Defects and deformities

The Poultry Club of Great Britain strives to promote adherence to the Standards, thereby encouraging the breeding of alert, healthy, active fowl, which reproduce well. Poultry Club of Great Britain judges are encouraged to consider these factors in addition to the Standards, to ensure that exhibition breeding does not affect the vigour of breeds. In this section, defects, deformities, and issues with specimens are highlighted, which should be considered from both a breeding and judging point of view. This section should be considered in addition to the *defects* or *serious defects* included in each Standard, although some Standards explicitly mention components included herein. This is due to common issues found in the breed, and both judges and breeders should be particularly vigilant when examining birds.

TO BE PASSED OR PENALISED

The following are given as deformities and defects for which judges must pass or penalise an exhibit according to the seriousness of the defect.

Head points

Crossed or deformed beak. Malformation of beak. Badly dished bill in ducks. Blindness. Defective eyesight. Defective pupils. Odd eye colour. Comb that closes the nostrils. Side

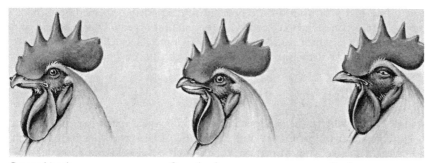

| Crossed beak | Open beak | Sunken eye |

Figure 7

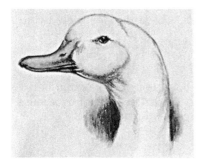

Figure 8   Dished bill

British Poultry Standards, Seventh Edition. Edited by J. Ian H. Allonby and Philippe B. Wilson.
© 2019 Poultry Club of Great Britain. Published 2019 by John Wiley & Sons Ltd.

sprigs or double end on a single comb. Excessive fall to side of rose comb, blocking vision. Split combs at blade. Fall-over comb that obstructs vision. Malformed combs. Defective serrations. Unusual head carriage. White in face for breed Standards demanding red. Wry neck. Indications of brain or nerve affection. Badly distended and sagging crop.

Back

Any deformity. Rounded or curved spine (roach back). Weak back formation. One bone higher than the other, giving the back a lopsided appearance.

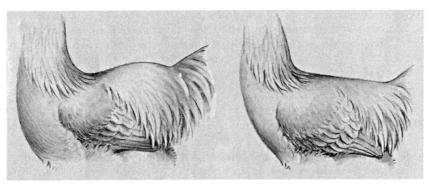

Roach back   Cut-away breast

Figure 9

Bone structure

Pigeon breast (abnormal protrusion of the breastbone). Seriously deformed breastbone. Malformation of breastbone that interferes with the internal organs. Down behind and curved end of breastbone, which leads to drooping abdomen. Dented breastbone from perching. Enlargement on breastbone of turkey. Broken or malformed pelvic bones. Faulty stance.

Wings

Badly twisted or curled wing feathers. Slipped or drooping wing. Split wing, in a serious form, with large gap between primaries and secondaries. Defective wing formation in waterfowl. Slightly defective wing formation, even if well positioned and carried, to be penalised.

Tail

Wry. Squirrel. Defective parson's nose. Split or divided tail feathers or badly twisted feathers in tail. High tail in excess.

Legs and feet

Enlarged bone. Curved thigh bones. Malformation of bone. Bow legs or 'out at hocks'. Badly in at hocks. Duck toes. Crooked toes. Turned toes. Twisted feet. Enlarged toe joints. Lack of spurs on adult male. Leg feathers on clean-legged birds.

Feathering

Soft or frizzled feathering in plain feathered breeds. Curled feathers on any part of body, including neck. Signs of slow feathering.

Figure 10 Comb faults

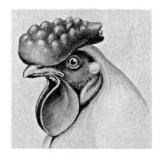 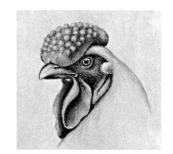

Left Ingrown leader

Right Short of leader, and uneven wattles

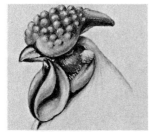 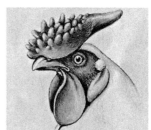

Left Rose comb falling to side and blocking vision

Right Bad leader and coarse worked comb

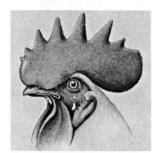 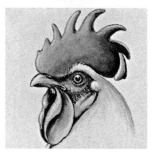

Left Beefy, and with part of blade too far forward

Right Badly curved at rear end with spikes falling over

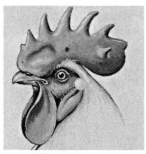 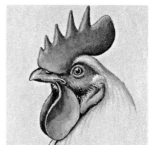

Left Thumb mark and side sprig

Right Flyaway comb

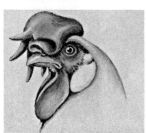 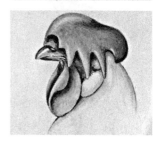

Left Double folded comb

Right Flop comb blocking vision

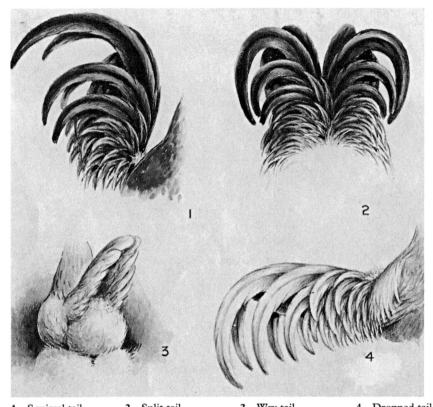

1 Squirrel tail	2 Split tail	3 Wry tail	4 Dropped tail

Figure 11

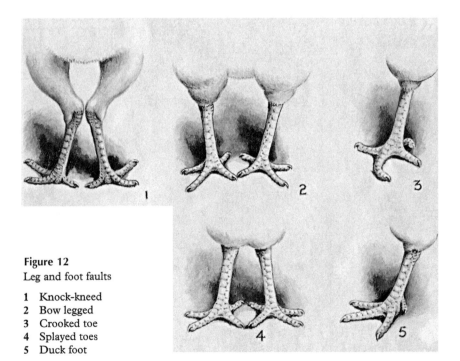

Figure 12
Leg and foot faults

1 Knock-kneed
2 Bow legged
3 Crooked toe
4 Splayed toes
5 Duck foot

Disease

Any disease or disorder not making for maximum health, condition, vigour, and breeding fitness, including colds, heartiness, abdominal dropsy, cysts, egg substance in oviduct, or abdomen. Sour crop. Impacted crop. External parasites. Any other disease symptom or deformity.

Lack of breed characteristics

Any exhibit deficient in breed or size characteristics, so that it is an unworthy specimen of the breed or variety intended, must be passed.

DISQUALIFICATIONS

Any bird that in the opinion of the judge has been faked or tampered with shall be disqualified.

Large fowl and bantams

ANCONA

LARGE FOWL

Origin: Mediterranean
Classification: Light: Soft feather
Egg colour: White

Named after the province of Ancona in Italy, specimens of this Mediterranean breed were imported into England in 1851, first the single then the rose comb. Controversy centres around the view that Anconas are akin to the original mottled Leghorn and, therefore, a member of the Leghorn family. However, the fact remains that breeders adhere to the name of Ancona. The breed has retained its popularity on the show bench not only for its laying propensities, but also because of its combination of breed type and characteristics of usefulness.

General characteristics: male

Carriage: Alert, bold and active.
Type: Body broad, close and compact. Back of moderate length. Breast full and broad, carried well forward and upward. Wings large and carried well tucked up. Tail full and carried well out.
Head: Deep, moderate in length, rather inclined to width, and carried well back. Beak medium with a moderate curve. Eyes bright and prominent. Comb single or rose. The single of medium size, upright and with five to seven deep, broad and even serrations forming a regular curve, coming well back and following the line of the head, free from excrescences. The rose resembles that of the Wyandotte. Face smooth and of fine texture. Ear-lobes medium, inclined to almond shape, free from folds. Wattles long, fine in texture, in proportion to comb.
Neck: Long, nicely arched and well covered with hackle.
Legs and feet: Legs of medium length, strong, set well apart, clear of feathers, thighs not much seen. Toes four, rather long and thin and well spread out.

Female

With the exception of the single comb, which falls gracefully to one side of the face without obscuring the vision, the characteristics are generally similar to those of the male, allowing for the natural sexual differences. The body, however, is round and compact, with greater posterior development than in the male. The back is rather long and broad, the neck of medium length and carried well up.

Colour

Male and female plumage: Good beetle-green ground tipped with white (the more V shaped the better). No inclination to lacing. The more evenly V-tipped throughout with beetle green and white the better, provided the ground colour is beetle green.

British Poultry Standards, Seventh Edition. Edited by J. Ian H. Allonby and Philippe B. Wilson.
© 2019 Poultry Club of Great Britain. Published 2019 by John Wiley & Sons Ltd.

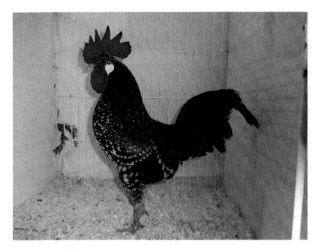

Ancona male, bantam

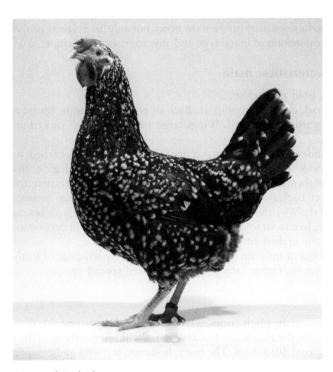

Ancona female, large

In both sexes: Beak yellow with black or horn shadings; a wholly yellow beak not desirable. Eyes, iris orange-red, pupil hazel. Comb, face and wattles bright red, face free from white. Ear-lobes white. Legs yellow, mottled with black, the more evenly mottled the better.

Weights

Cock 2.70–2.95 kg (6–6½ lb) Cockerel 2.50 kg (5½ lb)
Hen 2.25–2.50 kg (5–5½ lb) Pullet 2.00 kg (4½ lb)

Scale of points

Type and carriage	15
Texture (general)	10
Size	5
Purity of white, quality and evenness of tipping	20
Beetle-green ground colour dark to skin	15
Leg colour	5
Head (eye 5, comb 10, lobe 5)	20
Beak colour	5
Condition	5
	100

(*Note*: Eye points include brightness and prominence. Comb points include medium size and fine texture.)

Defects

	To lose
In-kneed	10
Squirrel tail	10
Crooked toes	10
White or light undercolour	10
Ground colour other than beetle green	10
Tail not tipped or not black to roots	10
Wings any other colour than black tipped with white	10
Bad comb	5
White in face	20
Lobe other than white	5
	100

(*Note*: Roach back or any bad structural deformity is a disqualification.)

BANTAM

Ancona bantams are to be exact miniatures of their large fowl counterparts and so Standard, colour and scale of points are to be used as for large fowl.

Weights

Male 570–680 g (20–24 oz)
Female 510–620 g (18–22 oz)

ANDALUSIAN

LARGE FOWL

Origin: Mediterranean
Classification: Light: Rare
Egg colour: White

Leonard Barber is believed to have been the first importer of chickens from the Andalucía region of Spain in 1846 and 1847, but these had an assortment of plumage colours. The Standard Blue Andalusian, with its characteristic sharp lacing, was developed in England. The two leading breeders in the 1850s who started this process were John Taylor, of Shepherd's Bush, London, and Mr Coles of Fareham, Hampshire. It took several decades of selective breeding by a succession of fanciers before birds with the perfect colour and lacing depicted by Victorian artists became a reality. In Spain the laced as we know them are recognised as English Andalusians, with all other colours known as Spanish Andalusians, and their blues are not laced. Andalusian bantams first appeared in the 1880s.

General characteristics: male

Carriage: Upright, bold and active.
Type: Body long, broad at the shoulders, and tapering to the tail, with the plumage close and compact. Breast full and round. Wings long, well tucked up and the ends covered by the saddle hackles. Tail large and flowing, carried moderately high but not approaching 'squirrel' or fan shape.
Head: Moderately long, deep and inclined to width. Beak stout and of medium length. Eyes prominent. Comb single, upright and of medium size, deeply serrated with spikes broad at the base, the back portion slightly following the line of the head but not touching the neck. Free from 'thumb marks' or side spikes. Face smooth. Ear-lobes almond in shape, medium size, free from wrinkles, and fitting closely to the face. Wattles fine and long.
Neck: Long and well covered with hackle feathers.
Legs and feet: Legs long. Shanks and feet free from feathers. Toes four, straight and well spread.

Female

With the exception of the comb, which falls with a single fold to one side without covering the eye, the general characteristics are similar to those of the male, allowing for the natural sexual differences.

Colour

Male and female plumage: Clear blue, edged with distinct black lacing, not too narrow, on each feather, excepting the male's sickles, which are dark (or even black), and his hackles, which are black with a rich gloss, while the female's neck hackle is a rich lustrous black, showing broad lacing on the tips of the feathers at the base of the neck. Undercolour to tone with surface colour.

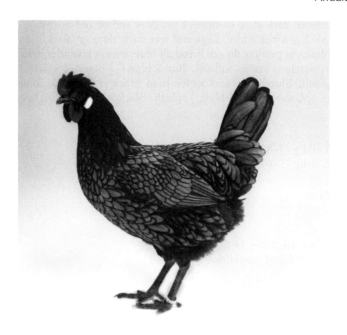

Andalusian female, large

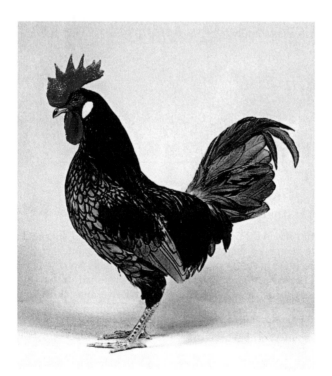

Andalusian male, bantam

In both sexes: Beak dark slate or horn. Eyes dark red or red-brown. Comb, face and wattles bright red. Ear-lobes white. Legs and feet dark slate or black.

(*Note*: Blue colours in poultry do not breed all blue, except lavender, which breeds true. The expected proportions are as follows: Blue × blue = $\frac{1}{4}$ black, $\frac{1}{4}$ splash, $\frac{1}{2}$ blue. Splash × splash = all splash. Blue-bred black × blue-bred black = all black. Blue-bred black × splash = all blue. Splash × blue = $\frac{1}{2}$ blue, $\frac{1}{2}$ splash. Black × blue = $\frac{1}{2}$ black, $\frac{1}{2}$ blue.)

Weights

Male   3.20–3.60 kg (7–8 lb)
Female   2.25–2.70 kg (5–6 lb)

Scale of points

Ground colour	30
Lacing	20
Head (comb 10, face 10, lobes 5)	25
Size, type, carriage, tail and condition	25
	100

Serious defects

In the male, much white in face or presence of red in lobes. White feathers. Sooty ground colour. Red or yellow in hackles. Any deformity and comb not upright. In the female any of these points apply, together with an upright comb.

BANTAM

Andalusian bantams are exact miniatures of their fowl counterparts and so Standard, colour and scale of points apply.

Weights

Male   680–790 g (24–28 oz)
Female   570–680 g (20–24 oz)

APPENZELLER

LARGE FOWL

Origin: Switzerland
Classification: Light (Spitzhauben); Light: Rare (Barthuhner)

The Appenzell Canton is in the north-eastern part of Switzerland. It is not known how long Spitzhaubens have been bred there, but the very similar Brabanter from The Netherlands was depicted in seventeenth century paintings, so Appenzeller Spitzhaubens may date from the same period. The Appenzeller Barthuhner was developed in the 1860s from crosses between Brown Leghorns, Russian Beardeds and Polveranas (now extinct, related to Bearded Polands). Kurt Fischer, of Stuttgart-Zuffenhausen, Germany, was a leading breeder involved in the revival of both breeds in the 1950s, as they had almost died out during the Second World War.

The Spitzhauben

Egg colour: White

General characteristics: male

Carriage: Neat and very active.

Type: Body medium long, tapering towards the tail (walnut shaped). Breast full and well rounded, carried high. Wings rather long, carried close. Tail well furnished, well spread, carried high, but by no means squirrel tail. Abdomen well developed. Back of medium length, slightly sloping with full hackle.

Head: Medium sized, held high, with typical raised skull. Medium-sized forward-pointing crest held tight and compact but with no inclination towards looseness or globular shape. Face smooth. Comb horn type consisting of two small rounded vertical spikes, separate and without side sprigs. Wattles moderately long and fine, free from folds. Ear-lobes medium sized, oval. Beak powerful, with strong, cavernous nostrils, and a prominent horseshoe ridge to the beak with a small fleshy knob at the front. Eyes prominent and alert.

Neck: Medium length, slightly arched with abundant hackle.

Legs and feet: Thighs slender and prominent; shanks medium length, fine. Toes four, well spread.

Plumage: Fairly hard and tight.

Female

General handling as befits a keen and active layer. Except for a more horizontal back line the general characteristics are the same as for the male, allowing for the natural sexual differences.

Colour

The silver spangled

Male plumage: Pure silvery white ground colour, with each feather ending in distinct black spangle free from an outer lacing of silvery white. The more V shaped the spangle, the better, with no inclination to lacing or circular shape. Spangling to be uniformly spread, fairly small so as to be surrounded as evenly as possible with silvery white ground colour. Less pronounced on the head and neck. Wing bows to be spangled evenly as on the body and forming two distinct and parallel bars running with the gentle curve across each wing. Primaries and secondaries silvery white, each feather ending with a black spangle. Tail pure silvery white ending with a defined spangle, as free as possible from any black or grey sootiness. Abdomen and fluff grey; undercolour dark grey.

Female plumage: Head, crest and the neck silvery white with black spangling. Breast, wing bows, primaries, secondaries, back and tail silvery white with distinct black spangling as for the male. Undercolour dark grey.

The gold spangled

Male plumage: Gold-red ground colour, spangling as for the silver spangled. Primaries and secondaries gold-red, each feather ending with a black spangle. Breast and flanks gold with black spangles. Abdomen and undercolour greyish-black. Tail gold-red, ending with a defined spangle, as free as possible from any black or grey sootiness is the ideal. A gold-red/blackish tail is permissible. The specimen with the least sootiness to be given the award where all else is equal.

Female plumage: Head, crest and neck golden-red with black spangling. Flights, breast, wing bows, back and tail golden-red with distinct black spangling as for the male. Undercolour dark grey.

The black

Male and female plumage: Black with lustrous beetle-green sheen throughout. Perfectly free from any other colour. Undercolour dark grey to black.

The blue

Male plumage: Head, neck, saddle and wing bows dark slate-blue. Remainder medium blue (pigeon blue preferred). Free from lacing, mealiness, sandiness or bronze. Undercolour grey-blue.

Female plumage: Medium blue (pigeon blue preferred) throughout. Free from lacing, mealiness, sandiness or bronze. A darker shade on the head and neck is permissible, but preference should always be given to those examples which are a uniform shade throughout. Undercolour grey-blue.

The Chamois spangled

Male plumage: Golden-buff ground colour, creamy white spangling as for the silver spangled. Uniform shade of golden-buff throughout allowing for the lustre on the wing bows, hackle and saddle of the male. Where all else is equal and definition of spangle is maintained from the ground colour, the exhibit with the lighter shade to take the award.

Flights golden-buff with a creamy white spangle. Breast and flanks golden-buff with creamy white spangles. Abdomen and undercolour creamy white. Tail golden-buff, ending with a defined spangle, as free as possible from any creamy white sootiness is the ideal. A golden-buff/creamy whitish tail is permissible. The specimen with the least sootiness to be given the award where all else is equal.

Female plumage: Head, crest and neck golden-buff with creamy white spangling. Flights golden-buff ending with a creamy white spangle. Breast, wing bows, back and tail golden-buff with a distinct creamy white spangling as for the male. Undercolour creamy white.

In both sexes and all colours

Beak bluish. Eyes dark brown. Comb, face and wattles bright red; ear-lobes bluish-white. Shanks blue.

Weights

Male   1.60–2.00 kg ($3\frac{1}{2}$–$4\frac{1}{2}$ lb)
Female   1.35–1.60 kg (3–$3\frac{1}{2}$ lb)

BANTAMS

Bantams should follow the large fowl Standard in all aspects apart from the size/weight difference.

Weights

Male   600–800 g (21–28 oz)
Female   500–700 g (17–24 oz)

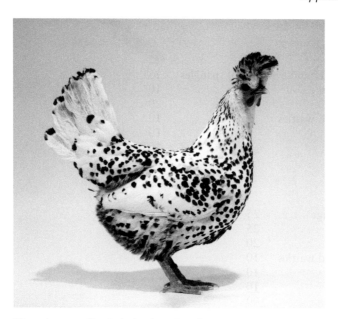

Silver Appenzeller Spitzhauben female

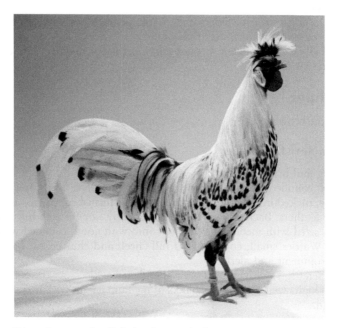

Silver Appenzeller Spitzhauben male, bantam

Scale of points

Spangled varieties

Type and carriage	25
Definition, clarity and evenness of spangles	15
Purity of ground colour	10
Crest	20
Head, comb and wattles	10
Legs and feet	10
Condition	10
	100

Self varieties

Type and carriage	25
Colour	25
Crest	20
Head, comb and wattles	10
Legs and feet	10
Condition	10
	100

Minor defects

Poor eye colour, where all else is equal, darkest eye should take preference.

Serious defects

Comb other than vertical horn. Side sprigs. Large comb – horns which are horizontal across front of crest. Narrow or roach back. Squirrel tail. Breast too deep or narrow. Low wing carriage. Tail lacking fullness. Crow beak. Nostril not cavernous. Bad stance. Any sign of feathering on shanks.

The Barthuhner

Egg colour: Light brown

General characteristics: male

Carriage: Strong and active.
Type: Body well rounded, medium long with broad shoulders. Breast full, carried high. Wings moderate, tucked in close to the body. Tail well furnished, carried like a fan with abundant sickle feathers. Back of medium length, slightly sloping with full saddle hackle.
Head: Medium sized with medium-sized rose comb with good, rounded working and a straight leader. Wattles small, covered by a full cheek and chin beard. Large beak and nostrils. Eyes prominent and alert.
Neck: Medium length, slightly arched with abundant hackle.
Legs and feet: Thighs well developed, shanks of medium length with no feathering. Toes four, well spread.
Plumage: Fairly tight.

Female

Except for a more horizontal back line, the general characteristics are the same as for the male, allowing for the natural sexual differences.

Colour

As in any of the recognised Game Fowl. The blue colour as per the Orpington Standard.

In both sexes and all colours

Comb and wattles red, ear-lobes white, beak black or horn, eyes as dark as possible, legs blue to black.

Weights

Male   2.26–2.94 kg (5–6½ lb)
Female   1.36–1.81 kg (3–4 lb)

Scale of points

Type and carriage	30
Colour	20
Head points	30
Legs and feet	10
Condition	10
	100

Serious defects

Comb other than rose. Narrow or roach back. Squirrel tail.
Missing beard or any sign of feathering on shanks.

ARAUCANA

LARGE FOWL

Origin: Chile
Classification: Light: Soft feather
Egg colour: Blue or green

When the Spaniards arrived in South America, bringing with them the light Mediterranean breeds, they found that the indigenous Indians had domestic fowl which soon cross-bred with the incomers. Notable for their fierce resistance to the Spaniards, however, were the Indians of the Arauca province of northern Chile, who were never conquered. The name Araucana for the breed is derived therefore from that part of the world where the South American and European fowls had the least opportunity to interbreed.

The Araucana breed Standard in the British Isles is generally as envisaged by George Malcolm, who created the true-breeding lavender Araucana, among other colours, in Scotland during the 1930s. Araucanas are prolific layers of strong-shelled eggs, blue or green eggs having been reported from South America from the mid-sixteenth century onwards. These are unique in that their colour permeates throughout the shell.

General characteristics: male

Carriage: Alert and active.
Type: Body long and deep, free from heaviness. Firm in handling. Back moderately long, horizontal. Wings large and strong. Tail well developed with full sickles carried at an angle of 45°.

Head: Moderately small. Beak strong and stout. Eyes bold. Comb small triple pea. Face covered with thick muffling and ear muffs abundant. Crest compact, carried well back from eyes. Ear-lobes moderately small and concealed by muffling. Wattles absent.
Neck: Of medium length, abundantly furnished with hackle feathers.
Legs and feet: Medium length, strong and well apart. Shanks free from feathers. Toes four, straight and well spread.

Female

The general characteristics are similar to those of the male, allowing for the natural sexual differences. Comb pea.

Colour

The lavender
Male and female plumage: An even shade of blue-grey throughout.

The blue
Male plumage: Breast, belly, thighs, tail and closed secondaries the colour of new slate. Hackle, saddle and shoulders and sometimes the tail coverts and the primaries two shades darker (like a slate after being wetted). Fluff slate-blue.
Female plumage: Blue slate colour with dark hackle like the male, often marked or laced all over with the darker shade. Fluff slate-blue.

The black-red
Male plumage: Breast, thighs, belly, tail and wings black. Wing bars green-black; secondaries when closed bay. Crest, head and neck orange-red striped black. Back, shoulders and wing bows red or mahogany. Saddle hackle to match neck hackle. Fluff grey.
Female plumage: Hackle rich golden-yellow broadly striped with black. Breast salmon. Muff salmon. Salmon and ash grey on thighs. Body colour brown pencilled black, each feather with a pale shaft. Tail brown spotted or grizzled with black. Fluff grey.

The silver duckwing
Male plumage: Resembles the black-breasted red in the black markings and blue wing bars; rest of the plumage clear silvery white. Fluff light grey.
Female plumage: Hackle white, lightly striped black. Body and wings even silvery grey. Breast pale salmon. Primaries and tail nearly black. Fluff light grey.

The golden duckwing
Male plumage: Hackle and saddle yellow straw. Shoulders deep golden. Wing bars steel blue; secondaries yellow or creamy straw when closed, remaining plumage black. Fluff light grey.
Female plumage: Breast deeper, richer colour and body slightly browner tinge than the silver duckwing female. Fluff light grey.

The blue-red
Male plumage: The same colour pattern as the black-red with slate replacing black. Breast, thighs, belly and tail slate. Secondaries when closed bay. Wing bars slate. Hackle and saddle feathers orange-red with blue centre stripe. Shoulders deep crimson-scarlet. Fluff dark slate.
Female plumage: Hackle golden striped. Breast and muff salmon. Body, wings and tail blue, finely peppered with golden-brown. Fluff dark slate.

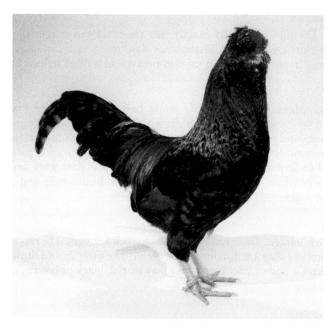

Crele Araucana male, bantam

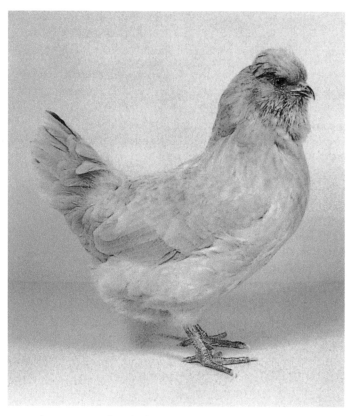

Lavender Araucana female, bantam

The pile

Male plumage: The pile is marked exactly like the black-red except that the black is exchanged for a clear cream-white. Secondaries bay.

Female plumage: Creamy white with salmon breast and golden striped hackle.

The crele

Male and female plumage: Neck hackle straw barred with gold or black. Back and shoulder bright gold-chestnut barred with straw-yellow. Wing bars dark grey barred with pale grey; primaries and secondaries dark grey barred with pale; outer web of secondaries chestnut, the chestnut only showing when wing closed. Saddle hackle pale straw barred gold. Breast and underparts dark grey. Tail and tail coverts dark grey barred with light grey. Legs and feet white, with some spotting allowed. Both single and double barred acceptable in the male.

The spangled

Male and female plumage: These have white tips to their feathers. The more of these spots and the more regularly they are distributed the better. The male should show white ends to the feathers on hackle and saddle. The colour may be red, black or brown, or a mixture of all three. Fluff white.

The cuckoo

Male and female plumage: Light grey-blue ground colour, each feather crossed with broad bands of dark blue-grey. In the male, a lighter shade is permissible. Undercolour banded but of a lighter shade. Beak light horn or bluish. Legs and feet white with blue spots.

The black

Male and female plumage: Black with green sheen.

The white

Male and female plumage: Snow white throughout.

In both sexes and all colours

Comb and face bright red. Eyes dark orange. Beak and nails horn. Legs in all colours except cuckoo and crele, willow to olive or slate.

Weights

Male   2.70–3.20 kg (6–7 lb)
Female 2.25–2.70 kg (5–6 lb)

Scale of points

Type and carriage	20
Colour	20
Crest and muffling	25
Comb	10
Other head points	5
Legs and feet	5
Condition	15
	100

Serious defects

Cut-away breast. Crest too small or too large, e.g. Poland type obscuring the sight. Comb lopped or twisted. Any comb other than minimal in female. Pearl or light-coloured eyes. Legs other than Standard colour. Uneven or splashed breast colour. In males white base in tail. In lavenders any straw or brassy tinge. Feet – duck footed or bent toes.

Disqualifications

Roach back. Wry or squirrel tail. Absence of crest or muffling. Comb other than of pea type. Presence of wattles. Feathered legs.

BANTAM

The Standard to be an exact miniature of the large fowl.

Weights

Male   740–850 g (26–30 oz)
Female   680–790 g (24–28 oz)

Serious defects

As large fowl.

RUMPLESS ARAUCANA

LARGE FOWL

Origin: Chile
Classification: Light: Soft feather
Egg colour: Blue or green

The Rumpless Araucana also has its origins in South America. It was introduced to Europe by Professor S. Castello in the early 1920s. The ear-tufts of feathers are unique to the breed in that they grow from a fleshy pad adjacent to the ear-lobe. Rumpless Araucanas lay a large egg in relation to body size and are as productive as the tailed Araucanas.

General characteristics: male

Carriage: Alert, active and assured.
Type: Body moderate in length, broad at shoulders. Back flat and slightly sloped. Rump well rounded with saddle feathers flowing over stern. Breast full, round and deep. Wings medium in length, carried close to the body and well up. Saddle hackle well developed. Tail entirely absent, with no uropygium (parson's nose).
Head: Moderately small. Beak medium stout, curved. Eyes bold and expressive. Comb small pea. Face moderate muffling. Ear-lobes small and concealed by ear-tufts. These originate from a gristly appendage arising from behind and just below the ear hole. The tufts of feathers, numbering from 5 to 15, grow from this pad. The tufts should be of a good length, matching in size and extending from the ears backwards in a well-defined sweep, or projecting horizontally. Wattles very small.
Neck: Medium length, well furnished with hackle feathers.
Legs and feet: Medium in length, straight and well set apart. Toes four, strong and well spread.

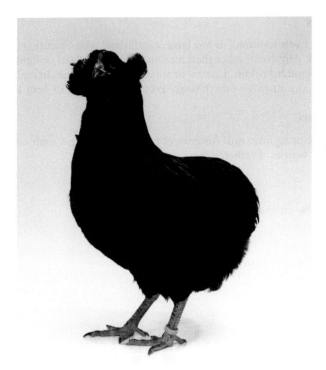

Black Rumpless Araucana, female

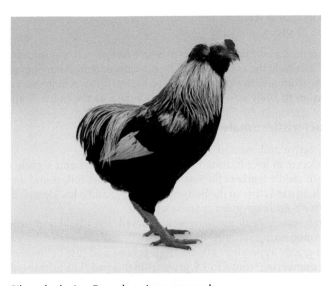

Silver duckwing Rumpless Araucana male

Female

The general characteristics are similar to those of the male, allowing for the natural sexual differences.

Colour

Standard colours as for tailed variety.

In both sexes and all colours

Eyes dark orange. Legs and feet willow to olive or slate.

Weights

Excess weight to be penalised

Male   2.25–2.70 kg (5–6 lb)
Female   1.60–2.00 kg (3.5 lb–4.5 lb)

Scale of points

Type and carriage	20
Ear-tufts	25
Comb	10
Other head points	5
Legs and feet	5
Colour	20
Condition and handling	15
	100

Serious defects

Unmatched ear-tufts. Shape other than Standard, e.g. narrow body. Any tail feathers (incomplete rumpless). Fluff showing below saddle hackle. Legs other than Standard colour. Pearl or light-coloured eye. No ear-tufts.

Disqualifications

Single ear-tuft, crest. Uropygium (parson's nose). Roach back, cut-away breast. Comb other than triple pea comb. Feathered legs. Presence of wattles.

BANTAM

These should be a true miniature of the large Rumpless Araucana. As the large Rumpless fowl is historically and naturally a small breed, it follows that great care must be taken to keep the bantams within the approved weight limits. Colours as tailed variety.

Weights

Excess weight to be penalised

Male   1.10–1.30 kg (38–46 oz)
Female   790–1020 g (28–36 oz)

ASIL

LARGE FOWL

Origin: India
Classification: Asian Hardfeather
Egg colour: Brown

This Standard refers to the small Asil (often called 'Reza' Asil, a term which applies only to birds of $3\frac{1}{2}$–4 lb, or 'Rajah' Asil, which is a term not used at all in India).

The Asil is probably the oldest known breed of gamefowl, having been bred in India for its fighting qualities for over 2000 years. The name Asil is derived from Arabic and means 'of long pedigree'. In different dialects it can be spelled 'Asil', 'Aseel' or 'Asli'. In its native land the Asil was bred to fight, not with false spurs, but rather with its natural spurs covered with tape, the fight being a trial of strength and endurance. Such was the fitness, durability and gameness of the contestants that individual battles could last for days. This style of fighting produced a powerful and muscular bird with a strong beak, thick muscular neck and powerful legs, together with a pugnacious temperament and stubborn refusal to accept defeat.

Never very numerous in Britain, the Asil has nevertheless always attracted a few dedicated admirers prepared to cope with its inborn desire to fight, a characteristic shared by the females, who are poor layers but extremely good mothers.

General characteristics: male

Type and carriage: Upright, standing firmly on strong legs. Sprightly and quick in movement. When seen in profile the eye should be directly above the middle toenail.
Body: Viewed from above, the body should appear to be heart shaped, with broad shoulders tapering to a fairly narrow but very well-developed stern, strong at the root of the tail. The body should be hard and muscular, feeling remarkably flat in the hand.
Breast: Wide and well thrown out.
Back: Broad and straight.
Wings: Carried well out from the body at the shoulders. Muscular where they join the body but otherwise carrying little flesh. Wing feathers hard and tough with rather short quills.
Tail: Sickle feathers narrow and scimitar shaped, drooping from the base. Saddle feathers pointing backwards.
Head: Skull broad with large square jaw bones, and large cheek bones covered in tough leathery skin. Beak short, thick and powerful, shutting tight. Eyes bright and bold set in oval pointed eyelids. Comb triple, very hard fleshed and set low. No wattles.
Neck: Medium length, carried slightly curved giving a short appearance. Thick and very hard to the touch, covered with short, hard, wiry feathers. Throat clean-cut with bare skin extending well down the neck.

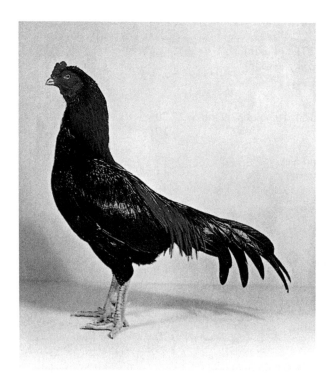

Black-red Asil male, large

Legs and feet: Shanks thick and square with a noticeable indentation down the front where the scales meet. Thighs not too long, but round, hard and muscular and when viewed from the front should be in line with the body, not the shoulders.

Plumage: Very short and wiry, difficult to break, and with little or no underfluff. Patches of bare skin showing red are to be seen on the breastbone, wing joints and thighs.

Handling: Extremely firm and muscular. Heavier in the hand than appearance would at first suggest.

Female

The general characteristics are similar to those of the male, allowing for the natural sexual differences.

Colour

Male and female plumage: There are no fixed colours. The principal colours seen today are light red and dark red, with grouse-coloured and red-wheaten females, but grey, spangle, black, white, duckwing and pile are not uncommon. No colour or combination of colours is disqualified.

In both sexes and all colours

Beak ivory, yellow burnish acceptable. Legs and feet ivory, or ivory with slight yellow burnish is preferred. Yellow or slate are acceptable. Comb, face, throat, ear-lobes and any exposed skin – red. Eyes pearl, yellowish tinge or slightly bloodshot appearance acceptable.

Weights

Male   1.80–2.70 kg (4–6 lb)
Female   1.35–2.25 kg (3–5 lb)

Scale of points

Head (skull and beak 10, eyes 5, comb 5)   20
Neck   10
Wings   5
Thighs, shanks and feet   15
Body shape and stern   15
Plumage   10
Carriage   15
Condition   <u>10</u>
                                           <u>100</u>

Serious defects

Lack of attitude. Any evidence of alien blood, e.g. red or dark eyes. Round shanks. Duck feet. High tail carriage. Wry tail. Roach back. Storklegged or in-kneed. Any other deformity.

BANTAM

Asil bantams should follow the large fowl Standards in all but weight.

Weights

Male   1130 g (40 oz)
Female   910 g (32 oz)

AUSTRALORP

LARGE FOWL

Origin: Great Britain
Classification: Heavy: Soft feather
Egg colour: Brown

The claim that the Australorp – an abbreviation of Australian black Orpington – is the prototype of the black Orpington, as originally made by Mr W. Cook, has never been questioned. Its breeders emphasised that its true utility type gives to poultrymen the Orpington at its best, an excellent layer and a good table fowl, with white skin. It was around 1921 that large importations of stock birds were made from Australia into this country and an Austral Orpington Club founded. Later the breed name of Australorp was adopted, and this remains today.

General characteristics: male

Carriage: Erect and graceful, denoting an active fowl, the head being carried well above the tail line.
Type: Body deep and broad, showing somewhat greater length than depth. Back broad across shoulders and the saddle, with a sweeping curve from neck to tail. Breast full and rounded, carried well forward without bulging; breastbone long and straight. Wings

compact and carried closely in, the ends being covered by the saddle hackles. Tail full and compact, rising gradually from the saddle in an unbroken line; the sickles gracefully curved, but not long and streaming.

Head: Finely modelled with skull rounded. Beak slightly curved, strong, of medium length. Eyes, large, prominent and expressive; high in skull standing out well when viewed from front or back. Comb single, medium in size, erect, evenly serrated (four to six serrations) and blade tending downwards without touching the neck, texture fine, but not of polished appearance. Face full, fine in texture, clean, free from feathers, wrinkles and overhanging brows. Ear-lobes small and elongated. Wattles medium in size, rounded at bottom and corresponding in texture to comb.

Neck: Fairly long, fine at the junction of head, with a gradual outward curve to the back, widening distinctly at the shoulders.

Legs and feet: Legs medium in length, strong, rounded in front and spaced well apart, the hocks nearly covered by body feathering, and the whole of the shanks showing below the underline. Shanks and feet (four toes) free from feathers or down.

Plumage: Feathering soft but close, with a minimum of fluff, the lower body fluff only sufficient to cover the thighs.

Skin: Fine in texture.

Female

The general characteristics are similar to those of the male, allowing for the natural sexual differences. The pelvic bones should be pliable, not showing an excess of fat or gristle; the abdominal skin being pliable without an excess of internal fat. All these parts to be of fine texture; any indication of coarseness should be discountenanced.

Colour

The black

Male and female plumage: Black with lustrous green sheen.

In both sexes: Beak black. Eyes black or dark brown iris, black preferred. Face, comb, ear-lobes and wattles bright red. Legs and feet black with white soles. Skin white.

The blue

Male plumage: Hackles, saddle, wing bows, back and tail a uniform dark slate-blue. Remainder medium slate-blue, each feather to show a wide band of lacing of a darker shade.

Female plumage: Head and neck dark slate-blue, remainder medium slate-blue, laced with a darker shade.

In both sexes: Undercolour to tone with surface colour in both sexes. Beak blue or black, black preferred. Eyes black or very dark brown, black preferred. Comb, face, wattles and ear-lobes bright red. Legs and feet black or blue. Toenails preferably white. Skin white. Soles of feet white.

The white

Pure white, free from straw tinge or brassiness. Beak bluish-white or (off) white. Eyes black or dark brown, black preferred. It is essential that the eyes are large and bold. Comb, wattles, ear-lobes and face bright red. Legs and feet slate blue. Soles of feet, toenails and skin white.

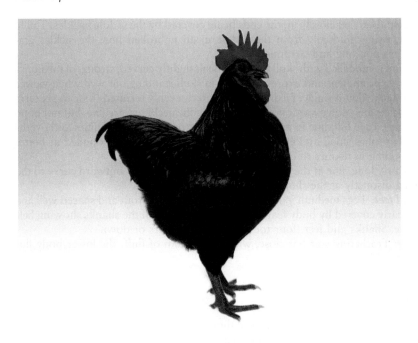

Australorp male, bantam

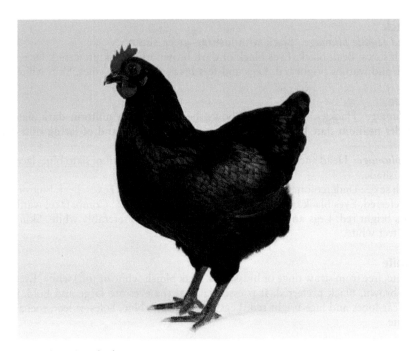

Australorp female, bantam

Weights

Cock   3.85–4.55 kg (8½ –10 lb)   Cockerel   3.40–4.10 kg (7½ – 9 lb)
Hen   2.95–3.60 kg (6½ –8 lb)   Pullet   2.50–3.20 kg (5½ –7 lb)

Scale of points

Type	30
Head (eyes 15, face, comb, wattles 10)	25
Plumage (colour, quality and character of feathering)	25
Condition	10
Legs and feet	10
	100

If all other points equal, large fowl and small bantams should be favoured.

Serious defects

Black and Blue: Red, yellow or white in feathers. Permanent white in ear-lobes.
White: Red eyes, white legs.

Defects (for which birds should be passed)

Any deformity such as wry tail, roach back, crooked breastbone, crooked toes, webbed feet. Yellow or willow colour in legs or feet. Yellow or pearl-coloured eyes. Feathering on shanks or feet. Side sprigs on comb. Split or twisted wing and slipped wing.

BANTAM

Australorp bantams are to be exact miniatures of their large fowl counterparts and so Standard, colour and scale of points to apply.

Weights

Male   1020 g (36 oz) max.
Female   790 g (28 oz) max.

AUTOSEXING BREEDS

An autosexing breed is one in which the chicks at hatching can be sexed by their down colouring. It was when crossing the gold Campine with the barred Rock in 1929 that Professor R.C. Punnett and Mr M.S. Pease discovered the basic principle in their experimental work at Cambridge, and made the Cambar.

Barring is sex-linked, there being a double dose in the male and a single dose in the female, the barring being indicated by the light patch on the head of the chick. This light patch is very similar in chicks of both sexes, having black down, but when the barring is transferred to a brown down there is a marked difference. The light head spot on the female chick (one dose) is small and defined, while on the male chick (double dose) it spreads over the body. For that reason, the down colouring in the day-old cockerel is much paler, and the pattern of markings more blurred, than in the newly hatched pullet chick, which has the sharper pattern of markings. Recently, the autosexing breeds have warranted enough popularity to reform the previously inactive Autosexing Breeds Association.

BROCKBAR

LARGE FOWL

Origin: British
Classification: Heavy
Egg colour: Brown

Created in the 1940s but extinct by 1950, the Brockbar was a cross between a female Buff Rock and a male barred Rock.

General characteristics: male

Carriage: Upright and graceful.
Type: Body large, deep and compact. Back broad, Breast well rounded. Wings carried well up. Tail rather small, rising from the saddle; sickles gracefully curved.
Head: Strong and refined, Beak short and stout. Eyes bright and prominent. Comb single, medium size, erect, evenly serrated and free from side sprigs. Ear-lobes and wattles fine, evenly shaped and well proportioned (i.e. not exaggerated).
Neck: Of medium length, thick and well covered with hackle feathers.
Legs and feet: Legs wide apart and stout. Thighs not more than 7.6 cm (3 in.) long, stiltiness to be avoided. Toes four, strong, straight, well spread and clean.
Plumage: Close and tight, not fluffy.

Female

The general characteristics are similar to those of the male, allowing for the natural sexual differences.

Colour

Male and female plumage: Even pale buffish all over, any shade from pale lemon to orange, but avoiding any suggestion of a red or rusty tinge. As free as possible from black markings or sootiness, and free also from white feathers. The male's plumage is paler than that of the female, though it should never be white. His feathers should be evenly and clearly barred throughout their length. In the female, the barring may be much less distinct, but the clearer the better; and some barring must be visible.
Male down colour: Cream, tinged salmon, even shade all over, free from sootiness.
Female down colour: Rich salmon buffish, even shade all over, free from sootiness.

In both sexes: Beak, legs and feet yellow or willow. Eyes red or orange. Comb, face, ear-lobes and wattles red.

Weights

Cock   4.10 kg (9 lb)   Cockerel   3.60 kg (8 lb)
Female   3.20 kg (7 lb)

Scale of points

Type	25
Colouring and feathering	10
Barring	10
Legs and feet	10
Condition	10
Size and weight	15
Head	5
Handling and capacity	15
	100

Serious defects

Much black in feathering. Legs other than yellow or willow: feathering on legs and feet. Other than four toes. White in ear-lobes or wattles.

BRUSSBAR

LARGE FOWL

Origin: British
Classification: Heavy
Egg colour: Brown

Crosses of Light Sussex with Brown Sussex led to the production of the Brussbar, from original matings of barred Rocks and Brown Sussex. Breeders of autosexing poultry felt that Brussbars were among the best dual-purpose birds in their inventory, however they never had a significant following. Standardised in 1952, the Brussbar – along with a number of other autosexing breeds – is beginning to gather interest. That said, the birds at – and from – Cobthorn are the only known pure flock.

General characteristics: male

Carriage: Graceful vigorous and well balanced.
Type: Body oblong shaped, deep, broad and long. Back broad. Long and flat, wide across the shoulders. Breast broad, full and well rounded; breast bone long, straight and well fleshed. Wings of medium length. Tail of medium size and carried at an angle of 45° to the body.
Head: Of medium size and quality. Beak short, strong and deep. Comb single, of medium size, firm, upright and fitting close to the head. Eyes prominent, full and bright, pupils clearly defined. Face smooth and free from coarseness. Wattles and ear-lobes of medium size and fine in texture.
Neck: Fairly long, profusely covered in hackle feathers.
Legs and feet: Legs of medium length and set well apart. Thighs short, stout and well fleshed. Toes four, long, straight and well spread.
Plumage: Of light silky texture, free from coarseness.
Flesh: Fine in texture.
Handling: Firm and compact with plenty of muscle.

Female

The general characteristics are similar to those of the male, allowing for the natural sexual differences.

Colour

Gold variety

Male plumage: Neck hackle dark gold, sparsely barred with dark grey, sooty generally, feathers gold tipped. Back and shoulder coverts dark gold-grey barred, rich brownish tinge. Feathers gold tipped. Wing bows dark gold-grey barred, gold predominating; primaries dark gold-grey barred; secondaries dark gold-grey barred, upper web with irregular gold markings. Saddle hackles dark gold barred, rich lustrous colour, feathers gold tipped. Breast black, barred, free from salmon colour. Tail evenly barred black or grey, sickles pale, but not white.

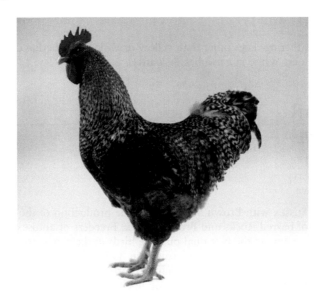

Brussbar male, large

Female plumage: Head and neck hackles dark gold, softly barred with dark grey. Breast salmon, clearly defined in outline. Body dark grey-gold with indistinct broad soft barring, feathers showing pale gold shaft and edging. Wing coverts dark grey-gold, barring soft and indistinct; primaries dark grey-gold, barring broad and soft; secondaries dark grey-gold, barring soft and broad, upper web with irregular gold mottling or peppering. Tail and saddle hackles dark grey-gold softly barred. Tail feathers on the whole darker.
Down colour: As for gold Legbars.

Silver variety
Male plumage: Neck hackle dark silver, sparsely barred with dark grey, but it will be noted that the tip of the hackle feather fades off to pure silver. Back and shoulder coverts silver, with dark grey barring, the feathers being silver tipped, as far as possible free from chestnut. Wing bows dark grey with silver-grey barring, as far as possible free from chestnut; primaries dark grey barred, some white permissible; secondaries dark grey barred, with the upper web white or grey mottled. Saddle hackles silver barred with dark grey, the feathers being silver tipped. Breast evenly barred dark grey and silver grey with well-defined outline. Tail evenly barred dark grey and silver grey, sickles paler. Tail coverts evenly barred dark grey and silver grey.
Female plumage: Head and hackle dark silver with black striping, softly barred grey. Breast salmon, clearly defined. Body dark grey with indistinct broad soft barring, the individual feathers showing lighter shaft and edging. Wing bows dark grey, as free from chestnut as possible; primaries dark grey as free from white as possible; secondaries dark grey, upper web lighter grey mottled or peppered. Tail dark grey with distinct soft barring.
Down colour: As for silver Legbars.

In both sexes and all colours
Beak white or horn. Eyes red or orange. Comb, face and ear-lobes red. Legs and feet white. Skin and flesh white.

Weights

All minimum

Cock   4.10 kg (9 lb)   Cockerel   3.60 kg (8 lb)
Hen   3.20 kg (7 lb)   Pullet   2.70 kg (6 lb)

Scale of points

Type	30
Colour	20
Legs	10
Condition	10
Head	20
Weight	10
	100

Serious defects

White in ear-lobe. Squirrel or wry tail. Feathers on legs and toes.

Defects for which a bird should be passed: Side sprigs on comb. Eye pupil other than round and clearly defined. Crooked breast or any other bodily deformity. In the gold female, excessive chestnut colour on the back or in the plumage generally. In the silver, gold feathers as distinct from chestnut.

CAMBAR

LARGE FOWL

Origin: British
Classification: Light
Egg colour: Cream

It was the accidental discovery of an autosexing characteristic that led to the further production of Cambars from Campines and barred Rocks. This resulted in the team from Cambridge showing the first Cambars at the Third World Poultry Congress in 1930. Unlike some of the other autosexing breeds, Cambars do not simply resemble another colour of Campine, but differ in type and weight. They are a dual-purpose breed of medium size, being intermediate between the cross of the light Campine and heavy barred Rocks. They were standardised in 1947, on the promise that the breeding would favour white lobes and a more Campine-like type.

General characteristics: male

Carriage: Upright and alert, with rangy body. A medium-sized breed.
Type: Body large, deep, broad at shoulders, compact. Back rather long, flat, narrowing slightly to saddle with a moderate slope. Breast well rounded, breast bone long and straight. Wings of medium size and neatly tucked into the body.
Tail medium length, carried well out 45° to the line of the body with nicely curved sickles; sickles and coverts broad and plentiful.
Head: Fine, deep and inclined to width. Beak short and stout. Eyes large and bright. Comb single, of medium size, erect, evenly and deeply serrated, free from side sprigs. Face smooth. Ear-lobes of medium length and fine texture. Wattles of medium size, fine and evenly matched.

Neck: Moderately long, profusely covered with feathers.

Legs and feet: Legs moderately long to hock, free from feathers. Thighs 5–7.6 cm (2–3 in.) long only. Toes four, strong, well spread and straight; stiltiness a fault.

Plumage: Tight and silky in texture.

Handling: Firm, with abundance of muscle, showing high qualities expected in a dual-purpose breed.

Female

The general characteristics are similar to those of the male, allowing for the natural sexual differences. Comb erect, not falling to one side, tail carried well out.

Colour

Gold variety

Male plumage: Grey and gold barred as regular as possible all over, except on the head, neck and saddle hackles, which should be gold, and as free from sootiness as possible. The gold as rich in tint as possible.

Female plumage: Generally darker than the male, gold on head, neck and saddle hackles rich and clear.

Male down colour: Much paler, washed out, pattern completely blurred without any well-defined light head patch.

Female down colour: Mottled chocolate brown on rich gold background, the mottling to be sharply defined in outline. Over the head and eyes there is thin black striping, breaking up into pinpoint black spots, giving the characteristic spotty appearance. White markings on the rump to be avoided. Light head patch showing up brightly.

Silver variety

Male and female: Same as for gold, but for 'gold' read 'silver'.

In both sexes and all colours

Beak white. Eyes rich bay. Ear-lobes white. Comb, face and wattles bright red. Legs and feet yellow.

Weights

Cock	3.60 kg (8 lb)	Cockerel	3.20 kg (7 lb)
Hen	2.50 kg (5½ lb)	Pullet	2.25 kg (5 lb)

Scale of points

Type and carriage	25
Colour	20
Dual-purpose qualities	10
Head	15
Size and symmetry	10
Condition	10
Legs and feet	10
	100

DORBAR

LARGE FOWL

Origin: British
Classification: Heavy
Egg colour: White

In 1941, the team at Cambridge attempted to create a heavy autosexing table breed from Dorkings and barred Rocks. Dorkings were well known at shows, but specimens had not been bred with utility values in mind for some time. By 1949, the decision was made to discontinue the breeding programme, as Dorbars were outperformed by Brussbars (table), Legbars (laying) and Cambars (dual purpose).

General characteristics: male

Carriage: Upright and alert.
Type: Body large, deep and moderately long. Back broad, saddle feathers of medium length and abundant. Breast broad and well rounded; keel bone long and straight. Wings moderately large and carried well up. Tail of medium size and carried well out, with curved sickles.
Head: Strong, deep and inclined to width. Beak stout. Eyes large and bright. Comb single, medium to large, evenly and deeply serrated, free from thumb marks or side sprigs. Face smooth. Ear-lobes moderately developed and pendant. Wattles of medium size and fine texture, evenly matched.
Neck: Rather short, tapering, abundant hackle feathers flowing well over the shoulders.
Legs and feet: Legs wide apart with moderately long hocks, free from feathers. Thighs short and well developed. Toes five, strong, hard, straight and well spread.
Plumage: Tight.

Female

The general characteristics are similar to those of the male, allowing for the natural sexual differences. Comb erect or lopped.

Colour

Gold variety
Male plumage: Barred all over head and neck, Breast black and barred. Wing coverts and saddle hackles gold, all as free from black markings as possible. Flights and tail grey-gold barred. In general the gold parts to be as rich in tint as possible.
Female plumage: Body colour silver-grey ground, softly barred. Hackle gold barred. Breast rich, even salmon-pink with sharply defined edges.
Down colour: *Male and female* – As for gold Legbar.

Silver variety
Male and female plumage: As for the gold, reading 'silver' instead of 'gold'. Gold feathers in the male to disqualify. Plumage of the male as far as possible free from chestnut smudges.
Down colour: Male *and female* – As for the gold, except that for the 'brown stripe' read 'silver-grey', and for 'the ground colour should be dark brown, though distinctly paler than the stripe' read 'ground colour silver-grey'.

In both sexes and colours
Beak white. Eyes red or rich bay. Comb, face, ear-lobes and wattles bright red. Legs and feet flesh colour.

Weights

Cock   3.60 kg (8 lb) min.   Cockerel   2.95 kg (7 lb) min.
Hen   2.70 kg (5½ lb) min.   Pullet   2.25 kg (5 lb) min.

Scale of points

Type	30
Colour	20
Head	20
Condition	10
Legs	10
Weight	10
	100

Serious defects (to lose points)

Narrow back or breast. Light weight. Side sprigs or thumb marks on comb and falling comb in the male. Exaggerated comb, lobes or wattles. Feathers on shanks or toes. Loose feathering.

Disqualifications

Any deformity. Gold feathers in male of silver variety.

LEGBAR

LARGE FOWL

Origin: British
Classification: Light
Egg colour: White or cream. Cream Legbar: blue, green or olive

These were one of the first autosexing breeds to be created at Cambridge, being based on the Leghorn as the name suggests. The Gold and Silver Legbars were standardised in the mid-1940s and early 1950s, respectively. These were based on utility strains of brown Leghorns which had managed to survive throughout the Second World War. Although relatively popular earlier on, both varieties of Legbar were covered by the Rare Poultry Society until recently, where the Autosexing Breeds Association reformed with only the Gold being seen occasionally. Cream Legbars have crests, varying plumage to the Legbar, and lay blue eggs. Interestingly, this breed was produced involuntarily. It was Mr Pease, attempting to improve on the Gold Legbars, who crossed them with White Leghorns. Because of the dominant white of the Leghorns, other colours were transferred to the offspring which, when mated again, led to 'interestingly cream-coloured' chicks. Evidently, these first Cream Legbars were crestless and laid white eggs, with the blue being later incorporated through Araucana crossing. Although not favoured by the markets of the day, Cream Legbars are now benefiting from renewed success through the work of dedicated fanciers.

General characteristics: male

Carriage: Very sprightly and alert, with no suggestion of stiltiness.
Type: Body wedge shaped, wide at the shoulders and narrowing slightly to root of tail. Back long, flat and sloping slightly to the tail. Breast prominent and breastbone straight.

Wings large, carried tightly and well tucked up. Tail moderately full at an angle of 45° from the line of the back.

Head: Fine. Cream variety: crest small, compact and carried well back from eyes, falling off the back of the head below the extended comb. Beak stout, point clear of the front of the comb. Eyes prominent. Comb single, perfectly straight and erect, large but not overgrown, deeply and evenly serrated (five to seven spikes broad at the base), extending well beyond the back of the head and following, without touching, the line of the head, free from 'thumb marks' or side sprigs. Face smooth. Ear-lobes well developed, pendant, smooth and free from folds, equally matched in size and shape. Wattles long and thin.

Neck: Long and profusely covered with feathers.

Legs and feet: Legs moderately long. Shanks strong, round and free of feathers. Flat shins objectionable. Toes four, long, straight and well spread.

Plumage: Of silky texture, free from coarse or excessive feather.

Handling: Firm, with abundance of muscle.

Female

The general characteristics are similar to those of the male, allowing for the natural sexual differences, except that the comb may be erect or falling gracefully over either side of the face without obstructing the eyesight, the tail should be carried closely and not at such a high angle. Cream variety: the crest of the female is somewhat fuller and larger than the male, but does not obstruct the eyes.

Colour

The gold

Male plumage: Neck hackle pale straw, sparsely barred with gold and black. Back, shoulder coverts and wing bows pale straw barred with bright gold-brown. Wing coverts (or wing bars) dark grey barred; primaries and secondaries dark grey barred, intermixed with white, upper web of secondaries also intermixed with chestnut. Saddle hackle pale straw barred with bright gold-brown, as far as possible without black. Breast and underparts dark grey barred. Tail grey barred; sickles paler. Tail coverts grey barred.

Female plumage: Hackle pale gold, marked with black bars. Breast salmon, clearly defined. Body dark smoky or slaty grey-brown with indistinct broad soft barrings, the individual feathers showing a paler shaft and slightly paler edging. Wings dark grey-brown. Tail dark grey-black with slight indication of lighter broad bars.

Male down colour: The down is much paler in shade, the pattern being blurred and washed out from head to rump.

Female down colour: Brown stripe type. The stripe should be broad and very dark brown, extending over the head, neck and rump. The edges of the stripe should be clearly defined rather than blurred and blending with the ground colour – the sharper the contrast, especially over the rump, the better. The ground colour should be dark brown, though distinctly paler than the stripe. A pale ground colour and a narrow or discontinuous stripe are to be avoided. A light head spot should be visible, though usually it is small. It should be well defined in outline and should show up as clearly as possible against the brown background.

The silver

Male plumage: Neck hackle silver, sparsely barred with dark grey but tips of feathers fade off to pure silver. Saddle hackle silver, barred with dark grey, the feathers tipped with silver. Back and shoulder coverts silver, with dark grey barring, the feathers tipped with silver. Wing bows dark grey with silver-grey barring; primaries dark grey, some white permissible; secondaries dark grey with tips of upper web white. Breast evenly barred dark grey and silver grey, with well-defined outline. Tail and tail coverts evenly barred dark grey and silver grey, sickles being paler.

Female plumage: Head and neck hackle silver, with black striping, softly barred grey. Breast salmon, clearly defined. Body silver grey, with indistinct broad soft barring, individual feathers showing lighter shaft and edging. Wings silver grey, as free from chestnut as possible; primaries silver grey, as free from white as possible; secondaries silver grey, upper web a lighter grey mottled. Tail silver grey with indistinct soft barring.

Male down colour: The down is much paler in tint, the pattern being blurred and washed out from head to rump; it may best be described as pale silvery slate.

Female down colour: Silver-grey type: the stripe should be very dark brown, extending over the head, neck and rump. The edges of the stripe should be clearly defined, not blurred and blending with the ground colour – the sharper the contrast, especially over the rump, the better. The stripe should be broad; a narrow or discontinuous stripe should be avoided. A light head patch should be visible, clearly defined in outline, showing up brightly against the dark background.

In both sexes: Beak yellow or horn. Eyes orange or red, pupils clearly defined. Comb, face and wattles bright red. Ear-lobes pure opaque white (resembling white kid) or cream, the former preferred. Slight pink markings and pink edging does not unduly handicap an otherwise good bird for utility purposes. Legs and feet yellow, orange or light willow in the female.

The cream

Male plumage: Neck hackles cream, sparsely barred. Saddle hackles cream barred with dark grey, tipped with cream. Back and shoulders cream with dark grey barring, some chestnut permissible. Wings and primaries dark grey, faintly barred, some white permissible; secondaries dark grey more clearly marked; coverts grey barred, tips cream, some chestnut smudges permissible. Breast evenly barred dark grey, well-defined outline. Tail evenly barred grey, sickles being paler, some white feather permissible. Crest cream and grey, some chestnut permissible.

Female plumage: Neck hackles cream, softly barred grey. Breast salmon, well defined in outline. Body silver grey, with rather indistinct broad soft barring. Wings and primaries grey peppered; secondaries very faintly barred; coverts silver grey. Tail silver grey, faintly barred. Crest cream and grey, some chestnut permissible.

Male and female down colour: As silver.

In both sexes: Beak yellow. Eyes orange or red. Comb, face and wattles red. Ear-lobes pure opaque, white or cream, slight pink markings not unduly to handicap an otherwise good male. Legs and feet yellow.

Weights

Male   2.70–3.40 kg (6–7$\frac{1}{2}$ lb)
Female   2–2.70 kg (4$\frac{1}{2}$–6 lb)

Scale of points

Type	30
Colour	20
Head	20
Condition	10
Legs	10
Weight	10
	100

Serious defects

Male's comb twisted or falling over. Ear-lobes wholly red. Any white in face. Legs other than orange, yellow or light willow. Squirrel tail.

Disqualifications

Side sprigs on comb. Eye pupil other than round and clearly defined. Crooked breast. Wry tail. Any bodily deformity.

BANTAM

Bantam Legbars should follow the exact Standard for the large fowl.

Weights

Male   850 g (30 oz)
Female   620 g (22 oz)

RHODEBAR

LARGE FOWL

Origin: British
Classification: Heavy
Egg colour: Brown

The Rhode Island Red was widely recognised to be one of the most commercially viable breeds, hence it was to be expected that an autosexing breed based on the Rhode Island Red would be created. A number of production efforts around the world were carried out in the 1940s and 1950s, each relying on slightly differing methods to produce the final Rhodebars. They are believed to be birds from a Mr B.de H. Pickard from Sussex that were shown to the Poultry Club of Great Britain in 1951 for standardisation. Mr Pickard created his strain from Rhode Island Red and barred Rock crosses, similar to an earlier team from Canada.

General characteristics: male

Carriage: Upright and graceful.
Type: Body large, fairly deep, broad and long. Back broad, long and somewhat horizontal in outline. Breast broad, full and well rounded. Wings carried well up, the bows and tips covered by the breast feathers and saddle hackle. Tail rather small, rising slightly from the saddle, the sickle of medium length, well spread and nicely curved, the coverts sufficiently abundant to cover the stiff feathers.
Head: Strong, but not thick. Beak moderately curved, short and stout. Eyes large and bright. Comb single, medium size, straight, upright, well set on, with well-defined serrations and free from side sprigs. Face smooth. Ear-lobes of fine texture, well developed and pendent. Wattles to correspond with size of comb and moderately rounded.
Neck: Of medium length and profusely covered with feathers flowing over the shoulders, but not too loosely carried.
Legs and feet: Legs wide apart and of medium length, stout and strong and free from feathers. Thighs large with well-rounded shanks of medium length. Toes four, strong, straight and well spread.
Handling: Firm, with abundance of muscle.
Plumage: Of silky texture, free from coarse or excessive feather.

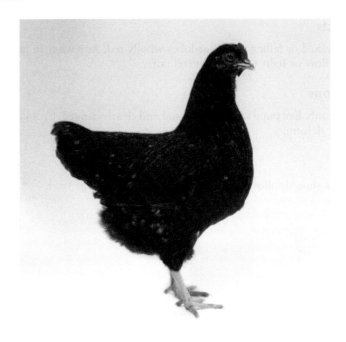

Female Rhodebar

Female

The general characteristics are similar to those of the male, allowing for the natural sexual differences.

Colour

Male plumage: Hackle deep red-gold barred, with centres black and grey-white barred, the black centre portions rather longer than the grey-white; the front of the cape showing less black, the feathers towards the tips of the cape lying on the back showing wider black and grey-white barring. Wing primaries lower web red-gold, faintly barred, upper grey and white barred, slightly gold tinted; secondaries the whole alternately black, white and gold barred, lower web showing more gold; flight coverts very bright red-gold and white barred; tips red-gold. Wings bows very brilliant chestnut-red and gold barred. Tail, including sickles, uniform black and white barring from tip to base, including the shaft; tips black. Saddle hackle deep red-gold and grey-white and narrower black barring towards the tips. Back and saddle deep red-gold barred, with occasional black bars towards the end of the feathers. Undercolour light creamy buff. Breast uniformly barred, deep red-gold and creamy white and black.

Female plumage: Hackle deep buff-red with bright chestnut edges, each feather with deep buff, gold, black and white narrow barring, the barring becoming narrower as it approaches the lower cape feathers. Tail feathers black with reddish tinge. Wing primaries upper web red-buff, lower black; secondaries buff-red. Remainder general surface dark buff-red barred with buff and buff-red, the tips of the feathers of the lighter colour. Undercolour creamy buff-red, as deep as possible. Quills yellow.

In both sexes: Beak red-horn or yellow. Eyes orange or red, pupils clearly defined. Comb, face, ear-lobes and wattles bright red. Legs and feet bright yellow.

Weights

Cock   3.85 kg (8½ lb) min.   Cockerel   3.60 kg (8 lb)
Hen   2.90 kg (6½ lb) min.   Pullet   2.50 kg (5½ lb)

Scale of points

Type   30
Colour   20
Head   20
Condition   15
Legs   10
Weight   __5__
           100

Serious defects

Male's comb twisted or falling over. Ear-lobes other than red. Legs other than yellow, orange or light willow. Squirrel or wry tail. Side sprigs on the comb. Eye pupils other than round and clearly defined. Crooked breast or any bodily deformity.

BANTAM

Bantam Rhodebars should follow the exact Standard for the large fowl.

Weights

Male   1020 g (36 oz)
Female   790 g (28 oz)

WELBAR

LARGE FOWL

Origin: British
Classification: Light
Egg colour: Brown

A breed now attracting a certain amount of interest, the Welbar was created not by the team at Cambridge but by a Mr Humphreys from Devon. Chicks were hatched from original Welsummer and barred Rock matings in 1941. The cockerels of these were then bred back to Welsummer hens. As can be expected, there was some variation between the early examples of the breed, but Mr Humphreys selected stock that most closely matched the size, shape and egg colour of Welsummers. This breed, along with Cream Legbars, is gaining support from dedicated fanciers and back-garden keepers alike.

General characteristics: male

Carriage: Upright, alert and active.
Type: Body well built on good constitutional lines. Back broad and long. Breast full, well rounded and broad. Wings moderately long, carried close to side. Tail fairly large and full, carried high, but not squirrel. Abdomen long, deep and wide.
Head: Refined. Beak strong, short and deep. Eyes large, bright. Comb single, medium size, firm and upright, free from any twists or excess, clear of the nostrils, fine texture, five to seven broad and even serrations, the back following closely, but not touching, the line of

the skull and neck. Face smooth and without overhanging eyebrows. Ear-lobes small and almond shaped. Wattles of medium size, fine texture, close together.

Neck: Fairly long, slender at top, finishing with abundant hackle.

Legs and feet: Thighs to show clear of the body. Shanks of medium length and bone, well set apart, free from feathers with soft sinews and free from coarseness. Toes four, long, straight and well spread out.

Plumage: Tight, silky, free from excess or coarseness and free from bagginess at the thighs.

Handling: Compact, firm and neat in bone throughout.

Female

The general characteristics are similar to those of the male, allowing for the natural sexual differences.

Colour

The silver

Male plumage: Head silver. Hackles silver, black ticking permissible. Back, shoulders, coverts and wing bows silver. Wings coverts (or bars) black barred; primaries and secondaries inner web black barred, outer web silver. Tail black barred. Breast black barred with silver mottling.

Female plumage: Head and hackle silver with black striping barred with white. Breast salmon. Back and wing bows and bars light grey, faintly barred, free from salmon smudges. Primaries and secondaries outer web silver, coarsely stippled with dark grey, inner web dark and faintly barred. Tail dark grey and faintly barred.

The gold

Male plumage: Head gold. Hackles gold, black ticking permissible. Back, shoulder coverts and wing bows gold. Wing coverts (or bars) black barred; primaries and secondaries inner web black barred, outer web gold. Tail black barred. Breast black barred with gold mottling.

Female plumage: Head and hackle gold with black striping barred with white. Breast rich salmon. Back and wing bows and bars mid-grey, faintly barred, free from salmon smudges.

Primaries and secondaries outer web gold coarsely stippled with dark browny grey, inner web brown-grey and faintly barred. Tail brown-grey and faintly barred.

In both sexes and colours

Beak yellow, eyes red. Comb, face, ear-lobes and wattles bright red. Legs and feet yellow.

Weights

Male   2.95–3.40 kg (6$\frac{1}{2}$–7$\frac{1}{2}$ lb)
Female   2.25–2.70 kg (5–6 lb)

Scale of points

Type	30
Colour	20
Head	20
Condition	10
Legs	10
Weight	10
	100

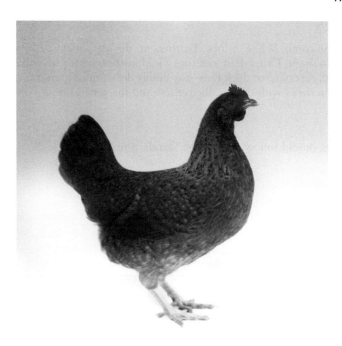

Welbar female, bantam

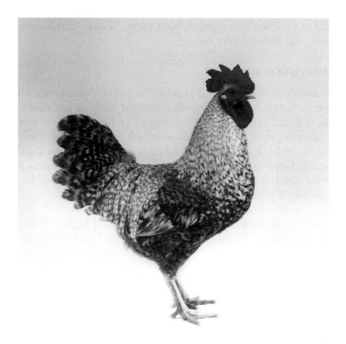

Welbar male, bantam

Serious defects

Side sprigs to the comb. White in lobe. Feathers on the legs, hocks or between the toes. Comb other than single. Other than four toes. Gold feathers on the silver male. Legs other than yellow. Badly crooked or duck toes. Any bodily deformity. Coarseness, beefiness and anything that interferes with the productiveness and the general utility of the breed.

BANTAM

Bantam Welbars should follow exactly the Standard for the large fowl.

Weights

Male   900 g (32 oz)
Female   745 g (26 oz)

WYBAR

LARGE FOWL

Origin: Great Britain
Classification: Heavy
Egg colour: Light brown

As the name suggests, this breed was created from the Wyandotte, by a dedicated fancier circa 1950. The principal aim of the Wybar was to fulfil a niche not covered by the majority of breeds: that of the triple-purpose fowl. It is true that some breeds are excellent layers, table birds and do well in the show pen; however, the Wybar sadly did not succeed in every aspect. Created from laced Wyandottes, barred Rocks and Brussbars, the Wybar laid adequately but did not particularly impress. Nowadays, Wybars can be seen at a couple of shows on occasion, but are still very rare.

General characteristics: male

Type: Body short and deep, well rounded at sides. Back short, with broad full saddle to tail with concave sweep. Breast full round, with a straight keel. Wings medium size closely folded to the side. Tail full but short, well developed and spread at the base, the true tail feathers carried rather upright, sickles medium length and gracefully curled.
Head: Broad and short, beak stout and curved. Comb rose firm, square and low in front, tapering evenly towards the back and ending in a well-defined leader following the curve of the neck. Top of the comb is evenly covered with small rounded points. Face smooth and fine. Ear-lobes oblong. Wattles medium, fine and rounded.
Neck: Well arched, medium length, with full hackle.
Legs and feet: Legs of medium length, thighs well covered with soft feathers, the fluff abundant, but close and silky. Shanks strong, well rounded and free from feathers. Toes four, straight and well covered.
Plumage: Fairly close and silky.

Female

The general characteristics are similar to those of the male, allowing for the natural sexual differences.

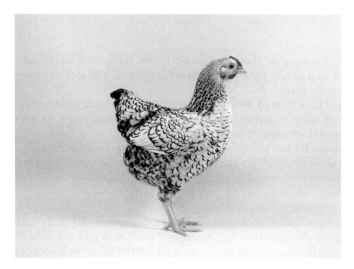

Wybar female, bantam

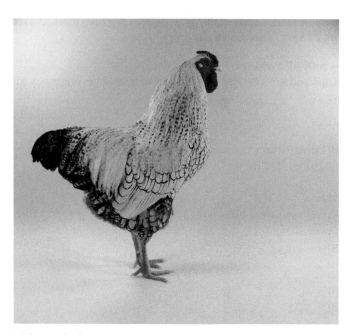

Wybar male, bantam

Colour

The silver

Male plumage: Evenly pale slate cuckoo on breast, belly and shoulders. Very silvery cuckoo on neck and saddle hackles and on wing coverts. Tail sickles even slaty cuckoo. Gold feathers to disqualify.

Female plumage: Evenly laced (but rather pale) on breast, back, saddle and wing coverts. Tail feathers and wing primaries silvery slaty and peppered. Neck hackles pale silvery cuckoo. Belly and thighs faintly (but certainly) cuckoo.

Male down colour: Rather pale silvery slaty with diffuse light head patch.

Female down colour: Dark silvery slaty, or dark silver-grey stripe, mottled over head. Light head patch, faint or very restricted in size.

The gold

Male plumage: Evenly slaty cuckoo on breast, mahogany tinged. Belly and tail feathers evenly slaty cuckoo. Wing coverts rich mahogany gold, neck and saddle hackles pale gold barred; wings indefinitely barred; primaries gold barred outer web cuckoo; secondaries similar but reversed.

Female plumage: Evenly dark gold laced (chestnut or mahogany tinged) on breast, back, saddle and wing coverts. Tail and wing primaries slaty chocolate, gold peppered. Belly and thighs faintly (but certainly) cuckoo.

Male down colour: Rather pale smoky gold, with diffuse light head patch.

Female down colour: Dark smoky gold, or dark brown stripe, mottled over head. Light head patch faint, or very restricted in size.

In both sexes and all colours

Comb, face, wattles and ear-lobes red. Beak yellow to horn. Eyes bright bay to orange. Legs and feet yellow.

Weights

Male   3–4.10 kg ($6\frac{1}{2}$–9 lb)
Female   2.50–3.20 kg ($5\frac{1}{2}$–7 lb)

Scale of points

Type	30
Colour	20
Head	20
Condition	10
Legs	10
Weight	10
	100

BANTAM

Bantam Wybars should follow exactly the Standard for large fowl.

Weights

Male   1020 g (36 oz)
Female   790 g (28 oz)

AYAM CEMANI

LARGE FOWL

Origin: Indonesia
Classification: Light: Soft feather, Rare
Egg colour: White

The Cemani fowl originates from the Indonesian archipelago. In 1998, the first examples came to The Netherlands, and in 2008 to Britain. There is some variety in type, but most look rather gamey, and all have single combs. The main characteristic of the breed is the intense black feather colour in combination with black skin colour, including face, ear-lobes and comb. Black skinned fowl are valued in many Asian countries for eating in ceremonial traditions.

General characteristics: male

Type and carriage: General appearance alert and quite gamey. Body medium sized, slim, firm and muscular, wings held strongly to body. Alert bearing. Breast fairly broad, full and firm. Back medium length, sloping from the neck; saddle hackle rather short. Wings long, large and strong, held slightly high at the shoulders. Held tight to the body, and not resting on the back. Shoulders wide and firm.

Tail held a little high; moderate spread with narrow, medium-length sickles. Rump moderately developed. Parson's nose small and firm, little fluff.
Head: Of medium size. Face black and smooth. Wattles medium, small black ear-lobes, eyes large and full of expression, dark brown to black with black pupils. Comb single, usually with five points, black. Back of comb not following down the line of the neck. Beak firm, well curved, black.
Neck: Long and firm; the neck hackle reaching to the shoulders.
Legs and feet: Thighs medium, powerful, set well apart, good bend of hock. Straight parallel medium-length shanks, black. Toes four, long, strong and well spread, with fourth toe standing well back and firm on the ground, black. Well-developed spurs in mature male birds.
Plumage: Feathers quite short and close-fitting.
Handling: Firm and muscular.

Female

The general characteristics are similar to those of the male, allowing for the natural sexual differences. The back line of the hen can be less angled, the face is often a more intensive black.

Colour

Male and female plumage: Black. Green sheen is not so obvious as in some black breeds.
In both sexes: Skin, face, comb and legs black.

Weights

Male   1.8–2 kg (4–4$\frac{1}{2}$ lb)
Female 1.2–1.5 kg (2$\frac{3}{4}$–3$\frac{1}{2}$ lb)

Scale of points

Colour (skin)	30
Colour (plumage)	20
Type	15
Condition	15
Legs	10
Head	10
	100

Serious defects

Carriage too horizontal. Tail carriage too high or too low.
Wings hanging down. Legs too short.
Too little black pigment in the skin colour.

BARNEVELDER

LARGE FOWL

Origin: The Netherlands
Classification: Heavy: Soft feather
Egg colour: Brown

This breed was originated in the district of Barneveld, The Netherlands, and stock was imported into this country in about 1921, with the brown egg as one of the chief attractions. At first the birds were very mixed for markings, some being double laced, others single, while the majority followed a partridge or 'stippled' pattern. Two varieties were standardised, namely double laced and partridge or 'stippled', but the former gradually came to the top, and is the popular variety of today.

General characteristics: male

Carriage: Alert, upright and well balanced, the body appearing compressed and the back concave.
Type: Body of medium length, deep and broad shoulders and high-set saddle. Breast and rump deep, broad and full. Wings rather short and carried high. Tail full, with graceful and uniform sweep.
Head: Carried high with neat skull. Beak short and full. Eyes very bold, bright and prominent. Comb single, upright, of medium size and well serrated, with a firm base, the heel to follow the neck. Face smooth and as free from feathers as possible. Ear-lobes long. Wattles of medium size.
Neck: Fairly long, full and carried erect.
Legs and feet: Thighs and shanks of medium length to give symmetry. Shanks and feet free from feathers. Toes four, well spread.
Plumage: Fairly tight and of nice texture.

Female

The general characteristics are similar to those of the male, allowing for the natural sexual differences.

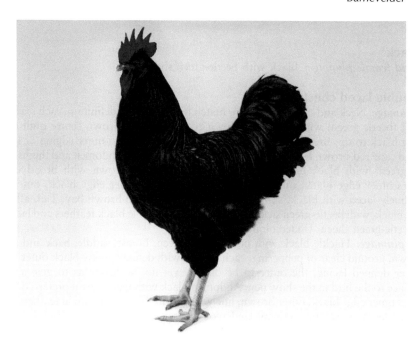

Double laced chestnut Barnevelder male, bantam

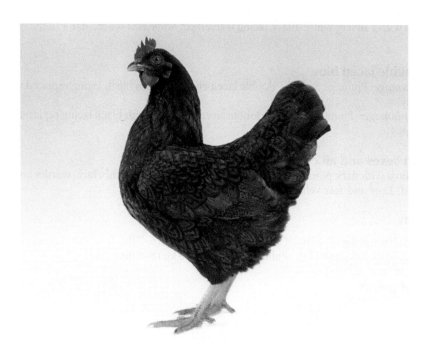

Double laced chestnut Barnevelder female, large

Colour

The black
Male and female plumage: Black with beetle-green sheen.

The double laced chestnut
Male plumage: Neck and saddle hackles to match for colour and definition, each feather to be black (beetle green) with slight red-brown edging and red-brown centre quill (stem) finishing black to tip. Breast red-brown with black (beetle green) outer edging or lacing. Back and cape red-brown feathers with very wide black lacing. Abdomen and thighs black (beetle green) with black down. Wing bows and bars red-brown with broad lacing; primaries inner edge black, outer red-brown; secondaries inner edge black, outer red-brown finely laced with black, showing when closed as a red-brown bay. Tail, all main feathers black, with beetle-green sickles and hangers. All visible black feathers and lacing to show beetle-green sheen. Undercolour slate grey.
Female plumage: Hackle black with beetle-green sheen. Breast, saddle, back and thighs red-brown, ground clear of peppering, each feather with defined glossy black outer lacing and inner defined lacing, the outer to be distinct yet not so heavy as to give a black appearance to the bird in the show pen. Abdomen black with black down preferred. Wing primaries inner edge black, outer brown, finely laced with black. Tail, main feathers black with laced feathers well up to them. Undercolour grey.

The double laced silver
Male plumage: Plumage as in the double laced chestnut, with chestnut ground colour replaced with a silvery white. Black lacing is retained. Laced chest preferred, however a solid black chest is acceptable.
Female plumage: Plumage as in the double laced chestnut, with chestnut ground colour replaced with a silvery white. Black lacing is retained. Some rust is acceptable in the ground colour.

The double laced blue
Male plumage: Plumage as in the double laced chestnut, with black lacing replaced with a blue-grey.
Female plumage: Plumage as in the double laced chestnut, with black lacing replaced with a blue-grey.

In both sexes and all colours
Beak yellow with dark point (in the silver, horn). Eyes orange. Comb, face, wattles and ear-lobes red. Legs and feet yellow.

Weights

Cock	3.20–3.60 kg (7–8 lb)	Cockerel	2.70–3.20 kg (6–7 lb)
Hen	2.70–3.20 kg (6–7 lb)	Pullet	2.25–2.70 kg (5–6 lb)

Scale of points

Type and size	30
Colour	25
Texture	15
Head	10
Legs and feet	10
Health and condition	10
	100

Minor defects

White in undercolour, flights, tails, wings, sickles or fluff.

Serious defects

White in lobes. Squirrel or wry tail. Feathered legs or toes. Side sprigs on comb. Crooked toes. High or roach back. Seriously deformed breastbones. More than four toes on either foot. Black legs.

BANTAM

Barnevelder bantams are exact replicas of their large fowl counterparts and so Standard, defects and scale of points apply.

Weights

Male   910 g (32 oz) max.
Female   740 g (26 oz) max.

BELGIAN BEARDED BANTAMS

The breeds of Belgian Bantams standardised in Britain are: Barbu d'Anvers, Barbu de Grubbe (Rumpless d'Anvers), Barbu d'Uccle, Barbu d'Everburg (Rumpless d'Uccle), Barbu de Watermael and Barbu de Boitsfort (Rumpless de Watermael). Each breed has its own unique characteristics but all are united in the requirement for a well-developed beard. Each of the six breeds has many colour variations, some of them intricate and all attractive. Not all colours are standardised in Britain.

Origin: Belgium
Classification: True Bantam
Egg colour: White or cream

BARBU D'ANVERS

General characteristics: male

(The Barbu d'Anvers is always rose combed and clean legged.)

Carriage and appearance: Small, proud, standing bold upright, with the head thrown well back; proud and provoking (appearing always ready to crow) with characteristic great development of neck hackle.
Type: Body broad and short, with arched breast carried well up. Back very short, slanting downwards to tail. Wings medium length, carried sloping towards ground. Tail carried almost perpendicularly, the main tail feathers strong and not hidden by the narrow sickle feathers; the two largest sickles slightly curved and sword shaped, the remainder in fan-like tiers to junction with saddle hackle.
Head: Appearing rather large. Beak short, strong and curved, carrying a longitudinal band of light or dark colour in keeping with the plumage. Comb curved broad in front, ending in a leader or spike at rear; for preference covered with small tooth-like points, or alternatively hollowed and ridged. Point or leader to follow line of neck. Eyes large and

prominent, as dark as possible, colour to vary in keeping with plumage. Face covered with relatively long feathers, standing away from the head, sloping backwards and forming whiskers which cover ears and ear-lobes. Brow heavily furnished with feathers. Beard composed of feathers turned horizontally backwards from both sides of the beak and from the centre vertically downwards, the whole forming a tri-lobe and giving a muffed effect. Ear-lobes small, wattles rudimentary only, but preferably none.

Neck: Of moderate length, the hackles thick and convexly arched (boule), entirely covering back and base of neck forming closely joined cape at front.

Legs and feet: Thighs short, with medium-length shanks free from feathers. Toes four, strong and straight, with nails of same colour as the beak.

Female

With certain exceptions the general characteristics are similar to those of the male, allowing for the natural sexual differences.

Carriage and appearance: A little bird, compact, plump, very lively, with characteristically full, rounded neck hackle and well-developed whiskers.

Head: Appearing broader than that of the male and more owl-like.

Neck: Hackle inclining backwards and forming a ruffle behind the neck, with feathers broader and more developed than in the male. The female hackle, contrary to that of the male, diminishes in thickness towards the bottom of the neck.

Tail: Short, carried sloping upwards, slightly curved towards the end and a little open.

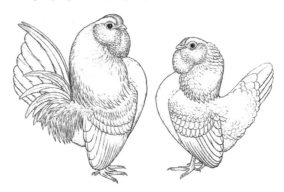

Black Belgian Barbu d'Anvers male

Weights

As small as possible. The British Belgian Bantam Club does not advocate a weight Standard for the breed but, purely as a general guide, suggests with the usual variations for age and maturity the following:

Male   680–790 g (24–28 oz) max.
Female   570–680 g (20–24 oz) max.

Scale of points

Type and carriage (beard, boule, wing and tail carriage)	60
Colour and markings	15
Size	10
General appearance and condition	15
	100

Serious defects

Wattles strongly developed. Conspicuous ear-lobes. Squirrel or wry tail. Excessive length of leg.

Disqualifications

Any trace of faking. Wattles cut or removed. Single comb. Absence of beard or whiskers. Feathers on shanks or feet. More than four toes. Yellow colouring of legs, feet or skin.

BARBU D'UCCLE

General characteristics: male

(The Barbu d'Uccle is always single combed and feather legged.)

Carriage and appearance: Typically male with a majestic manner, short and broad, with characteristic heavy development of plumage.

Type: Body broad and deep. Back very broad, almost hidden by enormous neck hackle. Breast extremely broad, the upper part very developed and carried forward, the lower part resembling a breast plate. Wings close, fitting tight to the body, sloping downwards and incurved towards but not beyond the abdomen; wing butts covered by neck hackle and tips (or ends of flights) covered by saddle hackle, which should be abundant and long. Tail well furnished, close and carried almost perpendicular to the line of the back, the two main sickles slightly curved, the remainder in regular tiers and fan-like down to the junction with the saddle hackle.

Head: Slender and small, with a longitudinal depression towards the neck. Beak short and slightly curved. Comb single, fine, upright, less than average size, evenly serrated, rounded in outline, blade following the line of the neck. Eyes round, surrounded with bare skin. Brow heavily covered with feathers becoming gradually longer towards the rear, with a tendency to join behind the neck. Beard as full and developed as possible, composed of long feathers turned horizontally from the two sides of the beak, and vertically under the beak downwards, the whole forming three ovals in a triangular group. Ear-lobes inconspicuous. Wattles as small as possible.

Neck: Furnished with silky feathers starting behind the beard at the sides of the throat, with a tendency to join behind the neck to form a mane; hackle very thick and convexly arched (boule), reaching to shoulder and saddle and covering the whole back.

Legs and feet: Legs strong and well apart, the hocks having clusters of long, stiff feathers close together, starting from the lower outer thigh, inclined downwards and following the outline of the wings. Front and outside of the shanks must be covered with feathers, short at the top of the shanks and gradually increasing in length towards the foot feather; footings turned outwards horizontally, with ends slightly curved backwards. Outer toe and outside of middle toe covered with feathers similar to shank feather.

Female

With certain exceptions the general characteristics are similar to those of the male, allowing for the natural sexual differences.

Carriage and appearance: A quiet little bird, short, thick and cobby.

Beard: Resembling that of the male but formed with softer and more open feathers.

Neck: Hackles very thick and convexly arched, composed of broad and rounded feathers, the shape of the mane resembling that of the male.

Tail: Short, flat in width and not high, the lower main feathers diminishing evenly in length.

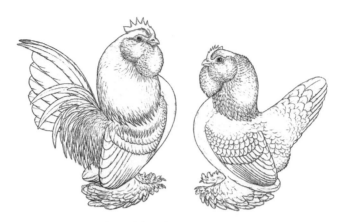

Barbu d'Uccle male and female

Weights

Dwarf, as small as possible. The British Belgian Bantam Club does not advocate a weight Standard but, purely as a general guide, suggests, with the usual variations for age and maturity:

Male   790–910 g (28–32 oz) max.
Female   680–790 g (24–28 oz) max.

Scale of points

Type and carriage (beard, boule, wing and tail carriage, hocks and footings)   60
Colour and markings   15
Size   10
General appearance and condition   <u>15</u>
                                                                               <u>100</u>

Serious defects

Strongly developed wattles. Conspicuous ear-lobes. Squirrel or wry tail. Excessive length of leg.

Disqualifications

Any trace of faking. Wattles cut or removed. Comb other than single. Absence of beard or whiskers. Poorly feathered shanks or feet. More than four toes. Yellow legs, feet or skin.

BARBU DE WATERMAEL

General characteristics: male

(The Barbu de Watermael is always crested and clean legged.)

Carriage and appearance: Proud little bantam characterised by its beard and small crest. Always on the move, perky.

Type: Breast rounded, carried forward and well up. Back short and sloping backwards. Wings medium length, carried sloping towards the ground, curving beneath the tail in the female, spread lower by the male. Tail slightly open and carried well off the perpendicular. The sickles quite short and only slightly curved.

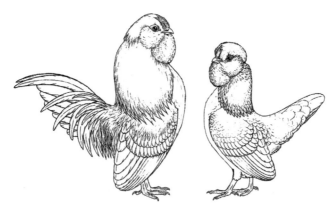

Barbu de Watermael male and female

Head: Appears large because of the crest and whiskers, skull normal. Rose comb, medium sized (length 3 cm ($1\frac{1}{4}$ in.), width 1 cm ($\frac{3}{8}$ in.)), covered with small tooth-like points, ending with three small leaders. Crest quite bushy, not too long, slightly erect and 'flying' backwards. Beak rather short, slightly curved. Ear-lobes and wattles rudimentary only and covered by muff and beard. Ear-lobes preferably white. Muff and beard well developed and forming a tri-lobe.

Neck: Hackles thick, forming a mane at the back.

Legs and feet: Thighs hidden by feathers of abdomen, shanks medium length (5 cm (2 in.)), fine. Toes four, smooth.

Female

Allowing for the natural sexual differences, the characteristics are the same as for the male except for the following.

Crest: Semi-globular, but much smaller than that of the Poland and not interfering with the sight of the bird.

Neck: Hackles not as thick as the male's but still forming a mane.

Back: A little longer than that of the male.

Tail: Closed, but carried at the same angle as that of the male.

Weights

Male   600–700 g (21–$24\frac{1}{2}$ oz) according to age
Female   450–550 g ($15\frac{1}{2}$–$19\frac{1}{2}$ oz) according to age

Scale of points

Type and carriage (beard, boule, crest, wing and tail carriage)	60
Colour and markings	15
Size	10
General appearance and condition	15
	100

Minor defects

Two leaders at end of comb instead of three. Gypsy face, or traces of dark pigmentation. Red ear-lobes.

Serious defects

Size too large. Light eyes. Wattles too developed. Beard insufficient or not trilobed. Tail open in hen or fan shaped in male, long sickles in male. Longitudinal furrow in the top of the comb.

Disqualifications

Poland-type skull or crest, crest too narrow. Yellow colouring of legs, feet or skin.

BARBU D'EVERBERG (Rumpless d'Uccle)

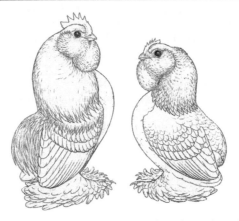

Barbu d'Everberg (Rumpless d'Uccle) male and female

BARBU DU GRUBBE (Rumpless d'Anvers)

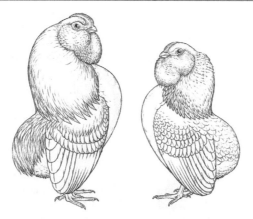

Barbu Du Grubbe (Rumpless d'Anvers) male and female

BARBU DE BOITSFORT (Rumpless de Watermael)

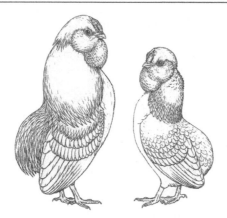

Barbu De Boitsfort (Rumpless de Watermael) male and female

The above three types should follow the types of the tailed varieties in every respect except for the following.

General characteristics: male

Tail completely absent, the whole of the lower back being covered with saddle feathers.

Female

The general characteristics are similar to those of the male, allowing for the natural sexual differences.

Colour

As for all Belgian bantam types.

Note: The scale of points for the rumpless varieties is the same as for the tailed versions, allowing for extra length of back with exclusion of tail within the Type and carriage section. The Barbu d'Everberg should include hocks and footings within the judgement of type and carriage. The Barbu de Boitsfort should include crest within the judgement of type and carriage.

Disqualifications

Any sign of tail.

Colours for all Belgian bantams

Standardised colours only are fully described. Belgian bantams exist in an extraordinary choice of colours, probably unequalled in any other breed, and much too numerous to be given in detail.

Comb, ear-lobes and rudimentary wattles are red in all colour varieties.

The millefleur

Male plumage: This is a very intricate and attractive colour scheme. Briefly, the head is orange-red with white points. The beard is of black feathers laced with very light chamois, each feather ending with a round black spot with a white triangular tip. Neck hackle black with golden shafts, and broadly bordered with orange-red, each feather having a black end tipped with a white point. The extraordinary abundance of neck hackle makes the main colour appear wholly orange-red, the black parts being scarcely visible. Back red, shading to orange towards saddle hackle. Wing bows mahogany-red, each feather tipped with white; wing bars russet-red with lustrous green-black pea-shaped spots at ends, finishing with silvery white triangular tips, the whole forming regular bars across the wings. Primaries black with a thin edging of chamois on outside; the visible lower third of each secondary feather chamois, upper two-thirds black. Remainder of wing a uniform chamois, each feather having at the end a large pea-shaped white spot on a black triangle, the tips spaced evenly to conform with shape and outline of wing. (Note the reversal of these pattern markings from the normal arrangement.) Tail feathers black with a metallic green lustre, having a fine edging or lacing of dark chamois, and terminating with a white triangle. Breast, foot feathering and remainder of plumage throughout of golden-chamois ground colour, each feather having a light chamois shaft and finished with a black pea-shaped spot tipped with a white triangle.
Female plumage: Ground colour uniform golden-chamois, each feather terminating with a black pea-shaped spot tipped with a white triangle. Tail feathers black, finely laced with chamois and with white tips. Wings markings and other plumage as described for the male, allowing for the natural sexual differences.

In both sexes: Eyes orange-red with black pupils. Beak and nails slate blue. Legs and feet slate blue.

Defects to be avoided: Ground colour too light or washed out. White markings excessively gay or unevenly distributed.

The porcelaine

Male and female plumage: This is an extraordinarily delicate colour pattern. Markings and patterns generally are as described for the millefleur in both sexes, with the exception that ground colour is light straw and the pea-shaped spots are pale blue, tipped with white triangles. Pale blue is substituted for the black of the millefleur in both sexes.

In both sexes: Eyes orange-red with black pupils. Beak and nails slate blue. Legs and feet slate blue.

Defects to be avoided: Ground colour too light or washed out. White markings too gay or unevenly distributed. Bareness or very poor quality feathering across the wing bows of the male.

The quail

Male plumage: This is a very striking colour scheme, with head feathers dark green-black, finely laced with gold. Crest of Watermael black ground colour with buff lacing and buff shafts. Beard golden-buff or nankin, shading darker towards the eyes, where plumage is black, finely laced with gold. Neck hackle with brilliant black ground, sharply laced with buff, having a golden lustre and yellowish-buff shafts. Back black ground colour with gold lacing, starting in the middle of the feathers and narrowing towards the tips, forming lance-like points with golden silky barbs and well-defined light ochre-coloured shafts from root to point. These feathers are relatively broad under the neck, but narrower and longer nearing the saddle hackle. Colour more intense and black ground more pronounced towards the saddle hackle. Wing bows light gold, lower half of each feather black and clearly defined from the upper half, which should be nankin; wing bars light ochre, each feather having black triangular tip, the triangles forming two regular bars across the wing; bottom third of secondaries chamois colour, other two-thirds dull black; primaries dull black, hidden when the wing is closed. Tail black with metallic green lustre, finely bordered with brown and with faintly defined light shafts. Sickles black, side hangers black, laced with chamois, with well-defined light shafts. Breast nankin, each feather finely laced with ochre (yellowish-buff), the shafts being distinct and clear. Thighs same colour as breast, abdomen and underparts greyish-brown, with silky, golden barb-shaped tips.

The general effect is that in this variety all the upper parts are dark and the lower parts light, giving the appearance of being covered with a dark chequered cloak. The dominating dark tint is chocolate-black, with a soft silvery lustre, known among artists as 'umber'. The general light tone is nankin or yellow-ochre, and well-defined light shafts are important.

Female plumage: Head, face and neck covered with feathers which increase in size as they near the body, ground colour umber with very fine gold lacing. Crest of Watermael umber ground colour, with gold lacing and shafts. Neck velvety, darker than the back and clearly detached from it. Shaft and lacing clearer and more golden towards the breast. Back covered with umber-coloured feathers having a silvery velvety lustre, each feather dark, finely laced with chamois and with bright nankin shafts showing in strong contrast. Wings the same colour as the back, dark umber finely laced with chamois, feathers broader and brighter towards the lower part of the wing; primaries are hidden when the wing is closed and are dark, intense umber. Tail plumage and cushion similar to the back and of the same character. Breast clear even nankin, the shafts pale and distinct, feathers nearing the wings finely and progressively bordered with dark umber, forming a distinctive colour pattern.

In both sexes: Eyes dark brown (nearly black) with black pupils. Legs and feet slate grey. Beak and nails horn.

Defects to be avoided: Salmon or brownish breast.

The blue quail
Male and female plumage: Similar to the quail in all respects except that black markings are replaced by blue.

The silver quail
Male plumage: Head covered with feathers of a dark greenish-black, finely laced with white. Beard white, going darker towards the eyes where the feathers assume a black ground colour finely laced with white. Neck hackle silky feathers with a brilliant black ground sharply laced with white, and having a light-coloured shaft. Breast deep solid white with shafts being very distinct and clear. Back black to umber with a lacing of white, which starts at the middle of the feather and gets narrower towards the top, forming a lance-like point with white barbs, clearer than the lacing, ending in the upper part of the feather. The shaft well defined. Light colour divides the feather from the root to the point. These feathers are relatively broader under the neck hackle, becoming narrower and longer. Towards the saddle hackle, the colours become more intense, the black ground more noticeable in proportion as it approaches the end of the saddle hackle feathers. Wing bows white, lower half of each feather black to umber and laced with white; wing bars white, each feather having a black triangular tip, the triangles forming two regular bars across the wing; bottom third of the secondaries white, the other two-thirds dull black; primaries dull black, hidden when the wing is closed. Tail black with metallic green lustre, finely bordered with dull black-umber and with finely defined light shafts. Sickles black. Thighs same as breast – white. Abdomen and underparts greyish-white with silky white barb-shaped tips.

The general effect is the same as for the normal, blue and lavender quail. The upper parts are dark and the lower parts are light, giving the appearance of being covered with a dark chequered cloak. The dominating dark tint is chocolate-black with a soft silvery lustre known as 'umber'. The light tone is white and well-defined light shafts are important.

Female plumage: Head, face and neck ground colour umber with fine white lacing. Beard as in male. Neck velvety, darker than the back and clearly detached from it. Shaft and lacing clearer and more white towards the breast. Breast clear even solid white. The shafts pale and distinct. Feathers nearing the wings finely and progressively bordered with dark umber, forming a distinctive pattern. Back covered with umber-coloured feathers having a silvery lustre, each feather dark, finely laced with white, with white/bright shafts showing in stronger contrast. Wings same as the back, dark umber finely laced with white feathers broader and brighter towards the lower part of the wing; primaries are hidden when the wing is closed and are dark intense umber. Tail and cushion similar to back and of the same character.

In both sexes: Eyes dark brown (nearly black) with black pupils. Legs and feet slate grey. Beak and nails horn.

Defects to be avoided: Salmon, brown or nankin on breast.

The lavender quail
In this colour the dark upper parts of the normal quail are replaced by pale silvery blue (uniform throughout the body) and the lower light parts are replaced by straw varying to cream according to the area of the body and the sex.

Male plumage: Head feathers laced with cream. Beard cream, darkening to straw towards the eyes, laced with gold. Neck hackle sharply laced in cream with golden lustre with lightish shafts. Back cream laced, golden-straw barbs, cream shafts. Wing bows light cream. The lower part of the feather clearly defined from the upper half, which should be straw. Wing bars light ochre; bottom third of secondaries cream. Tail bordered with golden-straw. Side hangers laced with chamois. Breast cream laced with ochre with distinct shafts. Thighs same as the breast. Abdomen and underparts silver/bluish-grey with straw barb-shaped tips.

Female plumage: Head, face and neck cream laced. Beard as in the male. Breast cream, shafts pale and distinct. Back feathers laced with cream or straw with light shafts. Wings same as back laced with cream, going lighter towards the bottom of the wing. Tail plumage and cushion similar to the back.

In both sexes: Eyes orange-red with black pupils. Beak, nails, legs and feet slate blue.

Defects to be avoided: Salmon, brown, nankin or white on breast.

The cuckoo

Male and female plumage: Uniformly cuckoo coloured, with transverse bands of dark bluish-grey on light grey ground. Each feather must have at least three bands.

In both sexes: Eyes orange-red. Legs, feet, beak and nails white, often spotted with bluish-grey in young birds.

Defects to be avoided: Feathers white or spotted with white, excessive number of black feathers, red on shoulders, wings and hackle.

The black mottled

Male and female plumage: All feathers black with metallic green lustre, regularly tipped with white, tips varying in size with the feather. Excessive white markings or uneven distribution to be avoided.

In both sexes: Eyes dark red. Legs and feet slate-blue or blackish. Beak and nails dark horn.

The lavender mottled

Male and female plumage: All feathers lavender, regularly tipped with white, the tips varying in size with the feather. Excessive white markings or uneven distribution to be avoided. Eyes orange-red with black pupils. Beak, nails, legs and feet slate blue.

The blue mottled

Male and female plumage: All feathers blue, regularly tipped with white, the tips varying in size with the feather. Excessive white markings or uneven distribution to be avoided. Eyes dark red. Beak, nails, legs and feet slate blue.

The black

Male and female plumage: Black all over with metallic green lustre, avoiding false colouring.

In both sexes: Eyes black, in Watermael dark brown. Legs and feet blue (blackish in young birds). Beak and nails black or very dark horn.

The white

Male and female plumage: Clear white throughout, avoiding false colours, straw tinge or yellow tint on back.

In both sexes: Eyes orange-red. Legs, feet, beak and nails white.

The lavender, or Renold's blue

Male and female plumage: This is a true-breeding pale silvery blue, all the feathers being of one uniform shade.

In both sexes: Eyes orange-red with black pupils. Beak and nails slate blue. Legs and feet slate blue.

Defects to be avoided: Any straw colouring in the hackles of the male.

The laced blue
Male plumage: Hackles, saddle, wing bows, back and tail dark slate blue, also the crest of Watermael. Remainder medium slate blue, each feather to show lacing of the darker shade.
Female plumage: Medium slate blue with darker lacing all through, except head and neck, dark slate blue.

In both sexes: Beak dark slate or horn. Eyes dark red or red-brown. Legs and feet slate. Nails dark slate or horn.

The Columbian (ermine)
Male and female plumage: Head pure white. Beard white. Neck hackle white with distinct broad black stripe down the centre of each feather, free from white shaft, such stripe to be entirely surrounded by a clearly defined white margin, finishing with a decided white tip, free from black outer edging, black tips and excess of greyness at the throat. Saddle hackle pure white. Tail main feathers black with beetle-green sheen; coverts black with beetle-green sheen either laced or not with white. Wings and primaries black or black edged with white; secondaries, black on the inner edge and white on the outer edge; remainder pure white, entirely free from ticking. Undercolour white, bluish-white or light slate, not to be visible when feathers are undisturbed. The female hackle bright intense black, each feather entirely surrounded by a well-defined white margin. Tail feathers black, except the top pair, which may or may not be laced with white. Legs and feet slate grey. Beak and nails horn coloured.

The buff Columbian (fawn ermine)
As Columbian but the white parts are replaced by buff.

The ochre white millefleur
Male plumage: Head buff with white points. Beard white laced with light buff, each feather ending with a white spot. Neck hackle white with buff shafts and broadly bordered with buff, each feather finishing in a white spot at the point. The abundance of neck hackle makes the main colour appear wholly buff, the white parts being scarcely visible. Back dark buff shading, lighter towards saddle hackle. Wing bows deep buff, each feather tipped with white; rich buff with white pea-shaped spots at ends, the whole forming regular bars across wings. Primaries white with a thin edging of light buff on the outside, the visible lower third of each secondary feather buff, with upper two-thirds white. Remainder of wing a uniform buff, each feather having at the end a large pea-shaped white spot, the tips spaced evenly to conform with the shape and outline of the wing. Tail feathers white, having a fine edging or lacing of buff, and terminating with a white tip. Breast, foot feathering and remainder of the plumage throughout an even buff ground colour, each feather having a light buff shaft and finished with a white pea-shaped spot.
Female plumage: Ground colour uniform buff, each feather terminating with a white pea-shaped spot. Tail feathers white, finely laced with buff and with white tips. Wing markings and other plumage patterns as described for the male, allowing for the natural sexual differences.

In both sexes: Eyes orange-red with black pupils. Beak and nails slate blue. Legs and feet slate blue.

The gold partridge
Male and female plumage: As in the Dutch bantam.

The silver partridge
Male and female plumage: As in the Dutch bantam.
Defects to be avoided: Ground colour too light or washed out, white markings excessively gay or unevenly distributed, and any black or blue feathers. Spotting in feathers.

BOOTED BANTAM

Origin: Europe
Classification: True Bantam
Egg colour: White or cream

These have a complex history which spreads over Great Britain, Germany (where they are named Federfußige Zwerghühner), The Netherlands (where they are named Sabel-poot) and Belgium (where they were crossed with Barbu d'Anvers to make Barbu d'Uccles). Although Black and White Booted bantams are believed to have been developed in the UK, all colours of Booteds have been rare here since they were overshadowed by Barbu d'Uccles when they were first imported in 1911. Fortunately, towards the late 1990s they were much more popular in Germany and The Netherlands, where large numbers in a wide range of colour varieties could be seen at the major shows. There has been a revival of interest in the UK since then, and, in 2014, the Booted Bantam Society UK was formed by an interested group of breeders from within the Rare Poultry Society. Booteds have tighter neck feathering than Barbu d'Uccles, with no beard or neck boule. Some young Booteds can seem too tall and narrow, but they usually become stocky, compact and full feathered when fully mature. As True Bantams, Booteds must be small, as befits their classification, and avoid the tendency towards large specimens sometimes seen at shows.

General characteristics: male

Type and carriage: Erect and strutting. Body short and compact. Full and prominent breast. Short back, the sweep of the neck, back and tail forming a clear 'U' shape, furnished with long and abundant saddle feathers. Large, long wings, carried at the same angle as, and more or less resting on, the vulture hocks. Large tail, full and upright; sickles a little longer than the main tail feathers and slightly curved. Coverts long, abundant and nicely curved.
Head: Skull small. Beak rather stout, of medium length. Eyes bright and prominent. Comb single, small, firm, perfectly straight and upright, well serrated, ideally with five to seven points. Face of fine texture, free from hairs. Ear-lobes small and flat, bright red. Wattles small, fine and well rounded.
Neck: Fairly short, but upright. Hackle feathering is full but straight, with no boule formation as seen on Barbu d'Uccles.
Legs and feet: Thighs powerful, well feathered with strongly developed vulture hocks, consisting of long rigid feathers which almost touch the ground. Fairly short shanks that are heavily furnished with long and rather stiff feathers on the outer sides. Toes four, straight and well spread, the outer and middle toes being very heavily feathered.
Plumage: Long and abundant.

General characteristics: female

The general characteristics are similar to those of the male, allowing for the natural sexual differences.

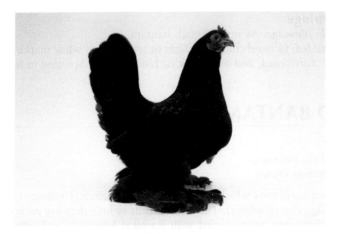

Black Booted Bantam female

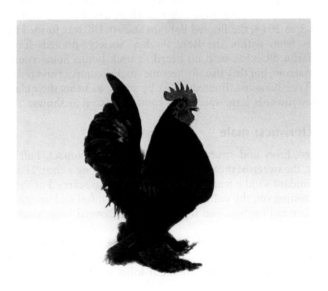

Black Booted Bantam male

Colour: self-coloured varieties

The black
Male and female plumage: Black, as lustrous as possible with a deep green sheen.

In both sexes: Beak black or horn. Eyes dark red or very dark brown. Comb, face, wattles and ear-lobes bright red. Legs and feet black, nails black.

The white
Male and female plumage: Pure snow white.

In both sexes: Beak white. Eyes red. Comb, face, wattles and ear-lobes bright red. Legs and feet white, nails white.

The blue
Male plumage: Hackles, saddle, wing bows, back and tail dark slate blue. Remainder medium slate blue, each feather to show lacing of darker shade.
Female plumage: Medium slate blue with darker lacing throughout, except head and neck – dark slate blue.

In both sexes: Beak dark slate or horn. Eyes dark red or red brown. Legs and feet slate. Nails dark slate or horn.

The lavender
Male and female plumage: This is a true breeding pale silvery blue, all the feathers being of one uniform shade.

In both sexes: Eyes orange-red. Beak and nails slate blue. Legs and feet slate blue.

Colour: the millefleur varieties

The gold millefleur
Male plumage: This is a very intricate and attractive colour scheme. Briefly, the head is orange-red with white tips. Neck hackle black with golden shafts, and broadly bordered with orange-red, each feather having a black end tipped with a white point. Back red, shading to orange towards the saddle hackle. Wing bows mahogany red, each feather tipped with white. Wing bars russet red with lustrous green black pea-shaped spots at the ends, finishing with silvery white triangular tips, the whole forming regular bars across the wings. Primaries black with a thin edging of chamois on the outside, the visible lower third of each secondary feather chamois, upper two-thirds black. Remainder of the wing a uniform chamois, each feather having at the end a large pea-shaped white spot on a pale black triangle, the tips spaced evenly to conform with the shape and outline of the wing. (Note the reversal of these pattern markings from the normal arrangement.) Tail feathers black with a metallic green lustre, having a fine edging or lacing of dark chamois, and terminating with a white triangle. Breast, foot feathering and remainder of the plumage throughout of golden-chamois ground colour, each feather having a light chamois shaft and finished with a black pea-shaped spot with a white triangle.
Female plumage: Ground colour uniform golden-chamois, each feather terminating with a black pea-shaped spot tipped with a white triangle. Tail feathers black, finely laced with chamois and with white tips. Wing markings as described for the male, allowing for the natural sexual differences.

In both sexes: Eyes orange-red. Beak and nails slate blue. Legs and feet slate blue.

The lemon millefleur
Markings and pattern as described for the gold millefleur, but with a delicate lemon-gold ground colour.

The silver millefleur
Markings and pattern as described for the gold millefleur, but with a pure silver white ground colour.

The porcelaine millefleur
Male and female plumage: Markings and patterns generally are as described for the gold millefleur in both sexes, with the exception that the ground colour is light straw and the pea-shaped spots are pale blue tipped with white triangles. Pale blue is substituted for the black in both sexes.

In both sexes: Eyes orange-red. Beak and nails slate blue. Legs and feet slate blue.

The buff white millefleur
Male and female plumage: Golden buff with a round white spangle at the end of each feather in all parts except for the tail, which is clear white.

In both sexes: Beak light blue. Eyes red. Comb, face, wattles and ear-lobes bright red. Legs and feet light blue. Nails light blue.

Colour: the birchen varieties

The silver birchen
In both sexes – face, wattles and ear-lobes dark red (but not gypsy face). Eyes orange or dark brown. Beak and nails dark horn. Legs and feet black.

Male plumage: Head silver-white. Hackle, back, saddle, shoulder coverts and wing bows silver-white, the hackles having narrow black shafts. Remainder of plumage a rich black, the breast having a narrow silver lacing gradually diminishing to black thighs.
Female plumage: Neck hackle similar to that of the male. Remainder of plumage a rich black with the breast delicately laced as in the cock.

The gold birchen
In both sexes – face, wattles and ear-lobes: dark red (but not gypsy face). Eyes orange or dark brown. Beak and nails dark horn. Legs and feet: black. Male and female plumage: As described for the silver birchen other than white or silver areas are a rich red-gold in colour.

Colour: the mottled varieties

The black mottled
Male and female plumage: All feathers black with metallic green lustre, regularly tipped with white tips, varying in size with the feather. Excessive white markings or uneven distribution to be avoided.

In both sexes: Eyes dark red, legs and feet slate blue or blackish. Beak and nails dark horn.

Lavender mottled
Male and female plumage: All feathers a pale silvery blue, regularly tipped with white, the tips varying in size with the feather. Excessive white markings or uneven distribution to be avoided.

In both sexes: Eyes are orange-red with black pupils. Beak, nails, legs and feet slate-blue.

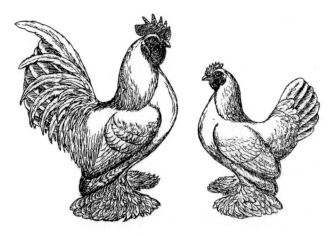

Line impression of Booted type

Other Standard colours

The cuckoo

Male and female plumage: Uniformly cuckoo coloured, with transverse bands or dark bluish-grey on a light grey ground. Each feather must have at least three bands.

In both sexes: Eyes orange-red. Legs, feet, beak and nails white, often spotted with bluish-grey in young birds.

Non-Standard colours

Many other colours are found in the UK, Germany, The Netherlands and France. These include barred, blue millefleur, blue partridge, blue mottled, buff, buff Columbian, Columbian, crele, gold duckwing, partridge, pyle, red, red mottled, and silver duckwing.

Weights

Male   750–850 g (27–30 oz)
Female   650–750 g (23–27 oz)

Scale of points

Type and size	25
Head	15
Colour (plumage)	15
Colour (legs and beak)	5
Leg and foot feathering	15
Weight	10
Condition	15
	100

Disqualifications

Any deformity.

Serious defects

Other than a single comb, gypsy face. Any sign of boule or beard. Other than four toes. Significantly overweight. Back too long/flat. Legs too short or too long. Missing toenails. Wrong leg/foot colour.

Defects to be avoided

White feathers in non-white self-coloured birds, purple barring in black birds, lacing or mottling in lavender birds, blue or slate legs in white birds, insufficient or poor white tipping in millefleur or mottled varieties, comb too large, wattles too large, vulture hocks too long.

RUMPLESS BOOTED BANTAM

Origin: Germany
Classification: True Bantam
Egg colour: Cream or white

The Rumpless Booted originates from the Thüringen Forest region of Germany, in particular the small industrial town of Ruhla in the district. It is a booted bantam, with a stocky, rumpless and rounded body and a lively and confident nature. Developed more recently than the Booted Bantam, the breed has its own Standard. They are known in the country of their origin as Ruhlaer Zwerg Kaulhuhner. Their first recorded appearances in the UK are at shows in 1901, shown as Rumpless Booted, however, there are references in articles taking them back to 1893.

General characteristics: male

Type: Body broad, short, stout and rounded. Back short and broad and only slightly sloping. Breast full and rounded. Keel well developed. Wings short and lying neatly. Shoulders broad and well rounded.
Head: Medium sized; rounded. Face red and smooth. Comb small, erect with three to five points. Wattles small and rounded. Ear-lobes red, but a little reddish-white colouring is permitted.
Neck: Short, full, not inclined backwards at all.
Legs and feet: Thighs powerful, well feathered with well-developed vulture hocks, consisting of long rigid feathers which almost touch the ground. Fairly short shanks which are heavily furnished with long and rather stiff feathers on the outer sides. Toes four, straight and well spread. The outer and middle toes being very heavily feathered.
Plumage: Wide and full. Saddle very full, saddle feathers forming a half ball rear. Tail completely absent.

Female

The general characteristics are similar to the male, allowing for the natural sexual differences. The hen's carriage is almost horizontal, with well-developed rump feathering. The comb and ear-lobes are smaller than in the male.

Colour

As per the Booted Bantams.

Weights

Male   625–700 g maximum (22–25 oz)
Female   525–600 g maximum (18.5–21 oz)

Scale of points

Type	25
Head	15
Colour (plumage)	15
Colour (legs and beak)	5
Leg and foot feathering	15
Size	10
Condition	15
	100

Disqualifications

Any sign of a tail, any deformity.

Serious defects

Other than a single comb, gypsy face. Any sign of boule or beard. Other than four toes. Significantly overweight. Back too long. Legs too short or too long. Missing toenails. Wrong leg/foot colour.

Defects to be avoided

White feathers in non-white self-coloured birds, purple barring in Black birds, lacing or mottling in Lavender birds, blue or slate legs in White birds, insufficient or poor white tipping in millefleur or mottled varieties, comb too large, wattles too large, vulture hocks too long.

BRABANTER

LARGE FOWL

Origin: The Netherlands
Classification: Light: Rare
Egg colour: White

Brabanters are known to have been bred in The Netherlands for at least 400 years because they were depicted in seventeenth century Dutch paintings. The bantam version was made comparatively recently however, and standardised in The Netherlands in 1934. They have a pointed crest, similar to crests on Appenzeller Spitzhaubens; however, Brabanters also have beards.

General characteristics: male

Carriage: Alert and active.
Type: Body moderately long with well-rounded breast. Back slightly sloping when standing normally. Large tail, well fanned and carried fairly high. Body plumage fairly tight. Head with small horned comb and a pointed crest. Beak of medium length with prominent nostrils as seen on other crested breeds. Well-developed tri-lobed beard and muffs, which cover the ear-lobes. Wattles preferably absent, or as small as possible. Neck medium length with well-developed hackles.
Legs and feet: Legs medium length. Toes four, well spread, with no trace of feather stubs.

Female

General characteristics are as for males, allowing for the natural sexual differences. Carriage is more horizontal, and crests tend to be bigger on females than males. Crests on females should not be so large that they lose their pointed shape.

Colour

The laced varieties
Gold with black lacing
Gold with blue lacing
Silver with black lacing
Silver with blue lacing
Buff with white lacing (chamois)

All of the laced varieties have markings similar to that of Polands. Brabanter lacing has always tended to be uneven, broad at feather ends, narrow up feather sides, approaching half-moon spangling. Judges should accept this, and not expect Sebright quality lacing.

The moorkop varieties
Black headed buff
Black headed white
Male and female plumage: Ideally all feathers on head and upper neck down to the bottom of the beard should be black. The next 5 cm (2 in.) of the neck has a mixture of black and buff or white (as applicable) feathers. The remaining plumage should be buff or white. This is a very difficult pattern to breed, and many birds have either some buff or white feathers on their head or solid black heads and black feathers elsewhere on their bodies.

The black
Male and female plumage: Rich metallic black throughout.

The blue
Male and female plumage: An even shade of blue throughout, darker and shiny on neck of females, neck and saddle of males.

The cuckoo
Male and female plumage: All plumage banded light and dark grey as clearly as possible. Males tend to be a generally lighter colour than females, but preference should be given to males which are reasonably uniform all over, i.e. not very light in neck, back and saddle.

The white
Male and female plumage: Pure white throughout.

In both sexes and all colours
Eyes orange to red. Beak colours range from horn, to bluish, to white, according to variety. Shanks and feet are slate blue on all varieties except cuckoos, on which they are white. Blacks may have black shanks/feet when young, usually lightening to slate blue with age.

Weights

Male   2–2.5 kg ($4\frac{1}{2}$–$5\frac{1}{2}$ lb)
Female   1.5–2 kg ($3\frac{1}{4}$–$4\frac{1}{2}$ lb)

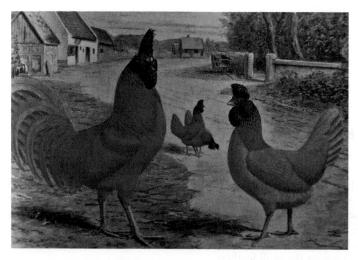

Artist's impression of Brabanter fowl

Scale of points

Head, including comb, crest and beard	30
Type and carriage	20
Legs and feet	10
Condition and show preparation	10
Colour and markings	30
	100

Serious defects

Crest too small (usually a problem on males) or too large (usually a problem on females). General size/weight: undersized large fowl, oversized bantams. Any deformity.

BANTAM

Brabanter bantams should follow the large fowl Standard.

Weights

Male   900–1000 g (32–35 oz)
Female   700–800 g (25–28 oz)

BRAHMA

LARGE FOWL

Origin: Asia
Classification: Heavy: Soft feather
Egg colour: Light brown

Although the name Brahma is taken from the river Brahmaputra in India, it is now generally agreed that they were created in America from large feather-legged birds imported from China in the 1840s known as Shanghais. These were crossed with

Malay-type birds from India, known as Grey Chittagongs, which introduced the pea comb and the beetle brow. Rivalry between breeders of various strains led to a wide variety of names and much confusion. A panel of judges meeting in Boston, MD, USA, in 1852 declared the official name to be Brahmapootras, later shortened to Brahma. After a consignment of nine birds was sent to Queen Victoria in 1852, the Brahma became one of the leading Asiatic breeds in this country. Both light and pencilled Brahmas were included in the Poultry Club's first *Book of Standards* in 1865.

General characteristics: male

Carriage: Sedate, but fairly active.
Type: Body broad, square and deep. Back short, either flat or slightly hollow between the shoulders, the saddle rising halfway between the hackle and the tail until it reaches the tail coverts. Breast full, with horizontal keel. Wings medium sized with lower line horizontal, free from twisted or slipped feathers, well tucked under the saddle feathers, which should be of ample length. Tail of medium length, rising from the line of the saddle and carried nearly upright, the quill feathers well spread, the coverts broad and abundant, well curved, and almost covering the quill feathers.
Head: Small, rather short, of medium breadth, and with slight prominence over the eyes. Beak short and strong. Eyes large, prominent. Comb triple or 'pea', small, closely fitting and drooping behind. Face smooth, free from feathers or hairs. Ear-lobes long and fine, free from feathers. Wattles small, fine and rounded, free from feathers.
Neck: Long, covered with hackle feathers that reach well down to the shoulders, a depression being apparent at the back between the head feathers and the upper hackle.
Legs and feet: Legs moderately long, powerful, well apart and feathered. Thighs large and covered in front by the lower breast feathers. Fluff soft, abundant, covering the hind parts, and standing out behind the thighs. Hocks amply covered with soft rounded feathers, or with quill feathers provided they are accompanied with proportionately heavy shank and foot feathering. Shank feather profuse, standing well out from legs and toes, extending under the hock feathers and to the extremity of the middle and outer toes, profuse leg and foot feather without vulture hock being desirable. Toes four, straight and spreading.
Plumage: Profuse, but hard and close compared with the Cochin.

Female

With the exception of the neck and legs, which are rather short, the general characteristics are similar to those of the male, allowing for the natural sexual differences.

Colour

The dark
Male plumage: Head silver-white. Neck and saddle hackles silver-white, with a sharp stripe of brilliant black in the centre of each feather tapering to a point near its extremity and free from white shaft. Breast, underpart of body, thighs and fluff intense glossy black. Back silver-white, except between the shoulders where the feathers are glossy black laced with white. Wing bows silver-white; primaries black, mixed with occasional feathers having a narrow white outside edge; secondaries part of outer web (forming 'bay') white, remainder ('butt') black; coverts glossy black, forming a distinct bar across the wing when folded. Tail black, or coverts laced (edged) with white. Leg feathers black, or slightly mixed with white.
Female plumage: Head silver-white or striped with black or grey. Neck hackle similar to that of the male, or pencilled centres. Tail black, or edged with grey, or pencilled. Remainder any shade of clear grey finely pencilled with black or a darker shade of grey than the ground colour, following the outline of each feather, sharply defined, uniform and numerous.

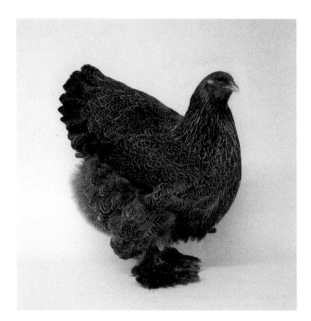

Gold Brahma female

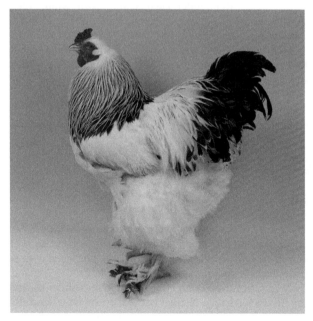

Light Brahma male

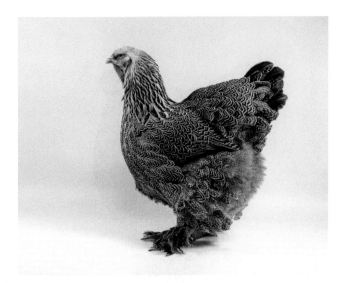

Dark Brahma female, large

The light

Male plumage: Head and neck hackle as in the dark variety. Saddle white preferably, but white slightly striped with black in birds having very dark neck hackles. Wing primaries black or edged with white; secondaries white outside and black on part of inside web. Tail black, or edged with white. Remainder clear white, with white, blue-white or slate undercolour, not visible when the feathers are undisturbed. Black-and-white admissible in toe feathering. Shank feathers white.

Female plumage: Neck hackle silver-white striped with black (dense at the lower part of the hackle), the black centre of each feather entirely surrounded by a white margin. In other respects the colour of the female is similar to that of the male.

The blue-light

Male and female plumage: As in the light, replacing black with pigeon blue.

The white

Male and female plumage: Pure white throughout.

The gold partridge

Male plumage: Head rich gold. Neck and saddle hackles rich gold, with sharp stripe of brilliant black in the centre of each feather tapering to a point near its extremity and free from gold shaft. Breast, underparts of body, thighs and fluff intense glossy black. Back rich gold except between the shoulders where the feathers may be laced with gold. Wing bows bright red; primaries black, with a narrow outer edge of rich bay; secondaries outer web (forming 'bay') partly bay, free from outer edge of black, remainder (forming 'butt') black. Wing coverts glossy black, forming a distinct bar across the wing when folded. Tail black or coverts edged with gold. Footings and leg feathers black, or slightly mixed with gold.

Female plumage: Head rich gold or striped with black. Neck hackle rich with sharp brilliant black striping free from shaftiness, the striping completely surrounded by gold. Tail black, edged with gold or pencilled. Remainder of plumage rich, even, clear gold, finely pencilled with black; the markings numerous, sharply defined and uniform, following the outline of the feather.

Blue partridge

Male and female plumage: Exactly the same as the gold partridge but with all black parts replaced with a clear even blue.

The buff Columbian

Male plumage: Head golden-buff. Neck and saddle hackles golden-buff, with a sharp stripe of brilliant black in the centre of each feather tapering to a point near its extremity and free from buff shaft. Saddle golden-buff preferably, but slightly striped with black in birds having very dark neck hackles. Wing primaries black or edged with golden-buff; secondaries golden-buff outside and black on part of inside web. Tail black, or edged with golden-buff. Remainder a clear golden-buff, with buff or slate undercolour. Black and buff in toe feathering. Shank feather buff.

Female plumage: Neck hackle golden-buff striped with black (dense at the lower part of the hackle), the black centre of each feather entirely surrounded by a golden-buff margin. In other respects the colour of the female is similar to that of the male.

In both sexes and all colours

Beak yellow or yellow and black. Eyes orange-red. Comb, face, ear-lobes and wattles bright red. Legs and feet orange-yellow or yellow.

Weights

Male   4.55–5.45 kg (10–12 lb)
Female   3.20–4.10 kg (7–9 lb)

Scale of points

Type, size and carriage	35
Colour (including purity and brilliance), markings and feather	30
Legs and feet (including foot feather and leg colour)	15
Head and eye	15
Condition	5
	100

Serious defects

Comb other than 'pea' type. Badly twisted hackle or wing feathers. Total absence of leg feather. Great want of size in adults. Total want of condition. White legs. Any deformity. Buff on any part of the plumage of light. Much red or yellow in the plumage, or much white in the tail of dark males. Utter want of pencilling, or patches of brown or red in the plumage of dark females. Split or slipped wings. Comb coarse or excessively large. White in flights of the colour varieties.

BANTAM

Brahma bantams are exact miniatures of their large fowl counterparts so all Standard points apply.

Weights

Male   1400 g (49 oz) max.
Female   1025 g (36 oz) max.

BRAKEL

LARGE FOWL

Origin: Belgium
Classification: Light: Rare
Egg colour: White

Brakel is a village near the market town of Aalst/Alost, north-west of Brussels in Belgium. The Brakel fowl was once kept on almost every farm and smallholding in its home area, and was generally more important in Belgium than the neighbouring breed, the Campine, which became better known in other countries. There is still an active Brakel Club in Belgium. Brakel males, which have normal cock feathering, are easily distinguished from the hen-feathered Campine males. The females of both breeds are very similar, but Brakel hens are heavier and stockier.

General characteristics: male

Carriage: Alert and graceful.
Type: Body proportionately long and deep, back moderately long, wide at the shoulders, narrowing to base of the tail, sloping slightly from shoulders to tail. Breast full, wide, deep, well rounded, carried well forward but not beyond a line drawn perpendicular with tip of beak. Wings moderately long and large, carried high, well above lower thighs, tips concealed by saddle feathers and ending short of stern. Main tail feathers broad, long, carried well back at an angle of 45° and well spread, sickles broad, long and well curved, lesser sickles, coverts and saddle hackles long and abundant.
Head: Medium size, broad and deep. Beak medium length, slightly curved. Comb single, upright, of medium size evenly serrated, the back carried well out just clear of the neck, slightly coarse in texture. Eyes full, round and bright. Face smooth and free from wrinkles. Ear-lobes medium sized, oval shaped and smooth. Wattles medium size, well rounded, free from wrinkles or folds.
Neck: Moderately long, gracefully arched and well covered with hackle feathers.
Legs and feet: Moderately long shanks, round and free from feathers. Toes four, medium length and well spread.

Female

With the exception of the single comb which falls gracefully over one side of the face, the general characteristics are similar to those of the male, allowing for the natural sexual differences.

Colour

The gold

Male plumage: Head, back and saddle hackles rich golden-bay, remainder beetle green-black barring on rich golden-bay ground. Each feather must be barred in a transverse direction with the end of the feather golden-bay, the bars being clear and with well-defined edges, running across each feather so as to form, as near as possible, rings around the body. The markings on the tail, wings, thighs and fluff are black, being twice as wide as the ground colour. The black on the breast and body is of equal width to the ground colour.
Female plumage: With the exception of the back and saddle, which should be barred with the black being twice the width of the ground colour, the rest of the plumage is as the male.

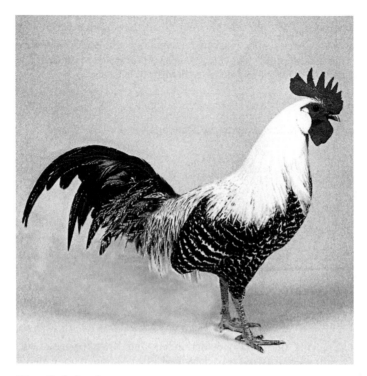

Silver Brakel male

The silver

Male plumage: Head, neck hackle, back and saddle hackles pure white, remainder beetle green-black barring on pure white ground, the markings being as in the gold.
Female plumage: Head and neck hackle pure white, remainder beetle green-black barring on pure white ground, the markings being as in the gold.

In both sexes and colours

Beak horn. Eyes dark brown with black pupil. Comb, face and wattles bright red. Ear-lobes white. Legs and feet leaden blue. Toenails horn. Undercolour slate.

Weights

Male   3.20 kg (7 lb)
Female   2.75 kg (6 lb)

Scale of points

Type	20
Markings	20
Colour	20
Head	15
Size	10
Legs and feet	10
Condition	5
	100

Serious defects

Lack of barring on breast, indistinct barring on female's back. White in face. Lack of size in adult birds. Excess ticking in neck hackle. Male's comb twisted, oversized or falling over. Dark pigmentation in comb of female. Any deformity.

BANTAM

Brakel bantams should follow exactly the Standard for the large fowl.

Weights

Male   790 g (28 oz)
Female   700 g (24 oz)

BREDA

LARGE FOWL

Origin: The Netherlands
Classification: Light: Rare
Egg colour: White or cream

This breed, also having the name Guelderlanders and Kraaikoppen (Dutch for crow headed) has been known at least as far back as the 1840s. Although not widely bred outside their homeland, Bredas have been described in many poultry books as they have a unique feature in having no comb at all.

General characteristics: male

Type and carriage: Moderately upright, the body and wings of a typical medium-weight breed, back fairly long. Breast rather full and well rounded. Tail large, full and well fanned, with the top line of the sickles carried at about 45° above the horizontal at the junction with the back. Head with beak rather long, strong, well hooked. Nostrils with a long structure similar to that found on crested breeds. Comb entirely absent. The feathers on top of the head usually stand upright, but there must be no crest. Ear-lobes and wattles moderately large. Neck medium length, well rounded and furnished.
Legs and feet: Legs of above average length, with long vulture hocks. Feet have four toes with moderate feathering down shanks and on middle and outer toes.
Plumage: Moderately abundant, but not too fluffy.

Female

Similar to the male, allowing for the natural sexual differences. However carriage is lower, and the breast is more prominent and rounded.

Colours

The black
Male and female plumage: A clear glossy green-black, beak horn colour black mixed. Feet black or slate grey.

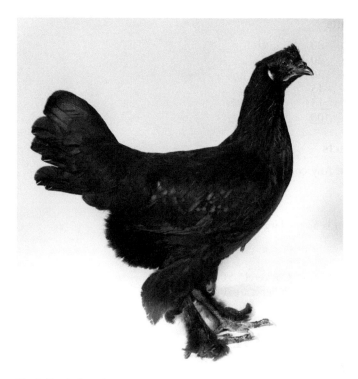

Black Breda female

The laced blue
Male and female plumage: A clear blue-grey with dark slate lacing and glossy dark slate or black hackles. Beak horn. Feet slate.

The blue
Male and female plumage: A bright clear blue-grey as free as possible from lacing. Beak horn. Feet slate.

The cuckoo
Male and female plumage: Evenly banded dark grey on silvery white. Wholly white feathers to be severely penalised. Beak white to horn shaded. Feet white to light blue-grey.

The white
Male and female plumage: Pure white throughout. Beak white to horn shaded. Feet white to light blue or grey.

In both sexes and all colours
Face and wattles bright red. Ear-lobes white. Eyes reddish-brown to orange-brown.

Weights

Cock	3 kg (6½ lb) or over	Cockerel	2.5 kg (5½ lb) or over
Hen	2.25 kg (5 lb) or over	Pullet	1.75 kg (4 lb) or over

Scale of points

Head	30
Type, carriage	20
Legs and feet	20
Colour	15
Condition	15
	100

Serious defects

Any deformity. Any comb or crest development.

BANTAM

The description is as for large fowl.

Weights

Cock	1000 g (36 oz)	Cockerel	900 g (32 oz)
Hen	800 g (29 oz)	Pullet	700 g (24 oz)

BRESSE-GAULOISE

LARGE FOWL

Origin: France
Classification: Light: Rare
Egg colour: White

The Bresse-Gauloise, deriving its name from the territory south of Burgundy, is a fairly firmly established favourite in France, renowned for its table qualities. There have been many attempts to popularise the breed in this country, and it is strange that a bird of such potential should fail to make its mark; for it is not to be despised as a layer, and it is quick maturing and hardy. As to its early failures as a table bird in Britain possibly an answer is to be found in the fact that it possesses shanks of a dark slate colour, and on this side of the Channel the prejudice against skin and legs of any colour other than white is extremely strong. It is however seeing a recent upsurge in keepers in recent years, and the fate of the breed in Britain may therefore be promising.

General characteristics: male

Carriage: Active and graceful.
Type: Body fairly broad and compact. Breast well rounded and deep. Moderately long back, broad shoulders and saddle. Long wings, carried closely to the body. Tail well developed and carried at an angle of 45° from the back. Well-rounded sickle feathers.
Head: Medium sized. Beak strong and fairly short. Eyes bold. Comb single, erect and of medium size, evenly serrated, fine texture, the back part of it (the heel) clear of the neck but following the curve of the head, free from 'thumb marks' and side spikes. Face smooth and free from feathers. Ear-lobes well developed and rather pendant. Wattles of medium length, fine in quality and rounded at the ends.
Neck: Of medium length, amply furnished with hackle feathers.
Legs and feet: Legs moderately long and well apart. Shanks free from feathers. Toes four, straight and well spread.

Female

With the exception of the comb, which falls gracefully over either side of the face, the general characteristics are similar to those of the male, allowing for the natural sexual differences.

Colour

The black

Male and female plumage: Black with a brilliant beetle-green sheen. Black undercolour.

In both sexes: Beak dark horn. Eyes black or dark brown. Comb, face and wattles bright red. Ear-lobes snow white. Legs and feet blue-grey.

The white

Male and female plumage: Pure white. Straw tinge objectionable.

In both sexes: Beak blue-white. Eyes black or dark brown. Comb and wattles bright red. Face red or sooty. Ear-lobes blue-white or white (a little red allowed). Legs and feet slate blue.

Weights

Cock 2.50–2.75 kg (5½–6 lb)   Cockerel 2.27–2.50 kg (5–5½ lb)
Hen 2.00–2.25 kg (4½–5 lb)   Pullet   1.81–2.00 kg (4–4½ lb)

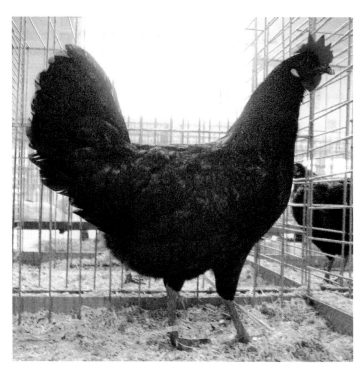

Black Bresse-Gauloise female

Scale of points

Type	25
Head	20
Colour	15
Legs and feet	10
Size	10
Quality	10
Condition	10
	100

Serious defects

Comb with white spikes. Black, white or yellow shanks or toes. White in face. White in plumage or undercolour of the black. Straw colour or cream tinge in the white. Any deformity.

BURMESE

Origin: Burma
Classification: True Bantam: Rare
Egg colour: White

These were imported by a British army officer stationed in Burma in about 1880. It was believed that they had died out before 1914, until Rare Poultry Society Founder Andrew Sheppy (1949–2017) was given a group by an elderly fancier in Wiltshire in 1970. A new 'facsimile' strain has been made in The Netherlands, but they do not yet fit the drawings made by J.W. Ludlow of the originals a century ago nearly as well as the strain that miraculously survived here. They are broadly similar to booted bantams but smaller with a lower tail carriage, which gives the Burmese a longer overall appearance, and a feathered crest in addition to a single comb. The original imports in 1880 were whites. Other colours of Burmese bantams, mentioned in old books, are believed to have been the result of crossing the few imports with Booted bantams in an attempt to increase numbers and vigour.

General characteristics: male

Carriage: Lively.
Type: Body deep, broad and long; breast broad, deep and full; back short and flat. Wings long and drooping, the ends touching the ground. Tail very large and profusely furnished with long, finely tapering sickles, carried moderately high.
Head: Skull small and fine. Crest full but falling over the back of the head. Beak short and strong. Eyes bright and prominent. Comb small single, well serrated, straight and erect, placed well forward, and in front of the crest. Ear-lobes very small and neat. Wattles rather long and pendant.
Neck: Short and thick, the hackle very abundant and long.
Legs and feet: Extremely short and heavily feathered. The outer foot feathering up to 12.5 cm (5 in.) long.
Plumage: Very abundant.

Female

The general characteristics are similar to those of the male, allowing for the natural sexual differences, except for having wattles as small as possible and the tail, which should be long and well spread.

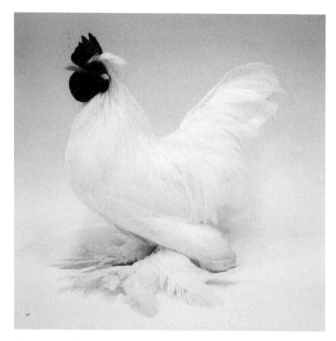

Burmese male

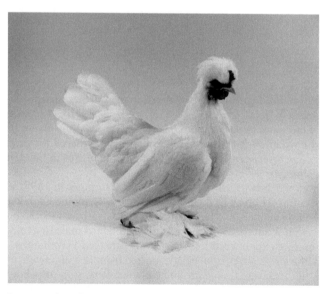

Burmese female

Colour

Male and female plumage: Pure white throughout, with no flecking or ticking of any other colour.

In both sexes: Beak yellow or horn. Eyes red or orange. Comb, face, wattles and ear-lobes bright red. Legs and feet rich yellow.

Weights

Male   570 g (20 oz)
Female   450 g (16 oz)

Scale of points

Type and size   30
Tail and foot feathering   30
Head, comb and crest   20
Colour   10
Condition   10
                                           100

Serious defects

Poor plumage quality and quantity, especially in the crest, feet and tail.
Any deformity.

CAMPINE

LARGE FOWL

Origin: Belgium
Classification: Light: Rare
Egg colour: White

The Campine (pronounced kam-peen) originated in the northern part of Belgium around Antwerp. It is closely related to the Brakel (also Belgium), Chaamse Hoen (The Netherlands) and Hergines fowl (northern France). Most Campine males bred in Belgium before 1900 had normal cock feathering, although hen-feathered males appeared occasionally. The difference between Brakels and Campines then was in build and weight, the Campines being slimmer.

British poultry expert Edward Brown wrote about Campines in 1897, soon leading to the first importation by Thomas Braken of Lancaster. A Campine Club was formed here about 1900. The club members had heard about the hen-feathered males, but did not have any at first. They were keen to adopt them as their Standard male to avoid the complications of double mating experienced by breeders of pencilled Hamburghs. The first hen-feathered male in the UK, a silver from eggs imported from Belgium, won at several shows in 1904. Sons of this bird were spread around club members, some of whom crossed them with gold females to produce hen-feathered gold males by 1911. Rosecombed Campines briefly appeared in the 1920s and 1930s. Campine bantams have appeared from time to time since the 1950s.

General characteristics: male

Carriage: Alert and graceful.

Type: Body broad, close and compact. Back rather long, narrowing to the tail. Breast full and round. Wings large and neatly tucked. Tail carried fairly high and well spread. Campine males are hen feathered, without sickles or pointed neck and saddle hackles. The top two tail feathers slightly curved.

Head: Moderately long, deep and inclined to width. Beak rather short. Eyes prominent. Comb single, upright, of medium size, evenly serrated, the back carried well out and clear of neck, free from excrescences. Face smooth. Ear-lobes inclined to almond shape, medium size, free from wrinkles. Wattles long and fine.

Neck: Moderately long and well covered with hackle feathers. The formation of the neck feathers in the Campine is called the cape.

Legs and feet: Legs moderately long. Shanks and feet free from feathers. Toes four, slender and well spread.

Female

With the exception of the single comb, which falls gracefully over one side of the face, the general characteristics are similar to those of the male, allowing for the natural sexual differences.

Colour

The gold

Male and female plumage: Head and neck hackle rich gold, not a washed-out yellow. Remainder beetle-green barring on rich gold ground. Every feather must be barred in a transverse direction with the end gold, the bars being clear and with well-defined edges, running across the feather so as to form, as near as possible, rings round the body and three times as wide as the ground (gold) colour. On the breast and underparts of the body the barrings should be straight or slightly curved. On the back, shoulders, saddle and tail they may be of a V-shaped pattern, but preferably straight.

The silver

Male and female plumage: Head and neck hackle pure white. Remainder beetle-green barring on pure white ground, the markings being as in the gold.

In both sexes and colours

Beak horn. Eyes dark brown with black pupil. Comb, face and wattles bright red. Ear-lobes white. Legs and feet leaden blue. Toenails horn.

Weights

Male   2.70 kg (6 lb)
Female   2.25 kg (5 lb)

Scale of points

Size and type	30
Head	15
Markings and colour	30
Tail	10
Legs and feet	5
Condition	10
	100

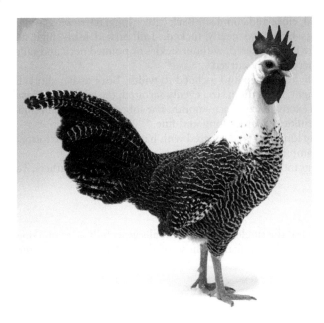

Campine male

Interpretation

The ideal is a bird clearly, distinctly and evenly barred all over with the sole exception of its neck hackle, which should be of the ground colour of the body. So that, taking the five main points of the bird – namely, neck hackle, top (including back, shoulders and saddle), tail, wing and breast – each is of as much importance as another, and judges are requested to bear in mind that a specimen excelling in one or two particulars but defective in others should stand no chance against one of fair average merit throughout. Special attention should be paid to size, type and fullness of front in breeding and judging Campines.

Serious defects

Sickle feathers or pointed hackles on the males. Bars and ground colour of equal width. Ground colour pencilled. Comb at the back too near the neck. Side spikes (or sprigs) on comb. Legs other than leaden blue. White in face. Red eyes. Feather or fluff on shanks. Dark pigmentation in combs of females. White toenails. Slate-blue beak. Black around the eyes. Any deformity.

BANTAM

Campine bantams should follow exactly the Standard for the large fowl.

Weights

Male   680 g (24 oz)
Female   570 g (20 oz)

COCHIN

LARGE FOWL

Origin: Asia
Classification: Heavy: Soft feather
Egg colour: Brown

The Cochin, as we know it today, originally came from China in the early 1850s, where it was known as the Shanghai, and later still as the Cochin-China. The breed created a sensation in this country in poultry circles because of its immense size and table properties. Moreover, it was an excellent layer. It was developed, however, for wealth of feather and fluff for exhibition purposes to the extent that its utility characteristics were neglected, if not made impossible, in winning types. There are no Cochin bantams.

General characteristics: male

General shape and carriage: Massive and deep. Carriage rather forward, high at stern, and dignified.
Type: Body large and deep. Back broad and very short. Saddle very broad and large with a gradual and decided rise towards the tail forming a harmonious line with it. Breast broad and full, as low down as possible. Wings small and closely clipped up, the flights being neatly and entirely tucked under the secondaries. Tail small, soft, with as little hard quill as possible, and carried low or nearly flat.
Head: Small. Beak rather short, curved and very stout at base. Eyes large and fairly prominent. Comb single, upright, small perfectly straight, of fine texture, neatly arched and evenly serrated, free from excrescences. Face smooth, as free as possible from feathers or hairs. Ear-lobes sufficiently developed to hang nearly or quite as low as the wattles, which are long, thin and pendant.
Neck: Rather short, carried somewhat forward, handsomely curved, thickly furnished with hackle feathers which flow gracefully over shoulders.
Legs and feet: Thighs large and thickly covered with fluffy feathers standing out in globular form; hocks entirely covered with soft curling feathers, but as free as possible from any stiff quills (vulture hocks). Shanks short, stout in bone, plumage long, beginning just below hocks and covering front and outer sides of shanks, from which it should be outstanding, the upper part growing out from under thigh plumage and continuing into foot feathering. There should be no marked break in the outlines between the plumage of these sections. Toes four, well spread, straight, middle and outer toes heavily feathered to ends. Slight feathering of other two toes is a good sign to breeders.

Female

With certain exceptions the general characteristics are similar to those of the male, allowing for the natural sexual differences. Comb and wattles as small as possible. The body more square than the male's and the shoulders more prominent. The back very flat, wide and short, with the cushion exceedingly broad, full and convex, rising from as far forward as possible and almost burying the tail. Wings nearly buried in abundant body feathering and the tail very small. Breast full, as low as possible. General shape is 'lumpy', massive and square. Carriage is forward, high at cushion, with a matronly appearance.

Colour

The black
Male and female plumage: Rich black, well glossed, free from golden or reddish feathers.

In both sexes: Beak yellow, horn or black. Comb, face, ear-lobes and wattles bright red. Eyes bright red, dark red, hazel or nearly black. Legs dusky yellow or lizard.

The blue
Male plumage: Hackle, back and tail level shade of rich dark blue free from rust, sandiness or bronze. Remainder even shade of blue free from lacing on breast, thighs or fluff and free from rust, sandiness or bronze.

Female plumage: One even shade of blue free from lacing; pigeon blue preferred.

In both sexes: Beak yellow, horn or yellow slightly marked with horn. Comb, face, ear-lobes and wattles bright red. Eyes dark. Legs and feet blue with yellow tinge in pads.

The buff
Male plumage: Breast and underparts any shade of lemon-buff, silver-buff or cinnamon provided it is even and free from mottling. Head, hackle, back, shoulders, wings, tail and saddle may be any shade of deeper and richer colour which harmonises well – lemon, gold, orange or cinnamon – wings to be perfectly sound in colour and free from mealiness. White in tail very objectionable.

Female plumage: Body all over any even shade, free from mottled appearance. Hackle of a deeper colour to harmonise, free from black pencilling or cloudiness, cloudy hackles being especially objectionable. Tail free from black.

In both sexes: Beak rich yellow. Comb, face, ear-lobes and wattles brilliant red. Eyes to match plumage as nearly as possible, but red eyes preferred although rare. Legs bright yellow with shade of red between the scales.

The cuckoo
Male and female plumage: Dark blue-grey bands across the feather on blue-grey ground, the male's hackle free from golden or red tinge, and his tail free from black or white feathers.

In both sexes: Beak rich bright yellow, but horn permissible. Comb, face, ear-lobes and wattles as in the black. Eyes bright red. Legs brilliant yellow.

The black mottled
Male and female plumage: Evenly mottled on a rich black with beetle-green sheen.

In both sexes: Beak yellow, horn or black. Comb, face, ear-lobes and wattles bright red. Eyes preferably bright red. Legs preferably yellow.

The partridge and grouse
Male plumage: Neck and saddle hackle rich bright red or orange-red, each feather with a dense black stripe. Back, shoulder coverts and wing bows rich red, of a more decided and darker shade than the neck. Wing coverts green-black, forming a wide and sharply cut bar across the wing; secondaries rich bay outside, black inside, the end of every feather black; primaries very dark bay outside and dark inside. Saddle rich red or orange-red, the same colour as, or one shade lighter than, the neck. Remainder glossy black, as intense as possible, white in tail objectionable.

Female plumage: Neck bright gold, rich gold, or orange-gold, with a broad black stripe in each feather, the marking extending well over the crown of the head. Remainder (including leg feathering) brown (darker in the grouse), distinctly pencilled in crescent form with rich dark brown or black, the pencilling being perfect and solid up to the throat.

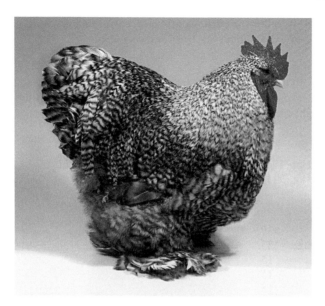

Cuckoo cochin male

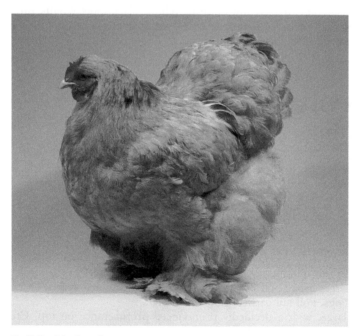

Buff Cochin female

In both sexes: Beak yellow or horn. Comb, face, ear-lobes and wattles as in the black. Eyes bright red. Legs yellow, but may be of a dusky shade.

The white

Male and female plumage: Pure white, free from any straw or red shade.

In both sexes: Beak rich bright yellow. Comb, face, ear-lobes and wattles as in the black. Eyes pearl or bright red. Legs brilliant yellow.

Weights

Cock   4.55–5.90 kg (10–13 lb)   Cockerel   3.60–5.00 kg (8–11 lb)
Hen   4.10–5.00 kg (9–11 lb)   Pullet   3.20–4.10 kg (7–9 lb)

Scale of points

Type and size	30
Colour and plumage	25
Head	15
Legs and feet	15
Condition	15
	100

Serious defects

Primary wing feathers twisted on their axes. Utter absence of leg feather. Badly twisted or falling comb. Legs other than yellow or dusky yellow. Black spots in buffs. Brown mottling (if conspicuous) in partridge males, or pale breasts destitute of pencilling in partridge females. White or black feathers in cuckoos. Crooked back, wry tail or any other deformity.

CRÈVECOEUR

LARGE FOWL

Origin: France
Classification: Heavy: Rare
Egg colour: White

The Crèvecoeur is an old French breed not unlike a Houdan, but having a horn-type comb, four toes and heavier, broad, square-built body and bold upright carriage.

General characteristics: male

Carriage: Bold and upright.
Type: Body large, broad and practically square. Well-rounded breast. Flat back. Large well-folded wings. Full tail carried moderately high.
Head: Skull large, with a decidedly pronounced protuberance on top. Crest full and compact, round on top and not divided or split, inclined slightly backwards fully to expose the comb, not in any way obstructing the sight except from behind, composed of feathers similar to those of the hackles, and at the ends almost touching the neck. Beak strong and well curved. Eyes full. Comb of the horn type (V shaped), of moderate size, upright and against the crest, each branch smooth (free from tines) and tapering to a point. Face muffed, the muffling full and deep, extending to the back of the eyes, hiding the lobes and face. Ear-lobes small but not exposed. Wattles moderately long.

Neck: Long and graceful, thickly furnished with hackle feathers.
Legs and feet: Wide apart, short and the shanks free from feathers. Toes four, straight and long.

Female

With the exception of the crest, which must be of globular shape and almost concealing the comb, the general characteristics are similar to those of the male, allowing for the natural sexual differences.

Colour

Male and female plumage: Lustrous green-black. No other colour is admissible, except a few white feathers in the crest of adults, which however are not desirable.

In both sexes: Beak dark horn. Eyes bright red, although black is admissible. Comb, face, wattles and ear-lobes bright red. Legs and feet black or slate-blue.

Weights

Male　　4.10 kg (9 lb)
Female　3.20 kg (7 lb)

Scale of points

Crest and muffling	30
Size	20
Comb	15
Colour	15
Type	10
Condition	10
	100

Serious defects

Coloured feathers. Loose crest obscuring sight. Any deformity.

BANTAM

Crèvecoeur bantams should follow the large fowl Standard.

Weights

Male　　1020 g (36 oz)
Female　790 g (28 oz)

CROAD LANGSHAN

LARGE FOWL

Origin: Asia
Classification: Heavy: Soft feather
Egg colour: Brown

The first importation of Langshans into this country was made by Major Croad and, as with other Asiatic breeds, controversy centred around it. Already there was the black

Cochin and then the black Langshan, some contending both were one breed, and others that they were quite separate Chinese breeds. As developed here the breed was called the Croad Langshan after the name of the importer. In 1904, a Croad Langshan club was formed to maintain the original stamp of the bird. The Modern Langshan has been developed along different lines and, in consequence, the two types are shown in separate classes at shows. Indeed, the Croad Langshan is successfully shown within its own breed classes at major shows, whereas the popularity of the Modern Langshan has dwindled, and is now shown in the Rare Poultry Society section.

General characteristics: male

Carriage: Graceful, well balanced, active and intelligent.
Type: Back of medium length, broad and flat across shoulders, the saddle well filling the angle between the back and the tail as seen in profile. In the male the back should appear shorter than in the female. Breast broad, deep and full (fuller in old bird) with long breastbone, the keel slightly rounded. Wings carried high, and well tucked up. Tail fan shaped, well spread to right and left and carried rather high; it should be level with the head when the bird stands in position of attention; side hangers plentiful, and two sickle feathers on each side projecting some 15 cm (6 in.) or more beyond rest. Abdomen capacious and resilient to touch, with fine pelvic bones. Saddle rather abundantly furnished with hackles.
Head: Carried well back, small for size of bird, full over the eyes. Beak fairly long and slightly curved. Eyes large and intelligent. Comb single, upright, straight, medium or rather small, free from side sprigs, thick and firm at the base, becoming rather thin, fine and smooth in texture, evenly serrated with five or six spikes (five preferred). Face free of feathers. Ear-lobes well developed, pendant and fine in texture. Wattles fine in quality and rather small.
Neck: Of medium length, with full neck hackle.
Legs and feet: Legs sufficiently long to give a graceful carriage to the body which should be well balanced, an adult bird neither high nor low on leg. Thighs rather short but long enough to let the hocks stand clear of fluff, well covered with soft feathers. Shanks medium length, well apart, feathered down outer sides (neither too scantily nor too heavily). Toes four, long, straight and slender, the outer toe feathered.
Plumage: Rather soft, neither loose nor tight.
Table merits: Size for table purposes must be a great consideration, consistent with type. Bone medium or rather fine, in due proportion to size, but subordinate to amount of meat carried. Male has higher proportion of bone than female. Skin thin and white. Flesh white.

Female

Hocks need not show in adult as she carries more fluff than the male. Cushion fairly full but not obtrusive. Tail may have two feathers slightly curved and projecting about 2.5 cm (1 in.) beyond rest. In other respects similar to the general characteristics of the male, allowing for the natural sexual differences.

Colour

The black

Male and female plumage: Surface dense black with beetle-green gloss free from purple or blue tinge. Undercolour dark grey, darker in the female. White in foot feather characteristic and not a defect.

In both sexes: Beak light to dark horn, preferably light at tip and streaked with grey. Eyes brown, the darker the better, but not black (ideal is colour of ripe hazel nut, a Vandyke brown). Comb, face, wattles and ear-lobes brilliant red. Shanks bluish-black (bluish in adult birds, scales and toes nearly black in young birds) showing pink between scales especially on back and inner side of shank. In male bird intense red should show through the skin along outer side at base of shank feathers. Toes the web and bottom of foot pinkish-white, the deeper the pink the better; black spots on soles a serious fault. Toenails white, dark colour or black a serious fault.

The white

The general characteristics are the same as for the original Croad above. Plumage is pure white, and the beak light horn. Eyes, comb, wattles and legs are as in the original Croad. Serious defects are black or coloured feathers, and black tips to the feathers.

Weights

Male   4.10 kg (9 lb) min.
Female   3.20 kg (7 lb) min.

Scale of points

Type and condition (shape 15, condition 10)	25
Body (girth 15, frame and bone 10)	25
Plumage (colour 15, furnishings and footings 10)	25
Head, feet and abdomen (head and feet 15, abdomen and pelvis 10)	25
	100

Note: It is left to the discretion of the judge to penalise any bad fault to the extent of 25 points.

Disqualifications

Yellow legs or feet. Yellow in face at base of beak or in edge of eyelids. Five toes. Other than single comb. Permanent white in ear-lobes. Grey (light slate colour) in webbing of flights. Black or partly black soles of feet as distinct from black spots. Vulture hocks.

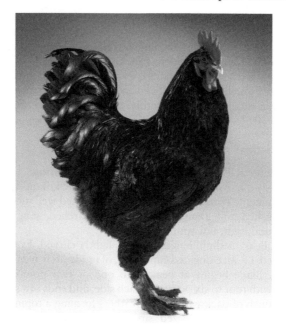

Black Croad Langshan male, large

Highly objectionable (to be firmly discouraged)

Appreciable amount of purple or blue barring. Decided purple or blue tinge. Light eye (make some allowance for age). Yellow iris. Wry or squirrel tail. Marked scarcity or absence of leg and foot feather.

Not objectionable (in stock birds and not seriously against birds in show pen, judges using their discretion)

Purple or blue barring in few feathers only where others are of good colour. Dark red in few feathers in neck hackle or on shoulders of male. White (not grey) in flights and secondaries. White tips on head of adult female. White tips or edging on breast in chicken feathers. Moderate amount of feathering on middle toe.

BANTAM

Croad Langshan bantams to follow large fowl Standard.

Weights

Male   770–910 g (27–32 oz)
Female   650–790 g (23–28 oz)

DANDARAWI

LARGE FOWL

Origin: Egypt
Classification: Light: Rare
Egg colour: White or cream

The Dandarawi is an old Egyptian breed hailing from the district in and around Dandera, where it is bred solely for egg production. It is one of the very few recognised breeds within Egypt. It has an unusual divided comb and may be related to ancient Bedouin fowl. Males are silver-grey in colour, females wheaten. Chicks are sex-linked, female chicks have a small black head spot. They are very hardy, extremely active, small boned and early maturing. They are an excellent layer of approximately 260 small eggs per year on a meagre diet. They have long been present in this country, and were accepted to the British Poultry Standards in 2017.

General characteristics: male

Carriage: Very alert and active with a proud and upright bearing.
Type: Body moderately narrow with a fine boned frame. Back of moderate length. Breast rounded but not prominent. Wings of moderate length carried well tucked up and close to body. Tail well furnished and abundant. Sickles well arched, long and flowing. Tail carriage well spread and high, not squirrel.
Head: Medium size. Beak medium length, strong, lightly curved. Eyes medium size and round. Comb is divided, i.e. an elongated cup shape, of moderately firm texture, of medium size and well set-on. Blade begins at beak with one or two points, divides into two corresponding sides, with four to six points on each side, and ends in a single blade. Behind the comb is a small bunch of backward facing feathers forming a topin or tassel. Face fine smooth texture. Ear-lobes medium-sized smooth ovals. Wattles medium sized, well rounded and of fine texture.
Neck: Long and gracefully arched with flowing abundant hackle.

Legs and feet: Thighs and shanks rather long and reachy. Fine round bone, free from feathers. Toes normally four, medium length, well spread. Five toes are sometimes present.

Female

General characteristics are similar to the male allowing for the natural sexual differences, with the exception of the comb, which is smaller and more cup-like.

Colour

The silver wheaten
Male plumage: Head and hackles white or straw, more or less striped with black. Back straw or white striped with black and lightly splashed with mahogany. Wing bows white with mahogany and black splashes. Wing bars black glossed beetle green. Secondaries outer web white, inner web black. Breast and under parts jet black. Tail a rich beetle green-black. Saddle hackles and primary sickles black laced with white.
Female plumage: Head and neck a creamy wheaten darkening to cinnamon laced grey-black on hackle. Underside of throat cream with black-grey flecks. Breast, body and thighs a delicate creamy wheaten. Wings varying shades of cinnamon, each feather with a cream shaft and a narrow lacing of cream. Flight coverts dark brown or black. Primaries outer web black, inner web pale cinnamon. Main tail nearly black. Tail and saddle cinnamon laced cream. Underfluff creamy grey.

In both sexes: Beak white. Eyes orange. Comb, face, ear-lobes and wattles bright red. Legs, feet and toenails white. Yellow legs are sometimes seen. Five toes are sometimes seen. Females often develop spurs. Tassels and topins are very common in both sexes.

Weights

Cock	1.60 kg ($3\frac{1}{2}$ lb)	Cockerel	1.36 kg (3 lb)
Hen	1.36 kg (3 lb)	Pullet	1.12 kg ($2\frac{1}{2}$ lb)

Scale of points

Type	30
Head	10
Colour	10
Legs	10
Condition	10
Tail	10
Size	10
Carriage	10
	100

Serious defects

Any specimen that does not bear the features of a productive layer with alert carriage.

DERBYSHIRE REDCAP

LARGE FOWL

Origin: Great Britain
Classification: Light: Soft feather
Egg colour: White

The Derbyshire Redcap is undoubtedly one of our oldest native breeds. Little appears to be known about its exact origin, but the consensus of opinion is that it is related to Pheasant Fowl and Gold Spangled Hamburghs, being descended from variations of localised crossbreeds that have been bred in the northern parts of England for a very long time. From the appearance and characteristics of the breed we need not for a moment doubt that the Old English Game played a prominent part in its composition. The breed is a good forager, a capital layer and has excellent breast meat. The unique feature of the breed is its immense comb, which is allocated 25 of the 100 judging points.

General characteristics: male

Carriage: Graceful action and well balanced.
Type: Back broad, moderate in length, falling slightly to tail and flat. Breast broad, full and rounded. Wings moderate in length, neat and fitting closely to the body. Tail full and carried at an angle of about 60°; broad, long and well-arched sickles.
Head: Of medium length and broad. Beak medium in length. Eyes full and prominent. Comb rose with straight leader, full of fine work or spikes, free from hollow in centre, set straight on the head and carried well off the eyes and beak; size about 8.25×7.0 cm ($3\frac{1}{4} \times 2\frac{3}{4}$ in.). Face smooth and of fine texture. Ear-lobes of medium size. Wattles of medium length, well rounded and fine in texture.
Neck: Of moderate length, nicely arched and with full hackle.
Legs and feet: Legs straight and wide apart. Thighs short and well fleshed, shanks moderately long. Toes four, well spread.

Female

The general characteristics are similar to those of the male, allowing for the natural sexual differences, with the exception of the comb, which is about half the size of the male's. The tail is large and full, and, like that of the male, carried at an angle of about 60°.

Colour

Male plumage: Neck, hackle and saddle to harmonise. Each feather to have a red quill with beetle-green webbing, very finely fringed and tipped with black (the feathers appear to be fringed with red, but if placed on paper they are seen to have a black fringe and tip; the fringe is almost as fine as a hair). Back rich red, tipped with black. Wing bows rich red; coverts rich red, each feather ending with a black spangle, forming a black bar across the wing; primaries and secondaries black on one side, red on the other side, heavily tipped with black. Breast and underparts black. Tail and hangers black.
Female plumage: Hackle as in the male, but nut-brown quill. Back and breast ground colour deep rich nut-brown, free from smuttiness, each feather ending with a half-moon black spangle. The markings on breast, back and wings to be as uniform as possible. Wing primaries and secondaries as in the male; wing coverts evenly spangled. Tail black.
  In both sexes: Beak horn. Eyes red. Comb, face, ear-lobes and wattles bright red. Legs and feet lead colour.

Weights

Cock 2.70–2.95 kg (6–6½ lb) Cockerel 2.50–2.70 kg (5½–6 lb)
Hen 2.25–2.50 kg (5–5½ lb) Pullet 2.00–2.25 kg (4½–5 lb)

Scale of points

Type and size	15
Head points (comb 25, eyes 5, ear-lobes and wattles 15)	45
Colour	25
Condition	10
Legs and feet	5
	100

Serious defects (for which birds should be penalised)

Comb over. White ear-lobes. Round back. Squirrel or wry tail. Feathers on legs. Legs other colour than lead. Other than four toes. Crooked breast. Coarseness. Excessive fat. Lacing. White-tipped feathers. Weight variations in excess of 8 oz or 227 g.

DOMINIQUE

LARGE FOWL

Origin: America
Classification: Heavy: Rare
Egg colour: Brown

This is perhaps the oldest of the distinctive American breeds, being mentioned in the earliest poultry books as an indigenous and valued variety, as an excellent layer, very hardy and good for the table. They were first seen in this country at the Birmingham Show of 1870 and re-imported in 1984.

General characteristics: male

Carriage: Erect and graceful, denoting an active fowl.
Type: Body broad, full, compact. Back medium length, moderately broad rising with concave sweep to the tail. Breast broad, round and carried well up. Wings rather large, well folded and carried without drooping, the ends being covered by the saddle hackle. Tail long, full, slightly expanded, carried at an angle of 45° above the horizontal, main tail broad and overlapping, sickles long, well curved.
Head: Medium size, carried well up. Beak short, stout, well curved. Face surface smooth, skin fine and soft in texture. Eyes large, full and prominent. Comb rose not so large as to overhang the eyes or beak, firm and straight on the head, square in front, uniform on both sides, free from hollow centre, terminating in a spike at the rear, the point of which turns slightly upwards, the top covered with small points. Ear-lobes oval, of medium size. Wattles broad, medium in length, well rounded, smooth, fine in texture, free from folds or wrinkles.
Neck: Medium length, well arched, tapering. Hackle abundant.
Legs and feet: Medium length legs, set well apart, straight when viewed from in front, shanks fine, round and free from feathers. Toes four, well spread.
Plumage: Feathering soft but close, body fluff moderately full.

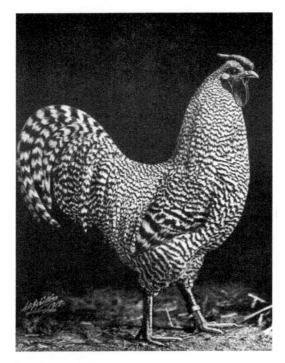

Dominique male

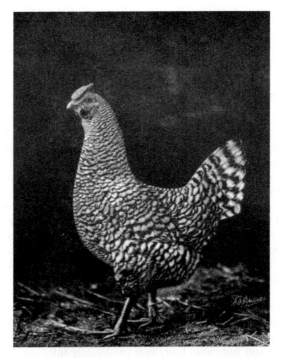

Dominique female

Female

The general characteristics are similar to those of the male, allowing for the natural sexual differences.

Colour

Male and female plumage: Slate. Feathers in all sections of the bird crossed throughout the entire plumage by irregular dark and light bars that stop short of positive black and white, the tip of each feather dark, free from shafting, brownish tinge or metallic sheen, excellence to be determined by distinct contrasts. The male may be one or two shades lighter than the female.

In both sexes: Beak, legs and feet yellow. Eyes reddish-brown. Face, comb, ear-lobes and wattles bright red. Undercolour slate.

Weights

Male   2.72–3.17 kg (6–7 lb)
Female   1.81–2.26 kg (4–5 lb)

Scale of points

Type	20
Colour	20
Markings	15
Head	15
Legs and feet	10
Tail	7
Size	7
Condition	6
	100

Serious defects

Coarse, over-refined and/or crow head. Low wing carriage. Flat and cutaway breast. Shallow and narrow bodied. Red or yellow in any part of plumage, completely white feathers. Any physical deformity.

BANTAM

Dominique bantams should follow exactly the Standard for large fowl.

Weights

Male   793 g (28 oz)
Female   566 g (20 oz)

DORKING

LARGE FOWL

Origin: Great Britain
Classification: Heavy: Soft feather
Egg colour: Brown

Its purely British ancestry makes the Dorking one of the oldest of domesticated fowls in lineage. A Roman writer, who died in AD 47, described birds of Dorking type with five toes, and no doubt such birds were found in England by the Romans under Julius Caesar. By judicious crossings, and by careful selection, the Darking or Dorking breed was established.

General characteristics: male

Carriage: Quiet and stately, with breast well forward.
Type: Body massive, long and deep, rectangular in shape when viewed sideways, and tightly feathered. Back broad and moderately long with full saddle inclined downward to the tail. Breast deep and well rounded with a long straight keel bone. Wings large and well tucked up. Tail full and sweeping, carried well out (a squirrel tail being objectionable) with abundant side hangers and broad well-curved sickles.
Head: Large and broad. Beak stout, well proportioned and slightly curved. Eyes full. Comb single or rose. Either kind is allowed in darks, single only in reds and silver greys, and rose only in cuckoos and whites. The single comb is upright, moderately large, broad at base, evenly serrated, free from thumb marks or side spikes. The rose is moderately broad and square fronted, narrowing behind to a distinct and slightly upturned leader, the top covered with small coral-like points of even height, free from hollows. Face smooth. Ear-lobes moderately developed and hanging about one-third the depth of the wattles, which are large and long.
Neck: Rather short, covered with abundant hackle feathers falling well over the back, making it appear extremely broad at the base, and tapering rapidly at the head.
Legs and feet: Legs short and strong. Thighs large and well developed but almost hidden by the body feathering. Shanks short, moderately stout and round (square or sinewy bone being very objectionable), free from feathers, the spurs set on the inner side and pointing inwards. Toes five, large, round and hard ('spongy' feet to be guarded against), the front toes (three) long, straight and well spread, the hind toe double and the extra toe well formed; namely, the normal toe as nearly as possible in the natural position, and the extra one placed above, starting from close to the other, but perfectly distinct and pointing upwards.

Female

The general characteristics are similar to those of the male, allowing for the natural sexual differences, except that the tail is carried rather closely. The single comb, too, falls over one side of the face. It is permissible for older hens to have small single spurs.

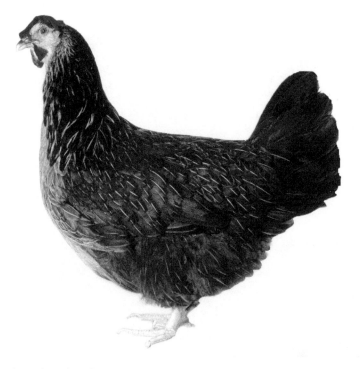

Dark Dorking female

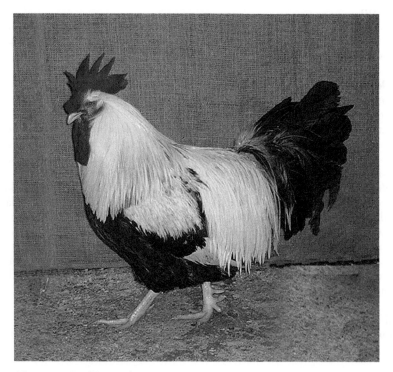

Silver grey Dorking male

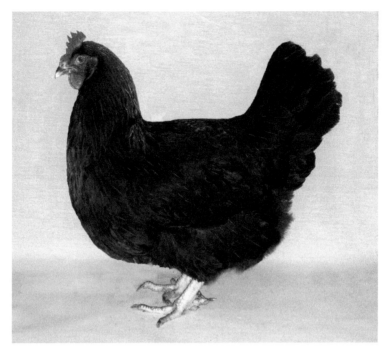

Red Dorking female

Colour

The cuckoo

Male and female plumage: Dark grey or blue bands on light blue-grey ground, the markings uniform, the colours shading into each other so that no distinct line or separation of the colours is perceptible.

The dark

Male plumage: Hackles (neck and saddle) white or straw more or less striped with black. Back various shades of white, black and white or grey, mixed with maroon or red (bronze objectionable). Wing bows white, or white mixed with black or grey; coverts (or bars) black glossed with green; secondaries outer web white, inner black. Breast and underparts jet black; white mottling not permissible. Tail richly glossed black, and a little white on primary sickles is permissible, but white hangers decidedly objectionable.

Female plumage: Neck hackle white or pale straw, striped with black or grey-black. Breast salmon-red, each feather tipped with dark grey verging on black. Tail nearly black, the outer feathers slightly pencilled. Remainder of plumage nearly black, or approaching a rich dark brown, the shaft showing a cream-white, each feather slightly pale on the edges, except on the wings, where the centre of the feather is brown-grey covered with a small rich marking surrounded by a thick lacing of the black, and free from red. Another successful colour is every feather over the body pencilled a brown-grey in the centre, with lacing round, and the breast as described above.

The red

Male plumage: Hackles (neck and saddle) bright glossy red. Back and wing bows dark red. Remainder of plumage jet black glossed with green.

Female plumage: Hackle bright gold heavily striped with black. Tail and primaries black or very dark brown. Remainder of plumage red-brown, the redder the better, each feather more or less tipped or spangled with black, and having a bright yellow or orange shaft.

The silver grey

Male plumage: Hackles (neck and saddle) silver-white free from straw tinge or marking of any kind. Back, shoulder coverts and wing bows silver-white free from striping. Wing coverts lustrous black with green or blue gloss; primaries black with a white edge on outer web; secondaries white on outer and black on inner web, with a black spot at the end of each feather, the corner of the wing when closed appearing as a bar of white with a black upper edge. Remainder of plumage deep black, free from white mottling or grizzling, although in old males a slight grizzling of the thighs is not objectionable.

Female plumage: Hackle silver-white, striped with black. Breast robin red or salmon-red ranging to almost fawn, shading off to ash grey on the thighs. Body clear silver-grey, finely pencilled with darker grey (the pencilling following the outer line of the feather), free from red or brown tinge or black dapplings.

Note: The effect may vary from soft dull grey to bright silver-grey, an old fashioned grey slate best describing the colour. Tail darker grey, inside feathers black.

The white

Male and female plumage: Snow white, free from straw tinge.

In both sexes and all colours

Beak white or horn, dark horn permissible in the dark. Eyes bright red. Comb, face, wattles and ear-lobes brilliant red. Legs and feet (including nails) a delicate white with a pink shade.

Weights

Cock   4.55–6.35 kg (10–14 lb)   Cockerel   3.60–5.00 kg (8–11 lb)
Hen   3.60–4.55 kg (8–10 lb)

Scale of points

	Dark	Silver grey and red	Cuckoo and white
Size	28	18	15
Type	20	12	20
Colour	12	24	15
Fifth toe	10	10	15
Condition	12	12	10
Head	10	16	17
Feet, condition of	8	8	8
	100	100	100

Disqualifications

Total absence of fifth toe. Legs other than white or pink-white, or with any sign of feathers. Spurs outside the shank. Single comb in cuckoo or white. Rose comb in red or silver-grey. White in breast or tail of silver-grey male. Any coloured feathers in white. Very long legs. Crooked or much swollen toes. Bumble feet. Any deformity.

BANTAM

Standards for large fowl to be used for Dorking bantams.

Weights

Male   1130–1360 g (40–48 oz)
Female   910–1130 g (32–40 oz)

DUTCH BANTAM

Origin: The Netherlands
Classification: True Bantam
Egg colour: Cream

The Dutch Bantam (or De Hollandse Krielan) in its country of origin has been around for a long time, though in The Netherlands a club was only formed on 1 December 1946. The breed first appeared in this country around the late 1960s, and a club was formed in 1982. Since then the breed has gone from strength to strength, with 13 colours standardised, although in the Netherlands many more varieties keep appearing.

General characteristics: male

Carriage: Upright and jaunty.
Type: Back very short, broad at shoulders, slightly sloping, saddle short and broad with abundant hackle running smoothly into tail coverts. Breast carried high, full and well forward. Wings relatively large and long, but not too pointed, carried low and close. Tail upright, full and well spread, with well-developed and curved sickles.
Head: Small, face smooth. Comb single, small with five serrations tending towards flyaway type. Beak short and strong, slightly curved. Eyes large and lively. Wattles fine, short and round. Ear-lobes small and fine, oval to almond shape.
Neck: Short, curved and finely tapered with plentiful hackle.
Legs and feet: Legs well spaced and straight, thighs short, shanks short and free of feather. Toes four, well spread.
Plumage: Luxuriant and lying close to body with plentiful sickles, side hangers and coverts.

Female

The general characteristics are similar to those of the male, allowing for the natural sexual differences.

Colours (British name followed by Dutch name in brackets where this differs)

The gold partridge (partridge)

Male plumage: Head orange-reddish-brown. Neck hackle a gradual transition from orange to light orange-yellow, each feather having a greenish-black middle stripe. Back deep reddish-brown. Side hackle corresponding with neck hackle, a little darker permitted. Breast black with green sheen, free from markings or spots. Wing bows black, shoulders deep reddish-brown; wing bars iridescent greenish-black; primaries inner web and tip black, outer web chestnut-brown; secondaries inner web black, outer web chestnut-brown; wing bag chestnut-brown when closed. Thighs deep black with green sheen, free from markings or spots. Abdomen black. Tail main feathers, sickles and tail coverts green iridescent black, the tail coverts nearest the side hangers with a brownish edge underneath at the tip. Undercolour greyish.

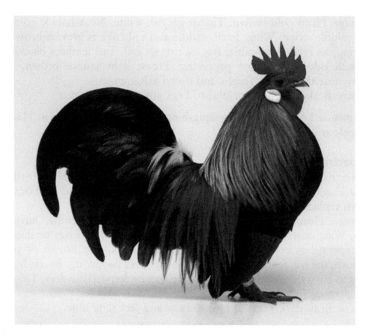

Gold partridge Dutch male

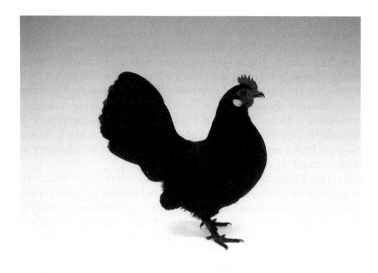

Black Dutch female

Female plumage: Head gold-brown. Throat greyish-white. Neck hackle goldish-yellow, with a black middle stripe. Wing, back, saddle and tail coverts greyish-brown with fine black peppering, as even as possible, free of rust or red. Tail feathers blackish, the top feather on each side with brown peppering. Breast light salmon-brown, shading to brownish-grey near the thighs. Thighs and down ash grey.

In both sexes: Beak dark horn or bluish. Legs and feet slate blue.

Faults: Any mismarked feathers. Any splashing or coloured feathers in black parts of male. Rusty colour in wings of female.

The silver partridge

Male plumage: Exactly the same as the gold partridge male in the black feathered parts and in the markings on the neck and saddle hackles. The orange and light orange-yellow and the brown replaced by a silvery white.

Female plumage: Head silver-white. Hackle silver-white, each feather having a black middle stripe. Wing coverts, back, saddle and tail coverts muted silver or slate grey with fine black peppering as even as possible, free from flecks, rust brown or yellow. Tail feathers blackish, the top feather on each side with silver peppering. Breast light salmon-brown, fading to ash grey underneath. Rump and rear underparts ash grey. Thighs ash grey with some peppering.

In both sexes: Beak dark horn or bluish. Legs and feet slate blue.

Faults: Any mismarked feathers. Any splashing or coloured feathers in black parts of the male. Red in plumage of male. Rusty colour in wings of female.

The yellow partridge

Male plumage: Head rich straw-yellow. Neck hackle light straw-yellow, each feather having a greenish-black middle stripe. Back deep golden-orange. Saddle hackle corresponding with neck hackle, a little darker permitted. Breast black with green sheen, free from markings and spots. Wing bows black. Shoulders golden-orange. Wing bars iridescent greenish-black; primaries black with the outer web of the feather having a narrow golden-yellow edge; secondaries inner web black which runs to the end of the feather into the outer web, which is cream coloured to straw-yellow; between the shaft and the straw-yellow of the outer web is a chestnut-brown edge that is clearly visible at the top of the wing triangle when the wing is folded. The wing triangle is creamy, straw-yellow. Thighs deep black with green sheen, free from markings and spots. Abdomen black. Tail main sickles and tail coverts green iridescent black, the tail coverts nearest the side hangers with a straw-coloured edge underneath at tip. Undercolour greyish.

Female plumage: Head greyish-yellow. Throat yellowy white. Neck hackle straw-yellow with a black middle stripe. Wing, back, saddle and tail coverts greyish/straw-yellow with fine black peppering, as even as possible, free from red rust. Tail main feathers blackish, the top feather on each side with yellow peppering. Breast rich salmon-yellow fading to greyish-yellow underneath. Rump and rear underparts grey-yellow. Thighs grey-yellow with some peppering.

In both sexes: Beak dark horn or bluish, Legs and feet slate blue.

Faults: Any mismarked feathers. Any splashing or coloured feathers in black parts of male. Red or silver plumage of male. Any rust or silver in wings of female.

The blue silver partridge

The blue yellow partridge

Male plumage: In both colours, exactly the same as the silver partridge and yellow partridge with the exception that all black parts are replaced with a clear even blue colour, free from lacing.

Female plumage: In both colours, exactly the same as the silver partridge and yellow partridge with the exception that all black is replaced with a clear even blue, free from lacing. This includes the peppering.

In both sexes and colours: Beak dark horn or bluish. Legs slate blue.

Faults: Any mismarked feathers, red in plumage of male blue silver partridge or red or silver in plumage of male blue yellow partridge. Rusty coloured wings in blue silver partridge females or rust or silver in wings of blue yellow partridge female. Wrong coloured legs.

The blue partridge

Male plumage: Exactly the same as the gold partridge male with the exception that all black parts are replaced with a clear even blue colour, free from lacing.
Female plumage: Exactly the same as the gold partridge female with the exception that all black is replaced with a clear even blue; this includes the peppering.

In both sexes: Beak dark horn or bluish. Legs and feet slate blue.

Faults: Any mismarked feathers. Any splashing or coloured feathers in the blue parts of the male. Rusty coloured wings of the female.

The pyle (white partridge)

Male plumage: Neck hackle orange-red, each feather having a white centre stripe. Back and shoulders carmine-red. Saddle hackle orange-red, each feather having a white centre stripe. Wing bars white-cream; primaries white-cream; secondaries outer web chestnut, inner web white-cream, the chestnut only showing when wing closed. Remainder of plumage white-cream.
Female plumage: Neck hackle gold-yellow, each feather having a white centre stripe. Breast salmon. Remainder of plumage white-cream.

In both sexes: Beak bluish-white or horn. Legs and feet light slate blue.

Faults: Any splashing or coloured feathers in white parts. Coloured parts of the male lacking depths of colour. Breast colour of female too pale and body colour other than white-cream.

The crele (cuckoo partridge)

Male plumage: Neck hackle straw colour banded with gold or black. Back and shoulders bright gold-chestnut banded with straw-yellow. Wing bars dark grey banded with pale grey; primaries and secondaries dark grey banded with pale grey; outer web of secondaries chestnut, the chestnut only showing when wing closed. Saddle hackle pale straw banded gold. Breast and underparts dark grey banded with light grey. Tail and tail coverts dark grey banded with light grey.
Female plumage: Neck hackle pale gold banded with black. Breast salmon. Body greyish-brown with indistinct soft banding. Wings dark greyish-brown with slightly lighter banding. Tail grey-black with slightly lighter bands.

In both sexes: Beak bluish-horn. Legs light slate blue or pearl grey.

Faults: White feathers in tail or wings.

The cuckoo

Male and female plumage: Light blue-grey ground colour with each feather banded across with broad bands of dark blue-grey. Banding to be distinct and uniform. In the male a lighter shade is permissible providing the banding is distinct. Undercolour banded but of a lighter shade. Beak light horn or bluish. Legs and feet white.
Faults: Black or white feathers. Unclear or uneven banding.

The black
Male and female plumage: Rich glossy black with beetle-green sheen throughout. Under-colour dark. Beak dark horn or bluish. Legs and feet dark slate.
Faults: Any white feathers. Purple banding. Light undercolour. Red in hackle of males. Tendency to gypsy face. Wrong leg colour.

The white
Male and female plumage: Pure snow white throughout, free from any yellow or straw tinge or any black splashes. Beak white or bluish. Legs slate blue or light slate blue.
Faults: Any yellow or straw tinge or any black splashes or peppering. Serious fault is white legs.

The blue
Male and female *plumage*: Of a clear even medium blue, free from lacing. Neck and saddle hackle in male a shade darker. Beak bluish or dark horn. Legs dark slate blue.
Faults: Unevenness of colour, black or white feathers in plumage. Any lacing. Wrong leg colour.

The lavender (pearl grey)
Male and female plumage: The lavender is not a lighter shade of blue, it is true breeding and genetically different. Lavender is light even blue with a very slight silver tint without the darker shading associated with the normal blue. The silver tint is most obvious in the male. Beak bluish or light horn. Legs slate blue.
Faults: Colour too dark or uneven. Gold or red in neck or saddle hackle in male. Wrong leg colour.

In both sexes and all colours
Eyes orange-red to brownish-red. Comb, face and wattles red. Ear-lobes pure white.

Weights
Male   500–550 g (18–20 oz)
Female   400–450 g (14–16 oz)

Scale of points
Type and carriage	35
Colour and markings	25
Head points	20
Legs and feet	10
Condition	10
	100

Serious defects
Long, narrow build. Carriage too sloping. Large glossy white or reddish ear-lobes. White in face. Wrong coloured legs or eyes. Whipped tail. Underdeveloped ornamental feathers in male. Any splashing or spotting in plumage.

BRITISH FAVEROLLES

LARGE FOWL

Origin: France
Classification: Heavy: Soft feather
Egg colour: Cream to light brown

Originating in the village of Faverolles, in northern France, this breed was created for its dual-purpose qualities. Its make-up includes such breeds as the Dorking, Houdan and Cochin, while Light Brahma blood as well as that of the Malines may be seen in some of the varieties. Imported into Great Britain in 1895, producers of table chickens crossed it freely with the Sussex, Orpington and Indian Game.

General characteristics: male

Carriage: Active and alert.
Type: Body thick, deep and cloddy. Sides deep. Back fairly long, flat and square, i.e. very broad across shoulders and saddle. Breast broad, keel bone very deep and well forward in front but not too rounded. Tail moderately long, somewhat upright with broad feathers. Wings small, prominent in front, carried closely tucked.
Head: Comb single, medium size, upright, with four to six serrations, smooth and free from coarseness or any side work.
Neck: Short and thick, especially near the body, which it should be well let into.
Serious defects: Squirrel tail or a flowing tail, either low or level with the back.

Female

Allowing for the natural sexual differences, the general characteristics are similar to the male with the following exceptions.

Type: Body and keel bone longer and deeper. Back longer in proportion. Tail carried midway between upright and drooping.
Head: Broad, flat and short, free from crest. Eyes prominent. Beak short, stout. Comb much smaller and neater. Ear-lobes and wattles small and of fine texture, both these with the face, are partly concealed by the muffling. The bird's vision should not be obscured. Face muffled. Muffling full, wide, short and solid.
Neck: Straighter than the male's.
Defects: Side sprigs in comb or badly lopped comb.
Serious defects: Deformed beak, little beard or muffs.
Serious defects (**in either** sex): Narrowness, hollow breast, crooked back or wry tail.
Disqualifications: Absence of muffling.
Legs and feet: Legs short and stout. Thighs and shanks: wide apart. Knees straight, shanks stocky, of medium length. Formation of feet and toes: toes five, the front three long, straight and well spread. The fourth, quite divided from the fifth, should be functional, on the ground and well back, the fifth turned up the leg. Foot feather: shanks sparsely feathered to the outer toe.
Defects: Excessive foot feather.
Serious defects: In-kneed. Pronounced vulture-hocks.
Disqualifications: Other than five toes on each foot, featherless shanks and outer toes.

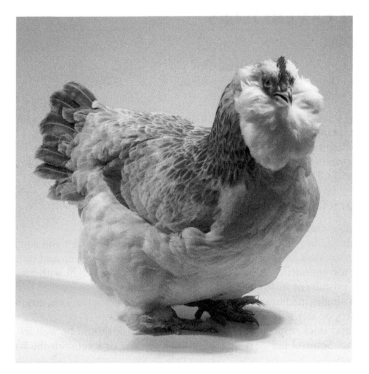

Salmon Faverolles female, large

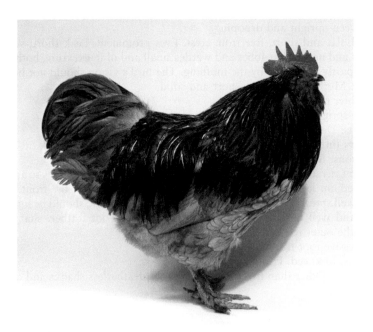

Blue Faverolles male, bantam

Table qualities

Handling qualities: The breast and thighs to be well fleshed with meat.
Disqualifications: Crooked breastbone.

General condition

Plumage quality, cleanliness, health and fitness of the bird to be good.

Serious defects (live poultry exhibits): Immaturity, significant or severe cases of inactivity, injury, illness, lameness, scaly leg, heavy infestations of lice or mites, heavily soiled or heavily moulting birds. Any bodily deformity.

Colour

(Please note that where explanations are given in brackets they are not strict Standard requirements.)

The black
Male and female plumage: A sound black showing rich beetle green.
Defects: White in foot feather.
Serious defects: White, brassiness or purple barring in hackle, wing or saddle.

The laced blue
Male plumage: Head, muffling, hackles, back, tail and wing bows a uniform dark blue. Remainder rich blue, each feather laced a dark shade.
Female plumage: A rich uniform blue, each feather laced a dark shade.
Defects: White in foot feather.
Serious defects: White or brassiness in hackle, wing or saddle.

The buff
Male and female plumage: Rich lemon-buff throughout.
Defects: Mealiness or any other colour than buff in any part of the plumage.

The cuckoo
Male and female plumage: Cuckoo throughout. Light or dark cuckoo is acceptable, uniformity of markings more important than an exact shade of colour. Ground colour pale to medium grey patterned with alternating horizontal bands of dark grey or dull black, the colours reasonably defined but shading into each other. Each feather to have at least three bands and end in a dark tip. Females tend to have fewer, wider and darker barring while the males have slightly angled/V-shaped markings in the tail and hackles.
Defects: Black or white feathers in wings or tail. Very indistinct markings or too distinct markings, i.e. barred with glossy black and smoky white bands.
Serious defects: Yellow or red in male hackles.

The ermine
Male and female plumage: Head and neck white striped with black, each feather having a solid black centre entirely surrounded by an even white margin. Wings white with black in flights. Tail and tail coverts black. Remainder of plumage pure white.
Serious defects: Smuttiness on back.

The salmon
Male plumage: Beard and muffs black. Breast, thighs, underfluff, tail and shank feathering black. Wing bars black; primaries black; secondaries white outer edge, black inner edge

and at tips. Hackles straw. In cockerels: back, shoulders and wing bows bright cherry-mahogany. In older males: a fringe of dark orange on the wing bows is permissible. (Typical undercolour is grey in the upper part of the fluff, fading paler towards the root.)

Defects: Straw colouring on wing bows, excessive thumb mark in neck hackle.
Serious defects: Extremely pale shoulders and wing bows of almost silver duckwing colouration. Very dark heavily striped hackles of almost partridge colouration.
Female plumage: Beard and muffs creamy white. Breast, thighs and underfluff cream. Remainder wheaten-brown, head and neck usually striped with a darker shade of the same colour but free from black. (*Note*: Most feathers of the head and neck also typically possess some cream lacing.) Wings similar to back but softer and lighter. Primaries, secondaries and tail wheaten-brown. (The usual colour of the inner edge of the primaries secondaries and tail is grey. Typical undercolour on the top of the body is grey in the upper part of the fluff, fading towards the root. On the front and undersides the typical undercolour is mostly creamy white.)
Defects: Dark blotchy breast, white in wing feathers.
Serious defects: Extremely pale back colour with almost white wing bows.

The white
Male and female plumage: Pure white throughout.
Serious defects: Brassiness on wings of male.

In all varieties

Comb, face, wattles and ear-lobes red. Skin colour white. Beak colour white or horn in the buffs, cuckoos, ermines, salmons and whites. Black in the black and laced blue. Legs and feet white or horn in the buffs, ermines, salmons and white. White or horn with dark markings or mottles in the cuckoo. Black in the black, black or blue in the laced blue.

Eye colour orange to yellow, grey or hazel in the buffs, cuckoos, ermines, salmons and whites. Black or brown in the black and blue.

Defects: Pale eyes a minor fault. Pure white in ear-lobe.
Serious defects: Other than Standard leg or skin colour in all colour varieties.

Weights

Large fowl

Cock	4.08–4.98 kg (9–11 lb)	Cockerel	3.4–4.53 kg ($7\frac{1}{2}$–10 lb)
Hen	3.4–4.30 kg ($7\frac{1}{2}$–9 lb)	Pullet	3.17–4.08 kg (7–9 lb)

Bantam

Male	1.13–1.36 kg ($2\frac{1}{2}$–3 lb)
Female	907–1133 g (2–$2\frac{1}{2}$ lb)

Serious defects

Any bird of an inappropriate size or weight *may* be passed. The general characteristics and recognised colour varieties detailed apply equally to large and bantam Faverolles.

Scale of points

Applies to all colours and both sizes.

Size	10
Type	20
Table qualities	10
Condition	15
Colour	20
Muffling	10
Comb	5
Formation of feet and toes	5
Foot feather (shanks and outer toes)	5
	100

Judging British Faverolles

It is accepted that a specimen excelling in one or two main areas but defective in other important features should stand no chance against a bird of fair average merit throughout. The following definitions are given for guidance to breeders and judges on how severe a penalty to award to any particular fault listed in the Standard.

Defects: Are failings which should be penalised by an appropriate deduction from the points given to that feature in the Standard.
Serious defects: Should exclude a bird from receiving a high prize card at a poultry show.
Disqualifications: Should exclude a bird from any prize or placing.

FAYOUMI

LARGE FOWL

Origin: Egypt
Classification: Light: Rare
Egg colour: White or cream

The Fayoumi is an ancient Egyptian breed from the district of Fayoum and has been selectively bred for egg production. They are hardy, very early maturing, strong fliers and vocal when handled. The Fayoumi is not genetically a barred breed but a pencilled breed. All chicks are born brown whether of the silver or gold variety. The plumage pattern is similar to that of the Brakel. They were introduced into the UK in 1984.

General characteristics: male

Carriage: Alert, graceful, very active, rather upright.
Type: Body wedge shaped, of moderate length and good depth, back moderately long, rather broad at shoulders narrowing towards tail. Breast moderately full and nicely rounded. Wings of moderate length carried well above lower thigh. Saddle full and flowing. Tail abundant, fairly large, well spread and carried high, but not squirrel.
Head: Medium size, rather broad. Beak medium length, strong and slightly curved. Eyes large, full and bright. Comb single, of medium size and evenly serrated. Face smooth and fine, free from wrinkles and folds. Ear-lobes elongated oval, smooth and fine. Wattles of medium length, well rounded.
Neck: Moderately long, gracefully arched. Hackle abundant, flowing down over back and shoulders.

Legs and feet: Thighs short and strong. Shanks medium length, round, free from feathers. Toes four, of medium length and well spread.

Female

The female has a smaller, upright comb and, allowing for the natural sexual differences, the general characteristics are similar to the male.

Colour

The silver pencilled
Male plumage: Head, hackles, back and saddle, pure silver-white. Saddle coverts black laced with silver. Tail solid black with beetle-green sheen. Remainder of plumage pure silver-white with coarse imprecise beetle green-black barring. Thighs and fluff barred. Every feather ends with a silver tip. Finer pencilling on wings to form a bar.
Female plumage: Head and hackle pure silver-white. Tail darkly barred or pencilled, main tail black. Remainder of plumage silver-white ground colour with coarse, imprecise beetle green-black barring. The bars appearing to form irregular rings around the body, approximately three times as wide as the ground colour. Thighs and fluff are barred. Every feather ending in a silver tip. Finer pencilling on wings to form a bar.

The gold pencilled
Male and female plumage: Except that the ground colour is gold, this variety is similar to the silver.

In both sexes and colours
Beak horn. Eyes dark brown. Comb, face, wattle and ear-lobes bright red. Legs and feet slate blue. Toenails horn.

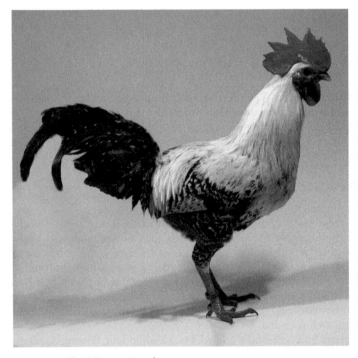

Silver pencilled Fayoumi male

Weights

Cock   1.81 kg (4 lb)   Cockerel   1.36 kg (3 lb)
Hen   1.36–1.58 kg (3–3½ lb) Pullet   900–1130 g (2–2½ lb)

Scale of points

Type   30
Head   10
Colour   10
Legs   10
Condition 10
Tail   10
Size   10
Carriage   10
          100

Serious defects

White ear-lobes. Black striping in neck. Laced body feathers. Any deformities in comb. Any specimen that does not bear the features of a productive layer with alert carriage.

BANTAM

Fayoumi bantams should follow exactly the Standard for large fowl.

Weights

Male   430 g (16 oz)
Female   400 g (14 oz)

FRIESIAN

LARGE FOWL

Origin: The Netherlands, Friesland province
Classification: Light: Rare
Egg colour: White

Friesian fowls are from the windswept northern coastal region of The Netherlands. This region was very isolated until modem times, so the breed is thought to be very similar to those bred in the area 1000 years ago. They are small, active and hardy birds, a characteristic they share with breeds from other parts of the world where chickens were expected to find most of their own food by foraging. Friesians have attracted several breeders in the UK since the 1980s, most choosing the chamois pencilled variety. As large Friesians are a small breed, they have frequently been entered in bantam classes at shows here by mistake. Friesian bantams are tiny, about the same size as Dutch bantams.

General characteristics: male

Carriage: Upright, bold and active.
Type: Body broad at the shoulders and moderately long, back sloping down slightly and narrowing to the tail. Breast carried high, full and forward. Back appears shorter with the high tail carriage. Wings are long and substantial and carried close above the thigh, slightly

sloping backwards. Tail is large and well spread and carried high. Saddle feathers well developed.

Head: Small to medium sized, somewhat oblong, fine hairy feathers on cheeks allowed. Comb single, small to medium in size, erect and evenly serrated (five or six), following the line of the skull but standing well clear of the neck. Eyes large. Beak medium length, slightly curved. Ear-lobes oval, small. Wattles medium length, round.

Neck: Long, slender near the head.

Legs and feet: Medium length legs, set well apart. Four well-spread toes.

Plumage: Full but close fitting.

Female

The abdomen is very well developed. The end of the comb may droop to one side. The other characteristics are the same as for the male, allowing for the natural sexual differences.

Colour

The gold pencilled

Male plumage: Head rich bright bay. Neck hackle, back and saddle rich lustrous bay. Front of neck rich reddish-bay. Main tail black. Sickles and lesser sickles lustrous greenish-black. Coverts greenish-black, edged with reddish-bay. Wing shoulders, front and bows lustrous reddish-bay; wing coverts rich bay, forming a distinct bar across the wing; primaries black, lower edge of lower feathers edged with bay; secondaries outer webs bay with black marking, inner web black with bay marking, exposed portion of webs forming wing bay bay. Breast rich reddish-bay. Body light bay. Abdomen fluff bay, shading to light bay at rear, some black marking. Lower thighs reddish-bay. Undercolour slate blue.

Female plumage: Head bright reddish-bay. Neck hackle bright bay. Front of neck golden-buff. Back, cushion, tail coverts and wings golden-buff marked with parallel rows of elongated black ovals, each oval extending slightly diagonally across web but not to edge. (The elongated ovals might also be called elongated spangles. The pencilling favours the description of the Sicilian Buttercup and is really not barred but has two or three pairs of small black spangles arranged in a parallel fashion.) Main tail black, lower webs barred with buff marking. Primaries buff splashed with black; secondaries golden-buff, barred with parallel black marking on outer web, forming wing bay, inner webs black edged with golden-buff. Upper breast golden-buff sparsely marked with small black ovals. Lower breast, body and lower thighs golden-buff marked same as back. Abdomen fluff buff. Undercolour slate blue.

The silver pencilled

The same as the gold pencilled except that the reds, bays and buffs are replaced with white.

The chamois pencilled

The same as the gold pencilled except that all the dark parts are a rich yellow or buff and all the other parts are white.

The lemon pencilled

The same as gold pencilled except that the gold ground colour is replaced by a light lemon.

The red pencilled

The same as gold pencilled except that the gold ground colour is replaced by a dark reddish-brown.

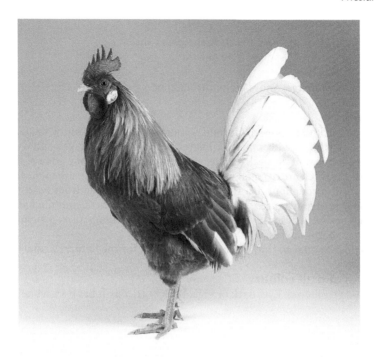

Chamois pencilled Friesian male

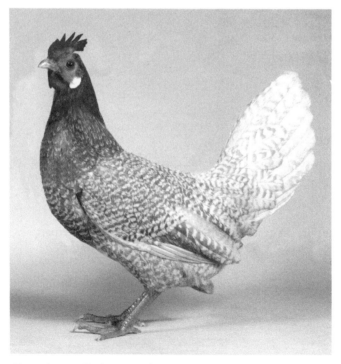

Chamois pencilled Friesian female

The black
Male and female plumage: Black with beetle-green sheen.

The white
Male and female plumage: Snow white throughout.

The cuckoo
Male plumage: Cuckoo feathered. Ground colour of body, thighs and wing feathers steel grey. The barring is black with a metallic lustre, that of the body, thighs and wing feathers straight across, but that of the neck hackle, saddle and tail slightly angled or V shaped. The alternating bars of black are of equal width and proportioned to the size of the feather. The bird should 'read' throughout, i.e. the shade should be the same from head to tail. The plumage should be free from red, black, white or yellow feathers, and the hackle, saddle and tail should be distinctly and evenly barred, while the markings all over should be rather small, even and sharply defined.
Female plumage: Similar to that of the male, allowing for the natural sexual differences.

In both sexes and all colours
Face, comb and wattles red. Eyes dark orange. Beak horn. Ear-lobes pure white. Legs slate-blue.

Weights
Male   1.40–1.60 kg (3–3½ lb)
Female   1.20–1.40 kg (2¾–3 lb)

Scale of points
Type	20
Colour and markings	30
Head	15
Condition	20
Legs and feet	5
Tail	10
	100

Serious defects

Too small, narrow frame, squirrel tail, tail carried too low. Fully folded comb in female. Black/brown eye colour.

BANTAM

Bantam Friesians are an exact miniature of the large fowl counterpart.

Weights
Male   550–650 g (19–22 oz)
Female   450–550 g (16–19 oz)

FRIZZLE

LARGE FOWL

Origin: Asia
Classification: Heavy: Soft feather
Egg colour: White

The Frizzle, a purely exhibition breed, is of Asiatic origin, and is notable for its quaint feather formation, each feather curling towards the head of the bird. It is more popular in bantams than in large fowls.

General characteristics: male

Carriage: Strutting and erect.
Type: Body broad and short. Breast full and rounded. Wings long. Tail rather large, erect, full but loose, with full sickles and plenty of side hangers. Lyre tails in males desirable but not obligatory.
Head: Fine. Beak short and strong. Eyes full and bright. Comb single, medium sized and upright. Face smooth. Ear-lobes and wattles moderate size.
Neck: Of medium length, abundantly frizzled.
Legs and feet: Legs of medium length. Shanks free from feathers. Toes four, rather thin, and well spread.
Plumage: Moderately long, broad and crisp, each feather curled towards the bird's head, and the frizzling as close and abundant as possible.

Female

The general characteristics are similar to those of the male, allowing for the natural sexual differences, except that the comb is much smaller and the neck is not so abundantly frizzled.

Colour

Male and female plumage: Black, blue, buff or white, a pure even shade throughout in the 'self-coloured' varieties; Columbian as in Wyandotte; duckwing, black-red, brown-red, cuckoo, pile and spangle as in Old English Game; red as in Rhode Island Red.

In both sexes and all colours

Beak yellow in the buff, Columbian, pile, red and white varieties; white in the spangle, black-red and cuckoo; and dark willow, black or blue in other varieties. Eyes red. Comb, face, wattles and ear-lobes bright red. Legs and feet to correspond with the beak. (There are variations in leg colour, and yellow legs are frequently seen in blacks, though not so standardised.)

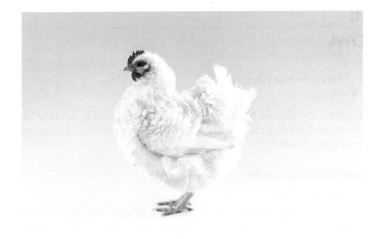

White Frizzle bantam female

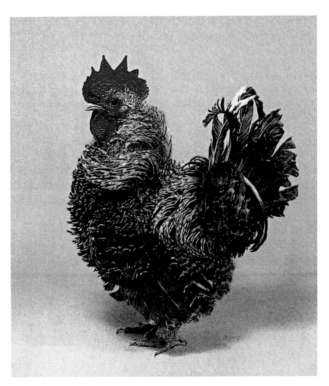

Cuckoo Frizzle bantam male

Weights

Cock   3.60 kg (8 lb)   Cockerel   3.20 kg (7 lb)
Hen   2.70 kg (6 lb)   Pullet   2.25 kg (5 lb)

Scale of points

Type   25
Colour   25
Curl of feather   30
Condition   10
Weight   <u>10</u>
                 <u>100</u>

Serious defects

Narrow feather. Want of curl. Long tail. Drooping comb. Other than single comb. White lobes. Deformity of any kind.

BANTAM

Frizzle bantams follow the large fowl Standard, although a slightly different scale of points is used.

Weights

Male   680–790 g (24–28 oz)
Female   570–680 g (20–24 oz)

Scale of points

Head and comb   5
Legs and feet   5
Plumage colour   15
Size   10
Curl   25
Feather quality   20
Type and symmetry   10
Condition   <u>10</u>
                    <u>100</u>

GERMAN LANGSHAN

LARGE FOWL

Origin: Germany
Classification: Heavy: Soft feather
Egg colour: White, cream to brown

Langshans were first imported into Germany and Austria in 1879 from Major and Miss Croad in England. German breeders kept to the Croad type, while others, led by Baron Villa-Secca of Vienna, developed their own Deutsches Langshan. A breed club was formed for their new type of Langshan in 1895. German Langshans are tall birds with unfeathered shanks and feet, and a rising tail and backline. These characteristics combine to give them their 'wine glass' outline when viewed in profile. Johann Heermann of Wedel, Holstein, developed German Langshan bantams circa 1902–1912.

General characteristics: male

Carriage: An upstanding, elegant and beautiful bird. With long extended body, leaning slightly forwards and with rising back line.
Type: Body strong, full and equally broad from front to back. Breast broad, arched and fairly deep. Belly broad, full and downy. Back long, lowest bearing starting directly under the neck hackle; from there, broad but not angular shoulders, the same width up the tail with smooth lines. Wings firmly set but carried high. Tail short, but carried in a continuing line with back, the coverts broad, soft and abundant, curved and covering the tail.
Head: Small, fairly narrow and slightly arched. Beak moderately long, strong and slightly curved. Eyes large and prominent. Comb small, single, erect, slightly arched and evenly serrated. Face smooth and slightly hairy. Wattles small, oval or round, of fine texture. Earlobes fairly long, narrow and slender.
Neck: Long, slightly curved, with moderately long hackles.
Legs and feet: Legs long, not too thick. Shanks unfeathered. Toes four, long, thin, straight and well spread with strong claws.

Female

The female displays the form of the male in a graceful manner but without marked cushion formation and with roomy hindquarters. The somewhat more loosely carried tail stands out only slightly from the coverts. Otherwise, the general characteristics are similar to those of the male, allowing for the natural sexual differences.

Colour

The black

Male and female plumage: Black with beetle-green sheen throughout.
   In both sexes: Beak black. Eyes brown-black. Legs and feet in the first year are black, later they are slate blue. Soles of feet light.

The white

Male and female plumage: Pure snow white throughout.
   In both sexes: Beak white. Eyes orange-red, Legs and feet slate blue.

The blue

Male and female plumage: Pigeon blue with dark lacing, undercolour dark grey, dark saddle and hackle feather.
   In both sexes: Beak black. Eyes brown-black. Legs and feet in the first year are black, later they are slate blue.

The birchen

Male plumage: Hackle, back, shoulder, coverts and wingbows silver-white. The neck hackle having narrow black striping, remainder rich black, the breast having a narrow silver margin around each feather, giving it a regular laced appearance gradually diminishing to perfect black thighs.
Female plumage: Hackle similar to the male, the remainder rich black, the breast very delicately laced as in the male.
   In both sexes: Beak black. Eyes brown-black. Legs and feet in the first year are black, later they are slate blue.

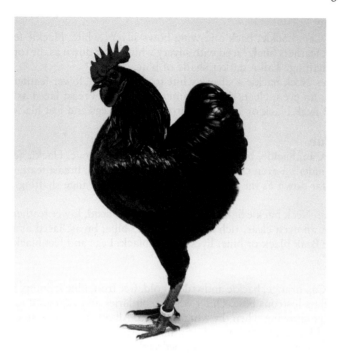

Black German Langshan bantam male

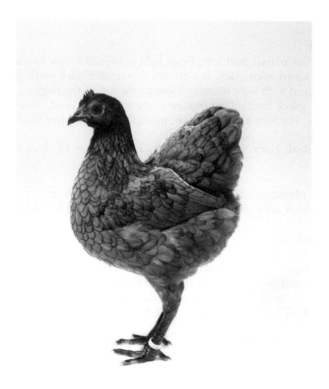

Blue German Langshan bantam female

The silver blue
Male plumage: Cap, hackle, back and wing bows silvery white. Hackle feathers striped with blue; breast feathers finely laced with silvery white as far down as the top of the thighs, with no silver shafting. Tail a darker shade of blue.
Female plumage: Neck hackle a silvery white to top of head, lower feathers striped with blue. Remainder an even, clear, rich medium to pale blue, breast laced as in the male.

In both sexes: Beak black or blue. Eyes brown-black. Legs and feet black or slate blue.

The lemon-blue
Male plumage: Cap, hackle, back and wing bows bright orange. Hackle feathers striped with blue, remainder an even clear, rich medium to pale blue; breast feathers finely laced with orange as far down as the top of the thighs, with no orange shafting. Tail a darker shade of blue.
Female plumage: Neck hackle light orange to top of the head, lower feathers striped with blue. Remainder an even clear, rich medium to pale blue; breast laced as in the male.

In both sexes: Beak black or blue. Eyes brown-black. Legs and feet black or slate blue.

The blue-red
Male plumage: Cap orange, hackle and saddle gold, free from blue striping, back and wing bows rich red. Bars lustrous blue. Outer edge secondaries and edging of lower primaries bay, the bay alone showing when the wing is closed. All other sections an even clear, rich medium to pale blue except tail, which is a darker shade of blue.
Female plumage: Hackle gold, slightly striped with blue. Breast light salmon running to slatey blue on the thighs. Remainder a rich to pale blue. Back, shoulders, wing bows, secondaries and top feathers of tail finely and evenly fringed with golden-brown.

In both sexes: Beak black. Eyes brown-black. Legs and feet willow.

The brown-red
Male plumage: Hackle, back and wing bows light orange, the neck hackle feathers being striped down the centre with black, not brown. Remainder black (with green sheen), the breast feathers edged with light orange as low as the top of the thighs.
Female plumage: Neck hackle light orange to the top of the head, lower feathers being striped with black. The breast laced as in the male, the shoulders free from ticking and the black from lacing.
In both sexes: Beak black. Eyes brown-black. Legs and feet black or slate blue.

The buff
Male and female plumage: Clear even buff to the skin throughout.
In both sexes: Beak light or horn. Eyes orange-red. Legs and feet white.

The barred (cuckoo)
Male and female plumage: Equal width of black (with green sheen) and white bars clear-cut and horizontal, carried to the skin and finished with a black tip. (Single coloured feathers, irregular and broken barring considered a defect.) V-shaped barring with the exception of the neck and saddle hackles of the male due to the natural shape of the barbs.
In both sexes: Beak light or horn. Eyes orange-red. Legs and feet slate blue.

In both sexes and all colours
Face, comb, wattles and ear-lobes red.

Weights

Male   3–4.5 kg (6½–10 lb)
Female   2.5–3.5 kg (5½–7¾ lb)

Scale of points

Type and carriage	35
Head	10
Thighs, legs and feet	20
Tail	15
Size and condition	10
Colour and plumage	10
	100

Defects

Long pointed beak. Body too high or too low in bearing. Flat breast. White in wings in coloured varieties. Stilty legs with no bend of hock.

Serious defects

Any deformity or weakness. Narrow breast. Little body depth. Stumpy loose feathers. Red, yellow or grey eyes in black or blue varieties. Saw-like comb. White in ear-lobes. Twisted feathers. Sloping shoulders with sharply set tail, cushion shape. Hollow or roached back. Coverts higher than tail feathers. In the black variety, dull colour and purple barring. In the blue variety, sooty tone or uneven colour, undefined lacing, very light beak or too light feet. In the white, any feathers that are not snow white. Feathered shanks.

BANTAM

Bantam German Langshans should follow exactly the Standard for the large fowl, including colour.

Weights

Male   1200 g (42 oz)
Female   900 g (31 oz)

GRONINGER

LARGE FOWL

Origin: The Netherlands, Groningen province
Classification: Light: Rare
Egg colour: Cream

The Groninger Meeuwen is a powerfully built farmyard fowl with a dense body, well-defined chest and slightly sloping back, making the posture almost horizontal. The tail should not be carried as high as in Friesian fowl, with a clear type difference between the two breeds.

General characteristics: male

Carriage: Almost horizonal.

Type: Back and saddle broad to medium, with faint slope to tail. Chest broad and full, carried slightly forward. Wings strong and fairly long, carried high and closed, resting on the flanks. Shoulders broad. Tail well developed, slightly fanned and carried backwards. Sickle feathers wide and well curved, tail coverts plentiful. Abdomen deep and full. Thighs of medium size, quite sturdy and well feathered.

Head: Medium sized, slightly long. Feather of the head quite fine. Face sparsely covered with fine hair-like feathers. Comb single, medium sized, not too high, even and not cut too deep, five or six serrations, fine texture, straight and standing upright. The comb does not follow the line of the neck, but is held horizontally. Beak short, only slightly bent at the tip. Wattles small to medium, quite short, thin and of fine texture and well rounded. Ear-lobes oval and quite small. Eyes rather large with a vivid expression.

Neck: Medium length, held erect with a slight curve. Hackle substantially developed on the front of the neck, shoulders and back partly covered by hackle.

Legs and feet: Straight and wide set under the body. Toes four, straight and well spaced.

Plumage: Well developed with rich decorative feathers. Wide saddle hackles in the cock, covering the wing tips.

Female

The characteristics are the same as for the male, allowing for the natural sexual differences.

Colour

The gold

Male plumage: Neck hackles glossy vivid golden-brown, feather at the front of the neck line matching that of the breast. Back and saddle glossy warm golden-brown. Shoulders shiny golden-brown; wing band golden-brown, inner web of the wing band feathers faintly spotted. Primary flights: inside web black, outer web golden-brown; secondary feathers: inside web golden-brown, transversely marked with glossy green or black dashes, outside web golden-brown, except for similar markings. Main tail feathers black. Tail coverts glossy green or black with narrow, sharply defined gold brown lacing. Chest, abdomen and thighs warm golden-brown. Rump grey or black with brown spots. Down colour dark to light blue or grey.

Female plumage: Hackle rich golden-bay, some spotting allowed on the bottom of the neck; feather at the front of the neck matching the breast, but slightly less strongly marked. Back rich golden-bay, each feather finely marked straight across with two green or black dots, forming three pairs of dots, three on each side of the shaft. Wing coverts and wing bands light golden-bay, each feather finely marked straight across with two green or black dots, forming three pairs of dots, three on each side of the shaft; primaries rich golden-bay, same markings as back. Main tail feathers rich golden-bay, same markings as back; tail coverts rich golden-bay, same markings as back. Chest rich golden-bay, each feather finely marked straight across with two green or black dots, forming three pairs of dots, three on each side of the shaft. The markings must continue uniformly upwards as far as possible. Keel and thighs rich golden-bay with black peppering. Down colour blue or grey.

Serious colour defects – male: Highly uneven ground colour, dark neck and saddle hackles, too broad or irregular wing markings, lack of sheen or bronze glow in the plumage.

Female: Too light, too dark, or uneven ground colour, coarse or very irregular markings, insufficient colour depth and sharpness of the markings; insufficient markings in the chest or markings continuing into the neck hackle.

The silver

Male and female plumage: This is, overall, similar to that of the gold, except that the golden-brown ground colour is replaced with silvery white.

Serious colour defects – male: A yellow tint in the neck or saddle hackle; rustiness in shoulders; black spots on chest, abdomen, thighs or wings; too wide or irregular lacing of sickles and tail coverts; lack of sheen.

Female: Yellow tint in the ground colour; coarse or very irregular markings; insufficient colour, depth or sharpness of markings; insufficient markings on the chest, or markings continuing into the neck hackle.

The citron

Male and female plumage: This is, overall, similar to that of the gold, except that the golden-brown ground colour is replaced with light straw-yellow.

Serious colour defects – male: Gold in the neck or saddle hackle; rustiness in shoulders; black spots on chest, abdomen, thighs or wings; too wide or irregular lacing of sickles and tail coverts; lack of sheen.

Female: Gold in the ground colour; coarse or very irregular markings; insufficient colour, depth or sharpness of markings; insufficient markings on the chest, or markings continuing into the neck hackle.

In both sexes and all colours

Face red. Comb and wattles bright red. Eyes orange-red to brown. Ear-lobes white. Beak blue or light horn-coloured blue. Legs and feet slate blue.

Weights

Male 1.8–2.1 kg (4–4¾ lb)
Female 1.6–1.8 kg (3½ – 4 lb)

Scale of points

Type	20
Colour and markings	30
Head	15
Condition	20
Legs and feet	5
Tail	10
	100

Serious defects

Too small in size, narrow build, back too long, tail held too low, too much red in the ear-lobe, light or yellow eye colour.

BANTAMS

The Standard to be an exact miniature of the large fowl.

Weights

Male 700–800 g (24–28 oz)
Female 600–700 g (22–24 oz)

HAMBURGH

LARGE FOWL

Origin: North Europe
Classification: Light: Soft feather
Egg colour: White

The origin of the Hamburgh is wrapped in mystery. The spangled were bred in Yorkshire and Lancashire 300 years ago as Pheasants and Mooneys, and there is a book reference to black Pheasants in the north of England in 1702. In its heyday, the Hamburgh was a grand layer and must have played its part in the making of other laying breeds. However, its breeders directed it down purely exhibition roads, until today it is in few hands.

General characteristics: male

Carriage: Alert, bold and graceful.
Type: Body moderately long, compact, fairly wide and flat at the shoulders. Breast well rounded. Wings large and neatly tucked. Tail long and sweeping, carried well up (but avoiding 'squirrel' carriage), the sickles broad and the secondaries plentiful.
Head: Fine. Beak short, well curved. Eyes bold and full. Comb rose, medium size, firmly set, square fronted, gradually tapering to a long, finely ended spike (or leader) in a straight line with the surface and without any downward tendency, the top level (free from hollows) and covered with small and smooth coral-like points of even height. Face smooth and free from stubby hairs. Ear-lobes smooth, round and flat (not concave or hollow), varying in size according to the variety. Wattles smooth, round and of fine texture.
Neck: Of medium length, covered with full and long feathers, which hang well over the shoulders.
Legs and feet: Legs of medium length. Thighs slender. Shanks fine and round, free of feathers. Toes four, slender and well spread.

Female

The general characteristics are similar to those of the male, allowing for the natural sexual differences.

Colour

The black

Male and female plumage: Rich black, with a distinct green sheen from head to tail, and especially on sickle feathers and tail coverts. Any approach to bronze or purple tinge or barring to be avoided.

In both sexes: Beak black or dark horn. Comb, face and wattles red. Ear-lobes white. Legs lead blue or black, lead blue preferred.

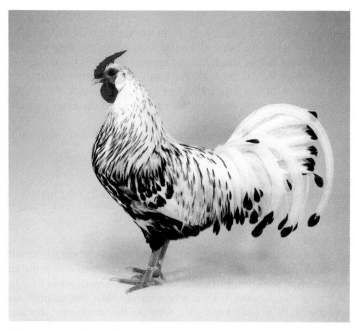

Silver Spangled Hamburgh male

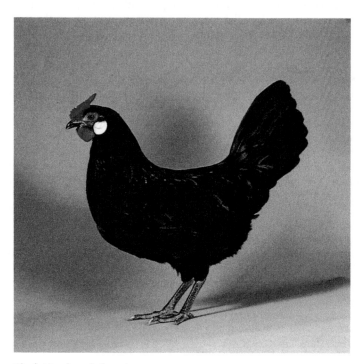

Black Hamburgh female

The gold pencilled

Male plumage: Bright red-bay or bright golden-chestnut, except the tail, which is black, the sickle feathers and coverts being laced all round with a narrow strip of gold.

Female plumage: Ground colour similar to the general colour of the male, and, except on the hackle (which should be clear of all marking), each feather distinctly and evenly pencilled straight across with fine parallel lines of a rich green-black, the pencilling and the intervening colour to be the same width, while the finer and the more numerous on each feather the better.

In both sexes: Beak dark horn. Comb, face and wattles red. Ear-lobes white. Legs and feet lead blue.

The silver pencilled

Male and female plumage: Except that the ground colour, and in the male the tail lacings, is silver, this variety is similar to the gold pencilled.

The gold spangled

Male plumage: Ground colour rich bright bay or mahogany; striping, spangling, tipping and tail rich green-black. Hackles and back each feather striped down the centre. Wing bows dagger-shaped tips at the end of each feather; bars (two), rows of large spangles, running parallel across each wing with a gentle curve, each bar distinct and separate; secondaries tipped with large round spangles, forming the 'steppings'. Breast and under-parts, each feather tipped with a round spot or spangle, small near the throat, increasing in size towards the thighs, but never so large as to overlap.

Female plumage: Ground colour and spangling are similar to those of the male. Hackle, wing bars and 'steppings' as in the male. Tail coverts black, with a sharp lacing or edging of gold on each feather. Remainder each feather tipped with a spangle, as round as possible, and never so large as to overlap, the spangling commencing high up the throat.

In both sexes: Beak, comb, face, wattles, ear-lobes, legs and feet as in the pencilled varieties.

The silver spangled

Male plumage: Ground colour pure silver; spangling and tipping rich green-black. Hackles, shoulders and back each feather marked with small, dagger-like tips. Wing bows dagger-shaped tips, increasing in size until they merge into what is known as the third bar; bars (two) and secondaries breast and underparts similarly marked to those of the gold spangled variety. Tail ending with bold half-moon-shaped spangles; sickles with large round spangles at the end of each feather; coverts similar, though spangles not so big.

Female plumage: Ground colour of each feather is black (not grey) with a gap of white before each spangle. Hackle marked from the head with dagger-shaped tips, which gradually increase in width until they merge into the spangles at the bottom. Wing secondaries as in the male, bars similar to those of the gold spangled female. Tail each feather with a half-moon-shaped spangle at the end; coverts reaching halfway up the true tail feathers to form a row across the tail (each side) of round spangles. Remainder marked as in the gold female.

In both sexes: Beak, comb, face, wattles, ear-lobes, legs and feet as in the pencilled varieties.

In all colours

Eyes red or dark, dark preferred.

Weights

Male   2.25 kg (5 lb) approx.
Female   1.80 kg (4 lb) approx.

Scale of points

Markings	60
Head, comb, lobes and face	20
Colour	10
Type, style and condition	<u>10</u>
	<u>100</u>

In pencilled males the points allotted for markings are to be awarded for the tail and colour.

Serious defects

White face. Single comb. Red ear-lobes. Squirrel or wry tail. White throated (bishop throated: silver spangled). Any other deformity.

BANTAM

Hamburgh bantams follow the large fowl Standard.

Weights

Male   680–790 g (24–28 oz)
Female   620–740 g (22–26 oz)

These weights are to be treated as maximums although the pencilled varieties are usually considerably larger.

HOUDAN

LARGE FOWL

Origin: France
Classification: Heavy: Rare
Egg colour: White

Introduced into England in 1850, the Houdan is one of the oldest French breeds, taking its name from the town of Houdan, and has been developed for table qualities. It is one of the few breeds carrying a fifth toe, a semi-dominant feature when crossed with other breeds.

General characteristics: male

Carriage: Bold and active.
Type: Body broad, deep and lengthy, as in the Dorking. Tail full with the sickles long and well arched.
Head: Fairly large, with a decidedly pronounced protuberance on top, and crested. Crest full and compact, round on top and not divided or 'split', composed of feathers similar to those of the hackle, inclining slightly backwards fully to expose the comb, in no way obstructing the sight except from behind. Beak rather short and stout, well curved and with wide nostrils. Eyes bold. Comb leaf type, somewhat resembling a butterfly placed at the

base of the beak, fairly small, well defined and each side level. Face muffled; muffling large, full, compact, fitting around to the back of the eyes and almost hiding the face. Ear-lobes small, entirely concealed by muffling. Wattles small and well rounded, almost concealed by beard.

Neck: Of medium length, with abundant hackle coming well down on the back.

Legs and feet: Legs short and stout, well apart, free of feathers. Toes five, similar to those of the Dorking.

Female

The general characteristics are similar to those of the male, allowing for the natural sexual differences, with the exception of the crest, which is full, compact and globular, not in any way obstructing the sight except from behind, and with the comb visible. Tail fairly full.

Colour

Male and female *plumage*: Glossy green-black ground with pure white mottles, the mottling to be evenly distributed, except on the flights and secondaries and in the male on the sickles and tail coverts, which are irregularly edged with white. *Note*: In young Houdans, black generally preponderates but what mottling there is should be even and clear. Mottling becomes gayer with age.

In both sexes: Beak horn. Eyes red. Comb, face and wattles bright red. Ear-lobes white or tinged with pink. Legs and feet white mottled with lead blue or black.

Weights

Male   3.20–3.60 kg (7–8 lb)
Female   2.70–3.20 kg (6–7 lb)

Scale of points

	Male	Female
Type	12	10
Size	18	20
Comb	15	8
Legs and feet	10	10
Colour	15	15
Crest	12	15
Muffling	8	12
Condition	10	10
	100	100

Serious defects

Red or straw-coloured feathers. Loose crest obstructing the sight. Spur outside the shank. Feathers on shanks or toes. Other than five toes on each foot. Any deformity.

BANTAM

Houdan bantams should follow the large fowl Standard.

Weights

Male   680–790 g (24–28 oz)
Female   620–740 g (22–26 oz)

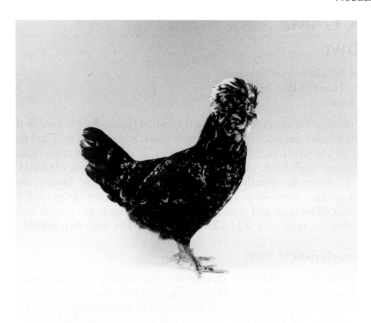

Female Houdan, large

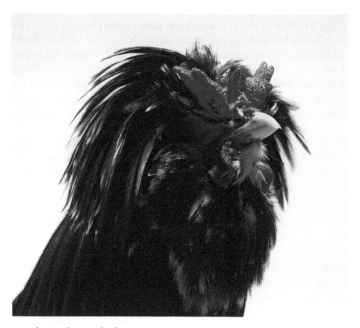

Head Houdan male, large

INDIAN GAME

LARGE FOWL

Origin: Great Britain
Classification: Heavy: Hard feather
Egg colour: Brown

To Cornwall must go the credit for giving us the Indian Game. Breeds used in the make-up were the red Asil, black-breasted red Old English Game and the Malay. The breed has been developed for its abundant quantity of breast meat, in which respect no other breed can equal it. When large table birds were the most popular in this country Indian Game males were chosen as mates for females of such table breeds as the Sussex, Dorking and Orpington, to produce extra-large crosses. The females chosen for mating belonged to breeds possessing white flesh and shanks. Jubilee Indian Game are similar to Indians, but the lacing is white; in Indians it is black. The two varieties are often interbred.

General characteristics: male

Carriage: Upright, commanding and courageous, the back sloping downwards towards the tail. A powerful and broad bird, very active, sprightly and vigorous.
Type: Body very thick and compact and very broad at the shoulders, the shoulder butts showing prominently, but the bird must not be hollow backed, the body tapering towards the tail. Back flat and broad at the shoulders, but the bird must not be flat sided. Elegance is required with substance. Breast wide, fairly deep and prominent, but well rounded, and rising to the vent. Wings short and carried closely to the body, well rounded at the points, closely tucked at ends and carried rather high in front. Tail medium length with short narrow secondary sickles and tail coverts, close and hard; carried in line with the back.
Head: Of medium length and thick, not so keen as in English Game, nor as thick as in the Malay; somewhat beetle browed but not nearly as much as in the Malay. Skull broad. Beak well curved and stout where set on the head, giving the bird a powerful appearance. Eyes full and bold. Comb pea type, i.e. three longitudinal ridges, the centre one being double the height of those at sides, small closely set on the head. Ear-lobes and wattles small, smooth and of fine texture.
Neck: Of medium length and slightly arched; hackle short, barely covering base of the neck.
Legs and feet: Legs very strong and thick. Thighs round and stout, but not as long as in the Malay. Shanks short and well scaled. The length of shank must be sufficient to give the bird a 'gamey' appearance. Feet strong and well spread. Toes long, strong, straight, the back toe low and nearly flat on ground; nails well shaped.
Plumage: Short, hard and close.
Handling: Flesh firm.

Female

The general characteristics are similar to those of the male, allowing for the natural sexual differences. The tail, however, which is well venetianed but close, is carried low but somewhat higher than the male's.

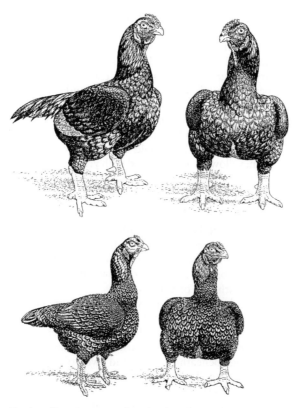

Dark Indian Game, cockerels above, hens below. These drawings form part of the Indian Game Standard

Colour

Dark Indian Game

Male plumage: Head, neck, breast, underfluff, thighs and tail black, with rich green glossy sheen or lustre, the base of the neck and tail hackles a little broken with bay or chestnut, which should be almost hidden by the body of the feathers. Shoulders and wing bows green glossy black or beetle green, slightly broken with bay or chestnut in the centre of the feather or shaft. Tail coverts green glossy black or beetle green slightly broken with bay or chestnut in the base of the shaft. Back feathers green glossy black or beetle green, also touched on the fine fronds at the end of the feathers with bay or chestnut, which gives the sheen so much desired. When the wing is closed there is a triangular patch of bay or chestnut formed of the secondaries, which are green glossy black or beetle green on the inner, and bay or chestnut on the outer web, and which when closed show only the bay in a solid triangle. The primaries 10 in number, are curved and of a deep black, except for about 6.25 cm ($2\frac{1}{2}$ in.) of a narrow lacing of light chestnut on the outer web.

Female plumage: The ground colour is chestnut-brown, nut-brown, or mahogany-brown. Head, hackle and throat green glossy black or beetle green. The pointed hackle that lies under the neck feathers green glossy black, or beetle green with a bay or chestnut centre mark; the breast commencing on the lower part of the throat, expanding into lacing on the swell of the breast, of a rich bay or chestnut, the inner or double lacing being most distinct, the belly and thighs being marked somewhat similarly and running off into a mixture of indistinct markings under the vent and swell of the thighs. The feathers of shoulders and back are somewhat smaller, enlarging towards the tail coverts and similarly marked with double lacing; the markings on wing bows and shoulders running down to the waist are most distinct of all, with the same kind of double lacing. Often in the best specimens there is an additional mark enclosing the base of the shaft of the feather and running to a point in the second or inner lacing. Tail coverts are seldom as distinctly marked but have the same style of marking. Primary or flight feathers are black, except on inner frond or web, which is a little coloured or peppered with a light chestnut. Secondaries are black on the inner web, while the outer web is in keeping with the general ground colour and is edged with a delicate lacing of green glossy black or beetle green. Wing coverts which form the bar are laced like those of the body and often a little peppered. The black lacing should be metallic green, glossy black or beetle green. This should appear embossed or raised.

In both sexes: Beak horn, yellow, or horn striped with yellow. Eyes from pearl to pale red. Face, comb, wattles and ear-lobes rich red. Legs rich orange or yellow, the deeper the better.

Jubilee Indian Game

Male plumage: Head, neck, breast, body, underfluff, thighs and tail white. Hackle feathers to have chestnut shaftings. Clear breasts are desirable. Wing bows and shoulders white, slightly broken with bay or chestnut; wing primaries and secondaries white with bay markings; triangular patch of bay or chestnut to show when wing is closed. Tail coverts white. Back white touched with bay or chestnut.

Female plumage: Ground colour chestnut-brown or mahogany. Head hackle and throat white. Breast commencing on the lower part of the throat and expanding to double lacing on the swell of the breast, mahogany laced with white. The inner, or double lacing, to be most distinct. The underparts and thighs are marked somewhat similarly and run into a mixture of indistinct markings beneath the vent and swell of the thighs. Feathers of the shoulders and back somewhat small, enlarging towards the tail coverts similarly marked with the double lacing; often in the best specimens there is an additional mark enclosing the base of the shaft of the feather and running to a point in the second or inner lacing. The tail coverts are seldom as distinctly marked, but with the same style of marking. Wing primaries white marked on inner web with chestnut; secondaries white inner web, chestnut outer web, edged with white. Main tail white. Remainder chestnut ground colour throughout, double laced with white, inner lacing should be quite distinct. Underparts and thighs may be less distinctly marked and wing coverts may be peppered.

In all other respects the Indian Game Standard should be followed.
In both sexes: Beak, eyes, comb and legs as described for Indians.

Double laced blue Indian Game

Male plumage: Lower throat, breast, thighs, belly fluff and tail even blue which can range from pigeon to dark blue, evenness of shade taking precedence. A slight edging of a darker shade round feathers permissible. Head, neck hackles, saddle, back and wing bows a darker shade of blue than the remainder of body, slightly broken with dark bay, this being mostly covered, giving an overall impression of dark slate blue. Undercolour pale blue-grey. Wing primaries blue to match main body colour with a fine chestnut outer edge; secondaries blue inner web, bay outer web, forming a solid bay triangle when the wing is closed; wing bars blue to match the main body.

Female plumage: Head, neck hackles and tail even dark slate blue. Lower neck hackles may be slightly broken in the centre with dark bay, but this not showing through. The remainder of the body to be chestnut to mahogany-brown ground colour, evenness of utmost importance. Each feather is to be laced with two concentric rings of clear even blue, lighter in shade to the neck and tail. Lacings to be as crisp as possible and encircle the feather completely, must not be crescent shaped, too heavy or run into each other. A third blue marking in the centre base of the feather producing triple lacing is desirable. Lacing to cover the whole remainder of the body, including tail coverts and extending to the thighs, but becoming indistinct into the belly fluff and round the vent, where it becomes even blue. Undercolour pale blue-grey. Wing primaries even blue with a little fine chestnut peppering on inner web; secondaries inner web blue, outer web to match body ground colour, with a clear lacing of blue round the outer web; wing bars double laced to match the remainder of the body.

In both sexes: Beak yellow, horn or horn striped with yellow. Eyes pearl to pale red. Face, comb, wattle and ear-lobes rich red. Legs rich orange or yellow, nails to match beak.

Weights

Male 3.60 kg (8 lb) min.
Female 2.70 kg (6 lb) min.

Scale of points

Type and colour (body and thighs 10; back, breast, wings, tail, legs 8 each; neck 3)	53
Carriage	12
Size	10
Head (skull, eyes and brows 3 each; beak, wattles, lobes, comb 2 each)	17
Condition	8
	100

Note: The Indian Game Fowl is in no way allied to the English Game Fowl. Hence, it is not recognised as a true Game bird in the Fancy; that is, unless classes are specially provided for the breed it must compete in the 'Any other variety' classes and not in those set aside for 'Game', see Poultry Club Show Rules.

Defects

Crooked breast or toes. Flat shins. Rusty hackles. Bad shape. Heavy feathering. White in hackles. Smallness of size. Long legs and thighs. Twisted hackle.

Disqualifications

In the male: Crooked back, beak and legs. Wry or squirrel tail, in-knees, bent legs and flat sides. Single or Malay comb. Red hackles. Additionally in the dark, female too light, too dark or mealy ground colour, and defective markings.

BANTAM

Dark, Jubilee and blue laced Indian Game bantams should follow the large fowl Standard, including the scale of points. Jubilees are similar to the Dark variety except that, where Darks are black, Jubilees are white. Both colours are frequently interbred.

Weights

The Indian Game Club does not issue definite weight Standards for bantams, and weights detailed below are suggestions only. These weights are often exceeded and excess size should be penalised.

Male 2.00 kg (4½ lb)
Female 1.50 kg (3½ lb)

Originally, British Bantam Association weights were below these. No characteristic of the breed must be developed or exaggerated to such an extent that Indian Game cannot effectively reproduce themselves.

IXWORTH

LARGE FOWL

Origin: Great Britain
Classification: Heavy: Rare
Egg colour: Cream

The all-white Ixworth was created by Reginald Appleyard in 1932, taking its name from the village in Suffolk, and was produced as an excellent table bird with good laying qualities. Breeds used in its make-up included white Sussex, white Orpington, white Minorca, Jubilee, Indian and white Indian Game. In 1938, Ixworth bantams were to follow and at the time their breeder said they were better than the large fowl. The breed is now kept by the dedicated few, in both large fowl and bantams.

General characteristics: male

Carriage: Alert, active and well balanced.
Type: Body deep, well rounded, fairly long but compact. Back long, flat, reasonably broad, without too prominent a slope to the tail. Breast broad, full, deep, well rounded, long and wide, low breastbone carried well forward; with unpronounced keel or keel point; well fleshed and rounded off for entire length. Wings strong, carried close, showing shoulder butts. Tail compact, of medium length and carried fairly low, the sickles close fitting.
Head: Broad and of medium length. Beak short and stout. Eyes full, prominent, keen expression, without heavy brows. Comb pea type. Face smooth and of fine texture. Ear-lobes and wattles medium size and fine texture.
Neck: Somewhat erect and of reasonable length. Hackle feathers short, close fitting and in no way excessive or loose.
Legs and feet: Legs well apart, and of reasonable length to ensure activity. Thighs well fleshed and of medium length. Shanks covered with tight scales, free from feathers. Toes four, straight, well spread and firm stance. Bone characteristic of a first-class table bird.
Plumage: Short, silky and close fitting; fluff likewise.

Female

The general characteristics are similar to those of the male, allowing for the natural sexual differences.

Colour

Male and female plumage: White.
   In both sexes: Beak white. Eyes red or bright orange. Comb, face, wattles, and ear-lobes brilliant red. Legs, feet, skin and flesh white.

Weights

Cock   4.10 kg (9 lb)   Cockerel   3.60 kg (8 lb)
Hen   3.20 kg (7 lb)   Pullet   2.70 kg (6 lb)

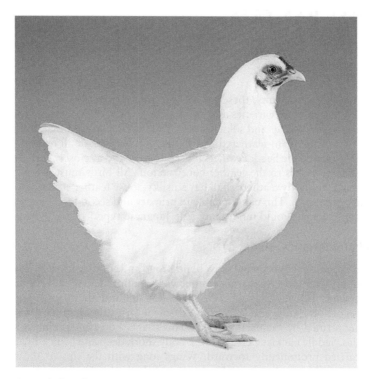

Ixworth female

Scale of points

Table merits	40
Shape and size	20
Colour (general)	20
Head	10
Plumage and condition	10
	100

Serious defects

Coarseness. Lack of activity. Loose feathers. Any point against table values or general usefulness. Any deformity.

BANTAM

Ixworth bantams should follow exactly the Standard for large fowl.

Weights

Male   1020 g (36 oz)
Female   790 g (28 oz)

JAPANESE BANTAM

Origin: Japan
Classification: True Bantam
Egg colour: White or cream

True Bantams of great antiquity, these are without counterparts in the large breeds. They are the shortest legged of all varieties and are standardised in three feather forms: plain or normal feather, frizzle feather and silkie feather. The frizzle feathered shall follow both the type and colours of the plain-feathered Standards, but the ends of all feathers are to curl back and point towards the head. Feathers must be broad and as closely curled as possible. The silkie feathered refers to the feather construction. All birds must follow closely the general Standard, but body feathers shall have a silky, loose feather structure (i.e. feathers have no main centre vein). This cannot apply to primary and secondary wing feathers or to true tail feathers, which would nullify any true Japanese type.

General characteristics: male

Carriage and appearance: Very small, low built, broad and cobby with deep full breast and full-feathered upright tail. Appearance somewhat quaint due to a very large comb, dwarfish character and waddling gait. Plumage very full and abundant.
Type: Back very short, wide, and seen from the side it forms the shape of a small letter U, the sides being formed by the neck and tail. This shape, however, is almost lost in fully feathered males. Saddle hackles rich and long. Body short, deep and broad. Breast very full, round and carried prominently forward. Wings long with the tips of the secondaries touching the ground immediately under the end of the body. Thighs very short and not visible. Tail very large and upright. The main tail feathers should rise above the level of the head by about one-third of their length, spreading well and with long sword-shaped main sickles and numerous soft side hangers. The tail may touch the comb with its front feathers, but must not be set so as to lean forward at too sharp an angle (squirrel tailed).
Head: Large and broad, beak strong and well curved, eyes large. Comb single, large (the larger the better), coarse grained, erect and evenly serrated with four or five points. The blade of the comb should follow the nape of the neck. Face smooth, ear-lobes medium size, red and free from all traces of white. Wattles pendant and large.
Neck: Rather short, curving backwards and with abundant hackle feathers which should drape the shoulders well.
Legs and feet: Shanks very short, clean (free from feather), strong and sharply angled at the joints. The shanks to be so short as to be almost invisible. Toes four, straight and well spread.

Female

The general characteristics should follow closely those described for the male regarding type. Breast should be as described for the male. Tail well spread and rising well above the head. The main tail feathers broad, the foremost part being slightly curved (sword shaped). Comb large, evenly serrated and preferably erect, although falling to one side being no defect.

Colour

The black-tailed white

Male and female plumage: Body feathers white, wing primaries and secondaries should have white outer and black inner webs, the closed wings look almost white. Main tail feathers black. Main sickles and side hangers black or black with white edges.
   In both sexes: Eyes red. Legs yellow.

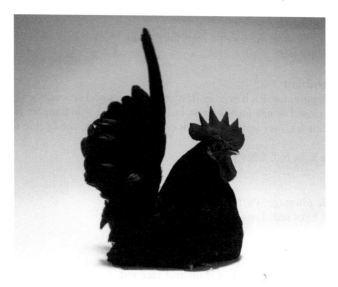

Black Japanese male

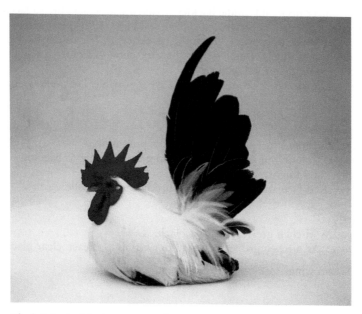

Black-tailed white Japanese male

The black-tailed buff
Male and female plumage: The same markings as the black-tailed white, except that the white is replaced by buff.

The buff Columbian
Male and female plumage: Rich even buff, wing primaries and secondaries buff with black inner webs, the closed wings look almost buff. Sickles and side hangers black with buff edges. Neck hackle feathers buff with black centre down each, the hackle to be free from black edges.

In both sexes: Eyes red. Legs yellow.

The white
Male and female plumage: Pure white without sappiness.

In both sexes: Eyes red. Legs yellow.

The black
Male and female plumage: Deep full black with a green sheen.

In both sexes: Eyes red or dark. Comb and face red. Legs yellow, black permitted on shanks but underside of feet must be yellow.

The greys

The birchen grey
Male plumage: Silver neck and saddle hackles streaked with black, breast laced to top of thighs, retaining light shaft to centre of feather. Tail black with green sheen.
Female plumage: Silver laced neck hackle to be clear-cut, back and tail black. Breast feathers laced to top of thighs retaining light shaft to centre of feather. Lacing to be clear-cut completely surrounding each feather.

In both sexes: Red face and eye, dark face and eye if possible. Legs yellow or dusky with yellow soles.

The silver grey
Male plumage: As birchen grey, lacing to be most pronounced.
Female plumage: Colour and lacing as in birchen grey, silvering to be allowed to extend over back, wings and thighs.

In both sexes: Red face and eye, yellow or dusky legs with yellow soles.

The dark grey
Male plumage: As birchen grey, but breast black.
Female plumage: As birchen grey female without lacing to breast, clear black breast.

All greys: tails and wings black with green sheen.

The mottleds

The black
Male and female plumage: All feathers should be black with white tips. The amount of white may vary, but the ideal is between 0.94 cm ($\frac{3}{8}$ in.) and 1.25 cm ($\frac{1}{2}$ in.). Tails and wings similar but more white permitted.

The blue
Male and female plumage: As above but blue instead of black.

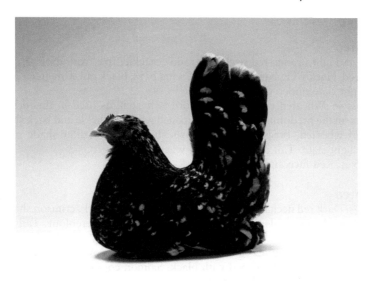

Mottled Japanese female

The red
Male and female plumage: As the black but red instead of black.

In both sexes and all mottleds
Beaks to match legs, which should be yellow or willow. Eyes red or orange.

The blues

The self
Male and female plumage: All feathers blue, neck feathers may be a darker blue than the remainder.
  In both sexes: Eyes orange. Legs slate or willow.

The lavender
Male and female plumage: All feathers a lavender blue to skin, even shade throughout.
  In both sexes: Eyes orange or dark brown. Legs slate or blue.

The cuckoo
Male and female plumage: The feathers throughout including body, wing and tail to be generally uniformly cuckoo coloured with transverse bands of dark bluish-grey on a light grey ground continuing to the root of the feather.
  In both sexes: Beak yellow marked with black. Eyes orange or red. Legs yellow.

The red
Male and female plumage: All feathers deep red, solid to skin and even shade throughout.
  In both sexes: Beak and legs yellow, both may be marked with red. Eyes red.

The tri-coloured
Male and female plumage: The colours white, black and brown or dark ochre should be as equally divided as possible on each feather.
  In both sexes: Eyes red or orange. Legs yellow or willow.

The black-red

Wheaten bred

Male plumage: Light orange-red neck and saddle hackle, free from dark striping, Wing bows bright red, black wing bars and light red wing bays, black tail with green sheen. Body black with light slate undercolour.

Female plumage: Wheaten coloured (the word 'wheaten' as used in this description is intended to mean the predominate colour of ripened wheat). Hackle and back should be an even shade of wheaten, breast and underparts should be a lighter shade of wheaten. Undercolour light slate. Tail dull black/dark wheaten.

In both sexes: Red face and eyes. Legs dusky yellow.

Partridge bred

Male plumage: Dark red neck and saddle hackle striped with black, crimson shoulders and dark, bay-coloured wing ends. Body black with light slate undercolour. Tail black with green sheen.

Female plumage: Back, shoulders and wings even partridge-brown stippled with fine dark markings, golden neck hackle striped with black. Salmon-coloured breast shading to ash grey belly; primary and tail feathers dark.

In both sexes: Face red. Eyes dark red. Legs yellow or dusky with yellow sole.

The brown-red

Male plumage: Gold neck and saddle hackles streaked with black, breast laced to top of thighs retaining light shaft to centre of feather. Tail and wings black with green sheen.

Female plumage: Gold laced neck hackle to be clear-cut, back, tail and wings black. Breast feathers laced to top of thighs retaining light shaft to centre of feather. Lacing to be clear-cut completely surrounding each feather.

In both sexes: Red face and eye, dark face and eye if possible. Legs yellow or dusky with yellow sole.

The blue-red, silver and gold duckwing

The latter three colours all as described for Old English Game.

The following secondary colours are permitted: ginger, blue dun, honey dun, golden hackled, furness.

Weights

Male   510–600 g (18–20 oz)
Female   400–510 g (14–18 oz)

Scale of points

Type and size	55
Head, beak and neck	10
Legs and feet	10
Colour and plumage	10
Condition	15
	100

Serious defects

Narrow build. Long legs. Long back. Wry or squirrel tail. Tail carried low. Deformed comb and lopped comb on males. High wing carriage. White lobes. Any physical deformity.

JERSEY GIANT

LARGE FOWL

Origin: America
Classification: Heavy: Rare
Egg colour: Brown

Originated in New Jersey in about 1880, this American breed took the name of 'Giant' because of the extra heavy weights that specimens could record. Its make-up accounts for such poundage as it includes black Java, dark Brahma, black Langshan and Indian Game. When introduced into this country it was claimed that birds from this breed were heavier than those of any other breed and that it was adaptable for farm range and for providing capons. Earlier specimens were of exceptional weights.

General characteristics: male

Carriage: Bold, alert and well balanced.
Type: Body long, wide, deep and compact; smooth at sides, with long keel, smooth and moderately full fluff. Back rather long, broad, nearly horizontal, with a short sweep to the tail. Breast broad, deep and full, carried well forward. Wings medium sized, well folded, carried at the same angle as the body, the primaries and secondaries broad and overlapping in natural order when the wings are folded. Tail rather large, full, well spread, carried at an angle of 45° above the horizontal, the sickles just sufficiently long to cover the main tail feathers, the coverts moderately abundant and of medium length, the main tail feathers broad and overlapping.
Head: Rather large and broad. Beak short, stout and well curved. Eyes large, round, full and prominent. Comb single, straight, upright, rather large and of fine texture, having six well-defined and evenly serrated points, the blade following the shape of the neck. Face smooth and fine in texture. Ear-lobes smooth and rather large, extending down one half of the length of the wattles. Wattles of medium size and fine texture, well rounded at the lower ends.
Neck: Moderately long, full and well arched.
Legs and feet: Legs straight and set well apart. Thighs large, strong, of moderate length and well covered with feathers. Shanks strong, stout, medium length and free from feathers; scales fine, bone of good quality and proportionate to size of bird. Toes four, of medium length, straight and well spread.

Female

With the exception of the tail, which is well spread and carried at an angle of 30° above the horizontal, the general characteristics are similar to those of the male, allowing for the natural sexual differences.

Colour

The black

Male and female plumage: The surface a lustrous green-black, and the undercolour slate or light grey.

In both sexes: Beak black, shading to yellow towards the tip. Eyes dark brown or hazel. Comb, face, wattles and ear-lobes red. Legs and feet black, with a tendency towards willow in adult birds, the underpart of the feet being yellow.

The white

Male and female plumage: The surface and undercolour white.

The blue
Male and female plumage: Modern Langshan blue laced preferred.

In both sexes and all colours
Beak willow (some yellow permissible at present). Eyes brown to black. Comb, face, wattles and ear-lobes red. Legs and feet willow, i.e. dark greenish-yellow, soles yellow. Skin nearly white.

Weights

Cock	5.90 kg (13 lb)	Cockerel	5.00 kg (11 lb)
Hen	4.55 kg (10 lb)	Pullet	3.60 kg (8 lb)

Scale of points

Shape and carriage	25
Colour	20
Quality	15
Head	10
Size and symmetry	10
Condition	10
Legs and feet	10
	100

Serious defects (in whites)

Smoky surface colour. Side sprigs to comb. More than 0.90 kg (2 lb) below Standard weight in mature stock.

Defects (in blacks and whites)

Overhanging eyebrows. Sluggishness. Coarseness. Excessive or superfine bone. In blacks: black or dull black undercolour extending to the skin of the hackle, back, breast, or body and fluff. Positive white showing on surface of plumage. Other than yellow under the feet. More than 0.90 kg (2 lb) below the Standard weight in mature stock.

BANTAM

Jersey Giant bantams should follow exactly the Standard of the large fowl.

Weights

Male	1.74 kg (3¼ lb)
Female	1.13 kg (2½ lb)

KO SHAMO

Origin: Japan
Classification: Asian Hardfeather. True Bantam
Egg colour: White to cream

Ko Shamo are the most popular of the small Shamo breeds, none of which have large fowl counterparts, and none of which should be referred to as 'Shamo Bantams'. They are strong, muscular little birds with very sparse plumage. Slightly differing types are considered to be correct in Japan, their country of origin, and there will probably always be some variation here too. The most important attributes should be character and attitude, strong head and beak, prominent shoulders, very short, hard feathers and a tiny 'prawn' tail.

General characteristics: male

Type and carriage: Upright stance. Alert, confident bearing. Full of character and attitude. The entire bird should comprise three equal parts: head and neck/body/legs.
Body: Extremely firm and muscular. Body narrowing gradually towards the tail. Rump firm.
Breast: Broad, deep, well rounded and muscular.
Back: Medium length and broad. Widest at the shoulders, gradually narrowing from above the thighs. Backbone straight, sloping down towards the tail. Saddle feathers should be sparse, narrow and short.
Wings: Short and strong with prominent shoulders. Wing tips should stop at the base of the saddle hackle and should not be carried over the back. Birds of the best type are usually found to have split wing. In the Ko Shamo this should never be judged a fault.
Tail: Very short. Main tail slightly fanned with sickles and tail coverts very short and curved, forming a 'prawn' tail, with feather tips pointing down and inwards. A tubular shape is also acceptable.
Head: Large with prominent eyebrows to suggest ferocity. Beak thick, short, well curved and deep from top to bottom. Comb triple, walnut or chrysanthemum: all types should be small and firm, closely set to the head. Eyes large and penetrating. Wattles very small or absent. Ear-lobes and throat skin thick and rather wrinkled with a dewlap of bare red skin (the wrinkled skin is not developed so much in the Ko Shamo as in the Yamato Gunkei).
Neck: Long, strong, curved slightly, almost erect. The bare skin of the dewlap extends well down the front of the neck. Neck hackle feathers are very short and narrow, hardly reaching the base of the neck.
Legs and feet: Thighs of medium length, well muscled and rounded. Legs well apart, accentuated by the general sparse plumage of body and legs. Shanks straight, thick and strong, with scales in four or more neat rows. Toes four, straight and well spread.
Plumage: Very hard and sparse. Bare red skin showing at keel, vent and point of wing.
Handling: Extremely firm fleshed and muscular.

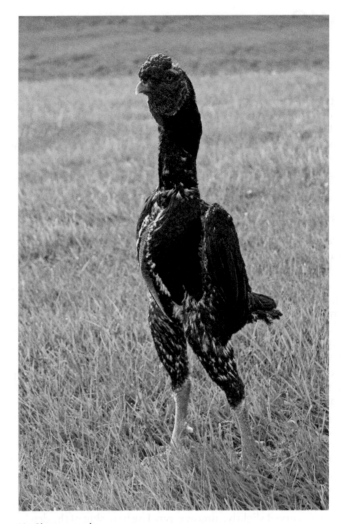

Ko Shamo, male

Female

The general characteristics are similar to those of the male, allowing for the natural sexual differences.

Colour

Black/red (the red may be any shade from yellow to dark red, with wheaten or partridge females which can be any shade from cream to dark brown with or without dark markings), duckwing, black, white, blue, ginger, splash, spangle and cuckoo are all recognised.

In both sexes and all colours

Beak yellow or horn, with dark markings acceptable. Legs and feet yellow, dusky markings acceptable in dark-coloured birds. Comb, face, ear-lobes, wattles and any exposed skin red. Eyes silver or gold. Darker eyes acceptable in young birds.

Weights

Cock	1000 g (2 lb 4 oz)	Cockerel	800 g (1 lb 12 oz)
Hen	800 g (1 lb 12 oz)	Pullet	600 g (1 lb 6 oz)

Scale of points

Type and carriage	30
Head and neck	20
Condition and plumage quality	20
Legs and feet	10
Eye colour	10
Legs and feet colour	5
Plumage colour	5
	100

Serious defects

Lack of attitude. Poor carriage. Overlarge comb. 'Duck' feet. Long tail. Any evidence of tail-plucking.

KRAIENKÖPPE

LARGE FOWL

Origin: The Netherlands and Germany
Classification: Light: Rare
Egg colour: White

Kraienköppe (pronounced Krai-en-kerper) is the German name, Twentse the Dutch name for this border area breed. The basic breed type began with crosses between Malays and local farmyard fowls in the late nineteenth century. Later, silver duckwing Leghorns were introduced. Kraienköppe were first exhibited in The Netherlands in 1920 and Germany in 1925. The bantams were developed from crosses of the large breed with Malay bantams. They were first exhibited in The Netherlands in 1940, in Germany in 1955 and in Britain around 1970.

General characteristics: male

Carriage: Upright and elegant with powerful appearance.
Type: Body extended, strongly built, becoming fuller towards the rear. Back fairly long, straight, rounded at the sides with wide and abundant saddle hackle. Shoulders powerful and fairly wide. Breast wide and full. Wings long and powerful, carried closely with the tips under the saddle hackle. Tail fairly long and carried at an angle of 30–40°, with full sickles.
Head: Short, wide, arched, with a visibly prominent nape. Face free from feathers. Comb narrow walnut, in the shape of an elongated strawberry (or acorn), well set. Wattles short. Ear-lobes small. Beak short, strong, the tip bent downwards. Eyes fiery, alert, set somewhat under beetling brows.
Neck: Powerful, wide between the shoulders, of good average length, carried upright, curved slightly backwards with abundant hackle falling over the shoulders and back.
Legs and feet: Thighs powerful, prominent with smooth feathering. Shanks slender, smooth, free from feathers. Toes four, fairly long, widely spread.
Plumage: Tight fitting.

Female

The general characteristics are similar to those of the male, allowing for the natural sexual differences. The back is carried almost horizontally. The tail is closed but not pointed. The comb is the size of a pea, very flattened. The wattles are small to the point of disappearance.

Colour

The silver

Male plumage: Head white, neck silvery white with black shaft stripe. Wing bows and back pure silvery white. Saddle silvery white with distinct shaft stripe. Wing bays silvery white, wide black wing bars with green sheen; primaries black with narrow white outer lacing; secondaries outer colour white, inner colour and tips black, so that the closed wing appears pure white. Breast, abdomen, thighs and hind part black, tail pure deep black with black sickles with green sheen.

Female plumage: Head silvery grey, hackle pure silvery white with black shaft stripe; back, shoulders and wings ash grey with silvery stippling and a whitish shaft. From hackle to tail every feather should show a narrow bright silvery grey lacing. Breast salmon to salmon-red, abdomen and hind part ash grey; tail black and greyish-black.

The gold

Male plumage: As for the silver, except that the silvery white is replaced by golden-red, lighter on head and neck.

Female plumage: Head and neck golden-yellow marked as the silver. Back, shoulders and wings light brown ground colour of even shade with fine black striping, peppering and stippling; yellow shaft. From hackle to tail every feather should show a narrow golden lacing. Breast salmon to salmon-red, abdomen and hind part brownish-ash grey. Tail black with brown markings.

The orange (lemon)

Same as for the gold, with the golden feathering replaced by a light orange.

The blue-gold

Same as for the gold, with the black plumage replaced by a bluish-grey.

The crele

Male plumage: Neck and saddle chequered (barred) orange. Back and shoulders deep chequered orange. Wing bows deep chequered orange with dark grey bar across; secondaries bay colour on the outer web; primaries dark grey. Tail dark grey with light grey bar.

Female plumage: Neck lemon chequered with grey. Breast and thighs chequered salmon. Back and wings chequered blue-grey. Tail dark grey with light grey bar.

The pile

Male plumage: Neck and saddle orange or chestnut-red. Breast and thighs white. Back and shoulders deep red. Wing bows red with a white bar across; secondaries bay colour on outer web; primaries white. Tail white.

Female plumage: Neck lemon. Breast salmon, lighter towards thighs. Back and wings white. Tail white.

The blue-silver

Male plumage: Neck, hackle, saddle silver streaked with blue. Back and shoulders silver. Breast and thighs blue laced with silver to top of thighs. Wing bows silver; secondaries and primaries blue. Tail blue.

Female plumage: Neck hackle silver striped with blue. Breast and thighs blue, laced with silver to top of thighs. Wings and back blue, free from silver. Tail blue.

The cuckoo

Male and female plumage: Neck, saddle, back, shoulders, wings and tail bluish-grey in colour, banded across the feathers with darker blue-grey or slate colour; the markings should be as even as possible throughout the plumage.

The silver cuckoo

Male plumage: Mainly white in neck and showing white on upper part of breast, also on top. Remainder banded throughout, with lighter ground colour than the dark cuckoo.

Female plumage: Mainly white in neck and showing white on upper part of breast. Remainder banded throughout, with lighter ground colour than the dark cuckoo.

In all sexes and colours

Beak yellow with dark tip. Eyes yellow-red to red. Face, comb, ear-lobes and wattles red. Legs and feet bright yellow.

Weights

Male	2.50–2.95 kg ($5\frac{1}{2}$–$6\frac{1}{2}$ lb)
Female	1.80–2.50 kg (4–$5\frac{1}{2}$ lb)

Scale of points

Type	25
Colour	25
Head	20
Legs and feet	15
Condition	15
	100

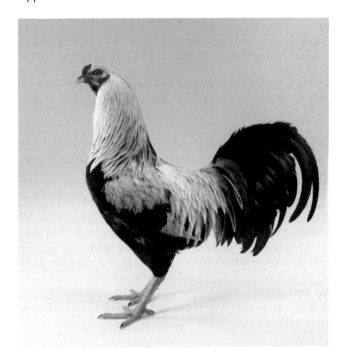

Silver Kraienköppe male

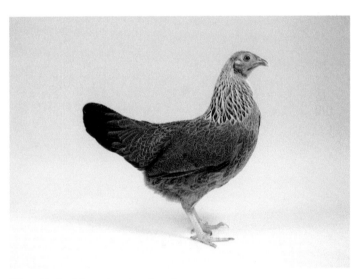

Silver Kraienköppe bantam female

Serious defects

Short or narrow body. Roach back. Upright or poorly furnished tail. Low stance. Drooping wings. Thin neck. Coarse, pointed or narrow head. Fish eyes. Fluffy plumage. Narrow sickles. Any other comb.

BANTAM

Kraienköppe bantams should follow the large fowl Standard in every respect.

Weights

Male   850 g (30 oz)
Female   740 g (26 oz)

KULANG

Origin: India and Pakistan
Classification: Asian Hardfeather. Large Fowl
Egg colour: White

The Kulang Asil is an Indian bird of Malayoid type, kept and fought in its country of origin for hundreds of years.

As Indian and Pakistani people migrated to Britain they brought these birds with them, and they have been kept here now for many years. The Standard is intended to preserve the original type, which does vary from area to area.

Their general appearance is very Shamo-like, the major differences being a rather less exaggeratedly upright stance and less prominent shoulders, and their development having been in India rather than the Shamo's development in Japan.

General characteristics: male

Type and carriage: General appearance powerful, alert and agile, balanced and full of aggressive spirit.
Body: Large, firm and well muscled.
Breast: Broad and full with deep keel.
Back: Long, broadest at shoulders, sloping down towards tail and gradually tapering from upper side of thigh. Backbone straight.
Wings: Short, big, strong and bony, carried close to the body, not showing on the back.
Tail: Carried horizontally or below, length to give balance to the bird.
Head: Strong, deep and broad with wattles and ear-lobes small or absent. Beak powerful, broad and curved downwards, but not hooked. Eyes deep-set under overhanging brows. Comb triple or walnut, set low on a broad base. Beard/muff acceptable.
Neck: Long, strong-boned and slightly curved or sometimes with a definite angle between head and neck.
Legs and feet: Thighs long, round and muscular. Legs medium to long, thick and strong with slight bend at hock. Square shanks preferred. Toes four, long and well spread. Hind toe straight and firm on the ground.
Plumage: Feathers short, narrow and hard, often showing red skin at throat, keel and point of wing. Henny feather is also acceptable in male birds.
Handling: Extremely firm fleshed, muscular and well balanced. Strong contraction of wings to body.

Female

The general characteristics are similar to those of the male, allowing for the natural sexual differences.

Colour

Black/red (wheaten) is the most common colour, but no colour or combination of colours is disqualified.

In both sexes and all colours

Beak yellow or horn. Legs and feet pale preferred, but any colour acceptable. Comb, face, throat, ear-lobes and any exposed skin brilliant red. Eyes pearl to gold. Darker eyes acceptable in young birds.

Weights

Male   3.5 kg (7 lb 12 oz) min.
Female   2.5 kg (5 lb 8 oz) min.

Scale of points

Type and carriage   40
Head   20
Feather/condition   20
Legs and feet   _20_
                     100

Serious defects

Lack of attitude. Overlarge comb. 'Duck' feet.

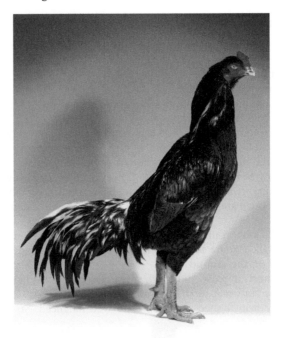

Kulang male

LA FLÈCHE

LARGE FOWL

Origin: France
Classification: Heavy: Rare
Egg colour: White

The La Flèche is a French breed which has never been widespread in Britain. A large black breed with two vertical spikes for a comb, it is related to the Crèvecoeur. In the middle of the nineteenth century it was used to produce white-skinned *petit poussin* for the Paris market.

General characteristics: male

Carriage: Bold and upstanding.
Type: Body general appearance large, powerful and rather hard. Back wide and rather long, slanting to the tail. Wings large and powerful. Breast full and prominent. Tail moderate in size.
Head: General appearance of the head long, slightly coarse and cruel. Beak large and strong with cavernous nostrils. Comb a double spike standing nearly upright with very small spikes in front. Wattles long and pendulous, ear-lobes large. Head should be quite free of crest.
Neck: Long and very upright, but not backward, with as much hackle as possible.
Legs and feet: Thighs and shanks long and powerful, the latter being free of feathers; toes large and straight.

Female

The general characteristics are similar to those of the male, allowing for the natural sexual differences.

Colour

Male and female plumage: Glossy black with bright green reflections.
    In both sexes: Beak black or very dark horn. Comb, wattles and face deep red. Ear-lobes brilliant white. Eyes bright red or black. Legs and feet very dark slate or leaden-black.

Weights

Male   3.60–4.10 kg (8–9 lb)
Female   2.70–3.20 kg (6–7 lb)

Scale of points

Type and carriage	25
Head	35
Colour	15
Size	15
Legs and feet	5
Condition	5
	100

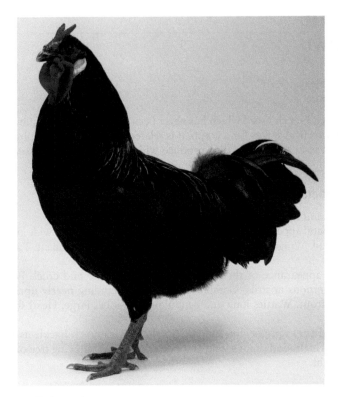

La Flèche male

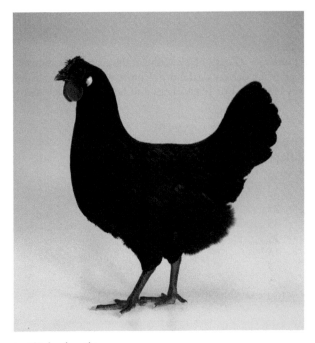

La Flèche female

Serious defects

Presence of crest. Entirely red ear-lobes. Feathers on legs. Incorrect leg colour. Coloured feathers. Wry tail or any deformity.

BANTAM

La Flèche bantams should follow exactly the Standard of the large fowl.

Weights

Male   1020 g (36 oz)
Female   790 g (28 oz)

LAKENVELDER

LARGE FOWL

Origin: Germany
Classification: Light: Rare
Egg colour: Cream

Lakervelt is a village near Utrecht, in the east of The Netherlands. It is also the place of origin of Lakenvelder cattle, which have a similar black and white colour pattern. The area where the chicken breed developed extended over the border to the Nordrhein-Westfalen region of Germany, where the breed name is Lakenfelder. These distinctively patterned chickens were recorded as far back as 1727. They were not imported to the UK until 1901 and then first exhibited at the 1902 Shrewsbury Show. Their popularity has been limited because very few birds have the desired completely black neck and tail with a white body.

General characteristics: male

Carriage: Upright, bold and sprightly.
Type: Body moderately long, fairly wide at the shoulders and narrowing slightly to the root of the tail. Full and round breast. Broad and apparently short back. Medium long wings, tucked well up, the bows and tips covered by the neck and saddle hackles. Long and full tail, the sickles carried at an angle of 45°, but avoiding 'squirrel' carriage.
Head: Skull short and fine. Beak strong and well curved. Eyes large, bright and prominent. Comb single, erect, evenly serrated, of medium size, and following the contour of the skull. Face smooth and of fine texture. Ear-lobes small and of almond shape. Wattles of medium length, well rounded at the base.
Neck: Of medium length and furnished with long hackle feathers flowing well on the shoulders.
Legs and feet: Of medium length. Thighs well apart. Shanks fine and round, free of feathers. Toes four, strong and well spread.

Female

The general characteristics are similar to those of the male, allowing for the natural sexual differences. (*Note*: The comb is carried erect, and not drooping.)

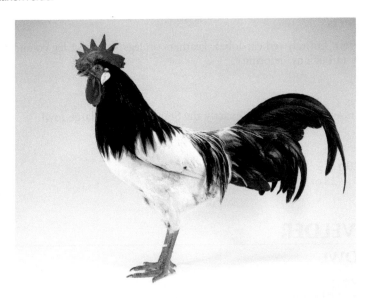

Lakenvelder male

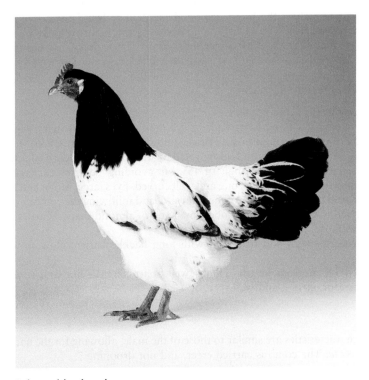

Lakenvelder female

Colour

Male and female plumage: Head, neck hackle and tail solid black, free of stripes, ticks or spots. Wing primaries and secondaries white outer web, black inner web. Remainder is white with light blue-grey undercolour. In the male the saddle hackles are white with black striping.

In both sexes: Beak dark horn. Eyes red or bright chestnut. Comb, face and wattles bright red. Ear-lobes white. Legs and feet slate blue.

Weights

Male   2.25–2.70 kg (5–6 lb)
Female   2.00 kg (4½ lb)

Scale of points

Colour	45
Size	20
Head	10
Type	10
Condition	10
Legs and feet	5
	100

Serious defects

Comb other than single. Feathers on shanks. Wry tail or any other deformity.

BANTAM

Lakenvelder bantams should follow the large fowl Standard.

Weights

Male   680 g (24 oz)
Female   510 g (18 oz)

LEGHORN

LARGE FOWL

Origin: Mediterranean
Classification: Light: Soft feather
Egg colour: White

Italy was the original home of the Leghorn, but the first specimens of the white variety reached this country from America around 1870, and of the brown two years or so later. These early specimens weighed not more than 1.6 kg (3½ lb) each, but our breeders started to increase the body weight of the whites by crossing the Minorca and Malay, until the birds were produced well up to the weights of the heavy breeds. In the postwar years, the utility and commercial breeders established a type of their own, and that is the one which is now favoured. In commercial circles the white Leghorn has figured prominently in the establishment of high egg-producing hybrids.

General characteristics: male

Carriage: Very sprightly and alert, but without any suggestion of stiltiness or in-kneed appearance. Well balanced.

Type: Body wide at the shoulders and narrowing slightly to root of tail. Back long and flat, sloping slightly to the tail. Breast round, full and prominent, carried well forward; breastbone straight. Wings large, tightly carried and well tucked up. Tail moderately full and carried at an angle of 45° from the line of the back; full, sweeping sickles.

Head: Well balanced with fine skull. Beak short and stout, the point clear of the front of the comb. Eyes prominent. Comb single or rose. The single of fine texture, straight and erect, moderately large but not overgrown, coarse or beefy, deeply and evenly serrated (the spikes broad at their base), extending well beyond the back of the head and following, without touching, the line of the head, free from 'thumb marks' and side sprigs or twist at the back. The rose moderately large, firm (not overgrown so as to obstruct the sight), the leader extending straight out behind and not following the line of the head, the top covered with small coral-like points of even height and free from hollows. Face smooth, fine in texture and free from wrinkles or folds. Ear-lobes well developed and pendant, equally matched in size and shape, smooth, open and free from folds. Wattles long, thin and fine in texture, free from wrinkles and creases.

Neck: Long, profusely covered with hackle feathers and carried upright.

Legs and feet: Legs moderately long. Shanks fine and round – flat shins objectionable – and free of feathers. Ample width between legs. Toes four, long, straight and well spread, the back toe straight and well spread, the back toe straight out at rear. Scales small and close fitting.

Plumage: Of silky texture, free from woolliness or excessive feather.

Handling: Firm, with abundance of muscle.

Female

With the exception of the single comb rising from a firm base and falling gracefully over either side of the face without obstructing the sight, and the tail, which is carried closely and not at such a high angle, the general characteristics are similar to those of the male, allowing for the natural sexual differences.

Colour

The black

Male and female plumage: Rich green-black and perfectly free from any other colour.

The blue

Male and female plumage: Even medium shade of blue from head to tail, free from lacing, a dark tint allowed in the hackles of the male, but no black, 'sand' or any other colour than blue, and the more even the better.

The brown

Male plumage: Head and hackle rich orange shading to lemon tips, striped with black, crimson-red at the front of hackles below the wattles. Back, shoulder coverts and wing bows deep crimson-red or maroon. Wing coverts steel blue with green reflections forming a broad bar across; primaries brown; secondaries deep bay on outer web (all that appears when wing is closed) and black on the inner web. Saddle rich orange-red with or without a few black stripes. Breast and underparts glossy black, quite free from brown splashes. Tail black glossed with green; any white in tail is very objectionable; tail coverts black edged with brown.

Female plumage: Hackle rich golden-yellow, broadly striped with black. Breast salmon-red, running into maroon around the head and wattles, and ash grey at the thighs. Body colour rich brown, very closely and evenly pencilled with black, the feathers free from light shafts, and the wings free from any red tinge. Tail black, outer feathers pencilled with brown.

The buff
Male and female plumage: Any shade of buff from lemon to dark, at the one extreme avoiding washiness and at the other a red tinge; the colour to be perfectly uniform, allowing for greater lustre on the hackle feathers and wing bows of the male.

The lavender
Male and female plumage: The lavender is not a lighter shade of the blue Leghorn, it is different genetically, and is of a lighter more silver tint, without darker shade associated with the normal blue feather. Shaft to be lavender and not dark (dilute blue). The silver tint is most obvious in the neck and saddle hackle feathers of the male.

The cuckoo
Male and female plumage: Light blue or grey ground, each feather marked across with bands of dark blue or grey, the markings to be uniform; the banding shading into the ground colour not cleanly cut but sharp enough to keep the two colours distinct.

The golden duckwing
Male plumage: Neck hackle rather light yellow or straw, a few shades deeper at the front below the wattles, the longer feathers striped with black. Back deep rich gold. Saddle and saddle hackle deep gold, shading in hackle to pale gold. Shoulder coverts bright gold or orange, solid colour (an admixture of lighter feathers is very objectionable). Wing bows the same as the shoulder coverts; coverts metallic blue (blue-violet) forming an even bar across the wing, sharp, cleanly cut and not too broad; primaries black, with white edging on the outer web; secondaries white outer web (all that appears when the wing is closed), black inner and end of feather. Breast black with green lustre. Tail black, richly glossed, with green-grey fluff at the base.
Female plumage: Head grey (a brown cap is very objectionable). Hackle white, each feather sharply striped with black or dark grey (a light tinge of yellow in the ground colour admitted). Breast and undercolour bright salmon-red (this point is very important), darker on throat and shaded off to ash grey or fawn on the underparts. Back, wings, sides and saddle dark slate grey, finely pencilled with darker grey or black. Tail grey, slightly darker than the body colour, inside feathers dull black or dark grey.

The silver duckwing
Male plumage: Neck hackle silver-white, the long feathers striped with black. Back, saddle and saddle hackle silver-white. Shoulders and wing bows silver-white, as solid as possible (any admixture of red or rusty feathers very objectionable). Wing coverts metallic blue (blue-violet) forming an even bar across the wing, which should be sharp and clearly cut, and not too broad; primaries black with white edging on outer parts; secondaries white outer edge (all that appears when the wing closed), black inner and end of feathers. Thighs and underparts black. Tail black richly glossed with green, grey fluff at the base.
Female plumage: Head silver-white. Hackle silver-white, each feather sharply striped with black or dark grey. Breast and underparts light salmon or fawn, darker on throat and shaded off to ash grey on underparts. Back, wings, sides and saddle clear delicate silver-grey or French grey, without any shade of red or brown, finely pencilled with dark grey or black (purity of colour very important). Tail grey, slightly darker than the body colour with the inside feathers a dull black or dark grey.

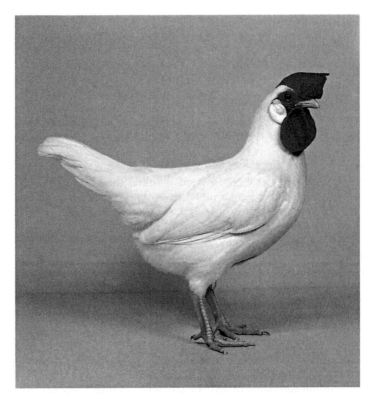

White Leghorn female, bantam

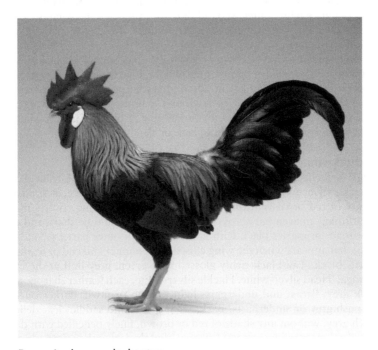

Brown Leghorn male, bantam

The exchequer

Male and female plumage: Black and white evenly distributed with some white in the undercolour, the white of the surface colour in the form of a large blob as distinct from V-shaped ticking. Wings and tail to appear white and black evenly distributed.

The mottled

Black mottled

Male and female plumage: Black with white tips to each feather, the tips as evenly distributed as possible. Black to predominate and to have a rich green sheen.

Red mottled

Male and female plumage: Light red to mahogany red with white tips to each feather, the tips as evenly distributed as possible. Red to predominate and to have a rich sheen.

The partridge

Male and female plumage: This colour is fully described under Wyandotte bantams and need not be repeated here.

The pile

Male plumage: Neck hackle bright orange. Back and saddle rich maroon. Shoulders and wing bows dark red. Secondaries dark chestnut outer web (all that appears when the wing is closed) and white inner. Remainder white.
Female plumage: Neck white tinged with gold. Breast deep salmon-red shading into white thighs. Remainder white.

The white

Male and female plumage: Pure white, free from straw tinge.

The Columbian

Male plumage: Head silver-white, neck and saddle hackles narrowly laced silver-white, centre of feather striped a lustrous greenish-black. Saddle preferably white, some ticking allowed. Wing primaries black with lower edge white, secondaries black inner web, white outer web. Tail lustrous greenish-black, coverts laced with silvery white. Remainder silver-white with white, light blue or slate undercolour.
Female plumage: As male except back silver-white and free from ticking. Tail black except top pair of feathers which are laced with white.

The buff Columbian

Male and female plumage: As Columbian with ground colour replaced by an even shade of buff.

The blue-red

Male plumage: Neck hackle bright orange, back and saddle rich marron. Shoulders and wing bows dark red; secondaries outer web dark chestnut, inner web blue, remainder blue.
Female plumage: Exactly the same as the brown female with the exception that all the black is replaced with a clear even blue.

  In both sexes: Blue to be an even, medium shade from head to tail, free from lacing. A darker tint allowed in the hackles of the male, with no black.

In both sexes and all colours

Beak yellow or horn. Eyes red. Comb, face and wattles bright red. Ear-lobes pure opaque white (resembling white kid) or cream, the former preferred. Legs and feet yellow or orange.

Weights

Cock   3.40 kg (7½ lb)   Cockerel   2.70–2.95 kg (6–6½ lb)
Hen   2.50 kg (5½ lb)   Pullet   2.00–2.25 kg (4½–5 lb)

Scale of points

Type	35
Head	25
Legs	10
Colour	20
Condition	10
	100

Serious defects in all colours (for which a bird should be passed)

Single comb: male's comb twisted or falling over, or female's erect. Ear-lobes red. Any white on face. Legs other than yellow or orange. Side sprigs on comb. Wry or squirrel tail, or any bodily deformity. Rosecomb: comb other than rose or such as to obstruct sight. Ear-lobes red. White in face. Wry or squirrel tail or any bodily deformity. Legs other than orange or yellow.

BANTAM

Leghorn bantams should follow the large fowl Standard in all respects.

Weight

Male   1020 g (36 oz) max.
Female   910 g (32 oz) max.

LINCOLNSHIRE BUFF

LARGE FOWL

Origin: British
Classification: Heavy
Egg colour: Brown

A dual-purpose utility breed found mainly in its native Lincolnshire. During the nineteenth and early twentieth centuries, it was supplied in vast numbers to the London markets as a white-fleshed table bird and was widely sold as a good winter layer. Standardisation of the buff Orpington, which many at the time considered to be a refined Lincolnshire Buff, led to its demise in name by the 1920s, although its genetic material still lived on in the Orpington albeit in a much modified form. In the 1980s, the breed was redeveloped in Lincolnshire using this genetic material, with the addition of that of the Cochin and Dorking.

General characteristics: male

Carriage: Alert, upright, with bold appearance.
Type: Body large, deep and moderately long. Back broad, saddle feathers medium length and abundant. Breast broad with well-rounded keel bone, long and straight. Wings moderately large and carried horizontally. Tail medium size and carried well out, with well-curved sickles.
Head: Head strong. Beak stout. Eyes large and bright. Comb to be single, upright and straight, medium size, free from side sprigs, smooth and fine in texture, with five or six evenly serrated spikes. Face smooth. Wattles medium size, rounded and of fine texture. Ear-lobes fine in texture.
Neck: Medium length with full hackle.
Legs and feet: Free from any feather. Legs set well apart, thighs large and medium length. Toes five, the three front toes to be large, round, long and straight but well spread. The fourth toe should be as near as possible to that of a four-toed bird, with the fifth toe quite separate, placed above, curving backwards and upwards.
Plumage: Close and free from unnecessary fluff. Feathers broad.

Female

The general characteristics are similar to those of the male, allowing for the natural sexual differences.

Colour

Male plumage: Back, neck and saddle hackles a rich orange, wing bow coverts copper, wing bar coverts chestnut. A degree of umber (very dark brown to dull black with no sheen) on some main wing feathers and axials. Tail side hangers bronze to copper, main feathers and sickles bronze to copper, shading into umber. Remainder of the plumage ginger-buff to the skin.
Female plumage: Back, neck, wings, saddle and tail ginger-buff. A small degree or no umber on some main wing feathers and axials. Neck hackle with sheen. Tail with darker shading up to umber at the end. Remainder of plumage a lighter shade of ginger-buff to the skin.

In both sexes: Beak white to horn. Eyes bright orange. Comb, face, lobes and wattles bright red. Legs and feet white, sometimes with horn shading on the front scales and, in males in breeding condition, a line of reddish pigment down the outer sides of the shanks.

Serious defects

Mealiness in surface colour. Grey undercolour. White in plumage, face or lobes. Lopped or beefy comb. Any green-black in plumage. Visible umber in the closed wing. Excess fluff.

Disqualifications

Any deformity. Absence of fifth toe. Leg colour other than as described. Any feathers on legs.

Weights

Cock	4.00–5.00 kg (9–11 lb)	Cockerel	3.10–4.00 kg (7–9 lb)
Hen	3.10–4.00 kg (7–9 lb)	Pullet	2.90–3.60 kg (6–8 lb)

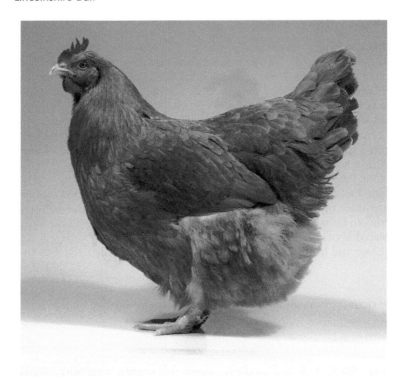

Lincolnshire Buff female

Scale of points

Type	20
Colour	20
Size	20
Head	10
Feet/legs and fifth toe	10
Dual-purpose utility qualities	10
Condition	10
	100

BANTAM

Lincolnshire Buff bantams should follow exactly the large fowl Standard.

Weights

Cock	1–1.3 kg (40 oz)	Cockerel	980 g (34 oz)
Hen	980 g (34 oz)	Pullet	850 g (30 oz)

MALAY

LARGE FOWL

Origin: Asia
Classification: Asian Hardfeather
Egg colour: Brown

At the first poultry show in England in 1845 the Malay had its classification, and in the first British *Book of Standards* of 1865 descriptions were included of both the black-red and the white Malay. One of the oldest breeds, the Malay reached this country as early as 1830 and our breeders developed it, particularly in Cornwall and Devon. At the turn of the twentieth century the Malay was the first breed to be bantamised, the bantams proving to be more popular than the large fowl. They were large in comparison with other bantams, and it is difficult to reduce size further without losing the typical large fowl characteristics. They should follow the large fowl Standard in every respect except weight.

General characteristics: male

Type and carriage: Fierce, gaunt and erect, high in front, sloping at stern. Hard, clean cut-up appearance. The profile of neck hackle, back and upper feathers of tail should form a succession of three curves.
Body: Extremely firm and muscular. Wide fronted, short and tapering. Shoulders broad and square.
Breast: Deep and full, generally devoid of feathers at point of keel.
Back: Short and sloping with convex outline. Saddle narrow and sloping.
Wings: Large, strong, carried high, held closely to the sides, and devoid of feathers at point. Wing butts prominent and well up.
Tail: Of moderate length, drooping but not whipped. Sickles narrow and only slightly curved.
Head: Very broad across the skull, with well-projecting overhanging eyebrows, giving a cruel expression. Beak short, strong and curved downwards, but not hooked. The profile of the beak should follow that of the skull; the two should resemble a semi-circle in shape. Eyes deep set. Comb shaped like a half walnut, small, set well forward and as free as possible from irregularities. Face smooth. Ear-lobes and wattles small and fine or absent.
Neck: Long and upright, with a slight curve, thick from gullet to back of skull. Bare skin on throat extending a long way down the neck, lightly covered with small hair-like feathers. Hackle full at base of skull, but very short and scant elsewhere.
Legs and feet: Legs long and strong boned, set well on the front of the body – in keeping with the balance of the bird. Thighs muscular with very little feather, leaving the hocks clearly exposed. Shanks free of feathers, neatly scaled, flat at the hocks and gradually rounding to the spurs, which should have a downward curve. Toes four, long and straight with powerful nails, hind toe firm on the ground.
Plumage: Very short, hard, narrow and scant.
Handling: Extremely firm fleshed and muscular.

Female

With the exception of the tail, which is carried slightly above the horizontal line, well 'played' as if flexible at the joint, rather short and square and neither fanned nor whipped, the general characteristics are similar to those of the male, allowing for the natural sexual differences.

Colour

The black
Male and female plumage: Glossy black all over with brilliant green and purple lustre, the green predominant. Free from brassy or white feather.

The black-red
Male plumage: Neck and saddle hackle, back and wing bows rich red. Secondaries bright bay. Flights black inner web, red outside edging. Remainder lustrous green-black.
Female plumage: Any shade of cinnamon with dark purple-tinted hackle, quite free of ticks, spangles or pencilling, or white in tail and wings. Partridge marked and clay females with golden hackle are also allowed.

The pile
Male plumage: Neck and saddle hackle, back and wing bows rich red. Secondaries bright bay. Flights white inner web, red outside edging. Remainder cream-white.
Female plumage: Hackle gold. Breast salmon. Remainder cream-white.

The spangled
Male plumage: Breast, underparts, thighs and tail an admixture of red and white. Remainder each feather somewhat resembling tortoiseshell in the blending of red or chestnut with black, and with a bold white tip or spangle. The flight feathers and tail as tri-coloured as possible.
Female plumage: Rich dark red or chestnut boldly marked with black and white.

The white
Male and female plumage: Pure white, free from any yellow, black or ruddy feathers.

In both sexes and all colours
Beak yellow or horn. Legs and feet rich yellow, although in the black a slight duskiness may be overlooked. Comb, face, throat, wattles and ear-lobes brilliant red. Eyes pearl, white or yellow with a green shade, but the lighter the better. A red or foxy tinge is very objectionable. However, it is acceptable for young birds to have slightly darker eyes than adults.

   Note: The foregoing are the principal colours, others not being kept or bred in sufficient numbers to warrant description. The above colours and markings are ideal, but type and quality are the most important points in the Malay.

Weights

Male   5 kg (11 lb) approx.
Female   4.1 kg (9 lb) approx.

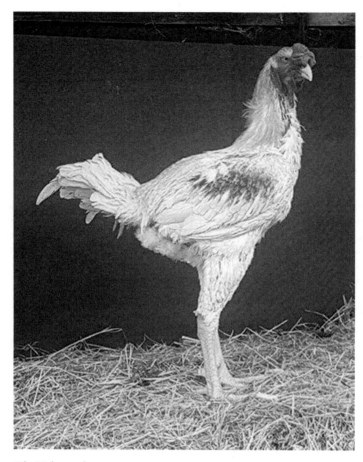

Pile Malay male

Scale of points

Type (shoulders 7, curves and carriage 16, reach 12)	35
Head	16
Eyes	9
Legs	10
Feathering	10
Colour	6
Tail	6
Condition	8
	100

Serious defects

Lack of attitude. Any clear evidence of an alien cross. Lack of size. Single, spreading or pea comb. Red eye, bow legs, knock knees, bad feet.

BANTAM

Malay bantams should follow the large fowl Standards in all but weight, oversize being a common but serious defect.

Weights

Male   1190–1360 g (42–48 oz)
Female   1020–1130 g (36–40 oz)

MARANS

LARGE FOWL

Origin: France
Classification: Heavy: Soft feather
Egg colour: Dark brown

Taking its name from the town of Marans in France, this breed has in its make-up such breeds as the Coucou de Malines, Croad Langshan, Rennes, Faverolles, barred Rock, Brakel and Gatinaise. Imported into this country around about 1929, it has developed as a dual-purpose sitting breed. Like other barred breeds the cuckoo Marans females can be mated with males of other suitable unbarred breeds to give sex-linked offspring of the white head-spot distinguishing characteristic.

General characteristics: male

Carriage: Active, compact and graceful.
Type: Body of medium length with good width and depth throughout; front broad, full and deep. Breast long, well fleshed, of good width and without keeliness. Tail well carried, high.
Head: Refined. Beak deep and of medium size. Eyes large and prominent; pupil large and defined. Comb single, medium size, straight, erect, with five to seven serrations, and of fine texture. Face smooth. Wattles of medium size and fine texture.
Neck: Of medium length and not too profusely feathered.
Legs and feet: Legs of medium length, wide apart and good-quality bone. Thighs well fleshed, but not heavy in bone. Shanks clean and unfeathered. Toes four, well spread and straight.
Plumage: Fairly tight and of silky texture generally.
Handling: Firm, as befits a table breed. Flesh white, and skin of fine texture.

Female

General characteristics similar to those of the male, allowing for the natural sexual differences. Table and laying qualities to be taken carefully into account jointly.

Colour

The black

Male and female plumage: Black with a beetle-green sheen.
Defects: Restricted white in undercolour. In both sexes: a little darkish pigmentation in white shanks.

The dark cuckoo

Male and female plumage: Cuckoo throughout, each feather marked across with bands of blue-black. A lighter shaded neck in both male and female, and also back in the male, is permissible if definitely banded. Cuckoo throughout is the ideal, as even as possible.

The golden cuckoo

Male plumage: Hackles bluish-grey with golden and black bands, neck paler than saddle. Breast bluish-grey with black bands, pale golden shading on upper part. Thighs and fluff light bluish-grey with medium black banding. Back, shoulders and wing bows bluish-grey with rich bright golden and black bands. Wing bars bluish-grey with black bands, golden fringe permissible. Wings, primaries dark blue-grey, lightly banded; secondaries dark blue-grey, lightly banded, with slight golden fringe. Tail dark blue-grey banded with black; coverts blue-grey banded with black. General cuckoo markings.

Female plumage: Hackle medium bluish-grey with golden and black bands. Breast dark bluish-grey with black bands, pale golden shading on upper parts. Remainder dark bluish-grey with black bands. Cuckoo markings.

The silver cuckoo

Male plumage: Mainly white in neck and showing white on upper part of breast, also on top. Remainder banded throughout, with lighter ground colour than the dark cuckoo.

Female plumage: Mainly white in neck and showing white on upper part of breast. Remainder banded throughout, with lighter ground colour than the dark cuckoo.

Weights

Black and cuckoo colour varieties

Cock	3.60 kg (8 lb)	Cockerel	3.20 kg (7 lb)
Hen	3.20 kg (7 lb)	Pullet	2.70 kg (6 lb)

The copper-black

General characteristics: male

Carriage: A well-built bird of average size. Plumage close to the body giving the impression of strength without looking too heavy.

Type: Strong body, back fairly long, wide and flat especially near the shoulders, which are held high. Back fairly concave towards the rear. Saddle large, slightly raised but not rounded and well feathered. Front broad, full, and deep. Breast strong and large, well fleshed and without pronounced keel. Tail carried well without going over 45°.

Head: Medium size, slightly flat and long. Face red coloured with or without down. Beak quite strong, slightly hooked and horn coloured. Eyes bright with an orangey-red iris. Comb single, medium size, straight, erect with five to seven serrations of a fairly rough texture and with sharp edges. Wattles of medium size, red with a fine texture. Ear-lobes medium size, red and long.

Neck: Of medium length and not too profusely feathered.

Legs and *feet*: Dark legs of medium length, wide apart and good-quality bone. Thighs well fleshed, but not heavy in bone. Shank feathers black. Toes four, well spread and straight.

Plumage: Fairly tight plumage held close to the body and of silky texture generally.

Handling: Firm, as befits a table breed. Flesh white, and skin of fine texture.

Female

General characteristics similar to those of the male although smaller body, but strong and more rounded having a straighter backline and well-developed abdomen. Comb of fine texture, straight or inclined only in the rear section. Table and laying qualities to be taken carefully into account jointly. Eggs should be large, ranging in size from about 65 g for a pullet to 70–80 g for an adult hen.

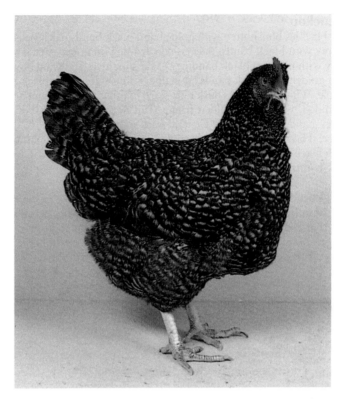

Dark cuckoo Marans female, large

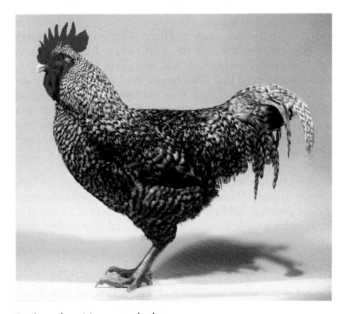

Dark cuckoo Marans male, large

Male plumage: Breast with red markings and a black wing triangle. Red markings not to be yellow or mahogany. Neck hackle and back black with copper-coloured pencilling. Shoulders deep red.

Female plumage: Neck and breast black with red hackle markings but without the typical Birchen breast lacing. Minor red breast marking is acceptable. Green sheen on black not required.

Weights

Copper-black

Cock	3.50–4.00 kg (7.8–8.8 lb)	Cockerel	3.00–3.50 kg (6.6–7.7 lb)
Hen	2.60–3.20 kg (5.7–7 lb)	Pullet	2.20–2.60 kg (4.9–5.7 lb)

In both sexes and all colours and varieties

Beak white or horn. Eyes red or bright orange preferred. Comb, face, wattles and ear-lobes red. Legs and feet white.

Scale of points

Type, carriage and table merits (to include type of breast and fleshing, also quality of flesh)	40
Size and quality	20
Colours and markings	15
Head	10
Condition	10
Legs and feet	5
	100

Serious defects

Feathered shanks in the black and cuckoo varieties, unfeathered shanks in the copper-black. General coarseness. Lack of activity. Superfine bone. Any points against utility or reproductive values. White in lobe.

Defects (for which a bird may be passed)

Deformities, crooked breastbone, other than four toes, etc. In the copper-black; any trace of colour other than black in flight feathers or yellow/straw colour in neck of males. Any brown pattern on body of female.

BANTAM

Marans bantams should be true miniatures of their large fowl counterparts. Copper-black Marans bantams have not yet been standardised.

Weights

Cock	910 g (32 oz)	Cockerel	790 g (28 oz)
Hen	790 g (28 oz)	Pullet	680 g (24 oz)

MARSH DAISY

LARGE FOWL

Origin: Great Britain
Classification: Light: Rare
Egg colour: Brown

The Marsh Daisy was created around the 1880s by a Mr J. Wright of Southport, using an Old English Game Bantam cock crossed on to cinnamon Malay hens. A cock produced from that cross was mated to hens which were a black Hamburgh/white Leghorn cross. A white rosecombed male produced from that cross was in turn crossed back to the hens of the Hamburgh/Leghorn cross. No other blood was introduced until 1913, when a Mr C. Moore purchased some hens from Mr Wright and crossed them on to a pure Pit Game cock. Desiring to secure the white lobe and willow leg stock, it was crossed with Sicilian Buttercups. The above were the basic ingredients for what we now know as the Marsh Daisy, a moderate layer and good forager. There are no known bantams in this breed.

General characteristics: male

Carriage: Upright, bold and active.
Type: Body long, fairly broad, especially at the shoulders, with square and blocky appearance. Almost horizontal back. Well-rounded and prominent breast. Full tail, carried at an angle of 45° from the vertical.
Head: Skull fine. Beak short and well curved. Eyes bold and prominent. Comb rose, medium size, well and evenly spiked, finishing in a single leader 1.25 cm ($\frac{1}{2}$ in.) long in line with the surface, not as high as the Hamburghs or following the nape of the neck as the Wyandottes. Face smooth. Ear-lobes almond shaped. Wattles of fine texture and in keeping with the comb.
Neck: Fairly long, fine. Hackle flowing and falling well on the shoulders to form the cape.
Legs: Moderately long. Shanks and feet light boned, free from feathers. Toes four, well spread.
Plumage: Semi-hard, of fine texture; profuse feathering to be deprecated.

Female

The general characteristics are similar to those of the male, allowing for the natural sexual differences.

Colour

The black
Male and female plumage: Black, with beetle-green sheen in abundance.

The buff
Male and female plumage: Golden-buff throughout and buff to the skin. (*Note*: The male's tail is often black to bronze but the ideal is a whole buff bird.)

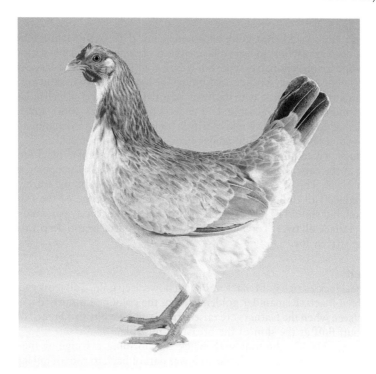

Wheaten Marsh Daisy female

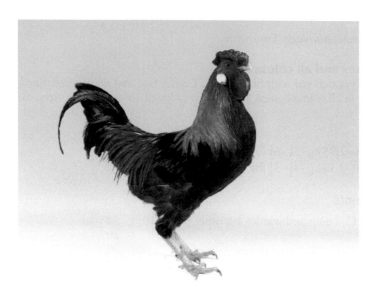

Wheaten Marsh Daisy male

The brown

Male plumage: Neck hackle rich gold, back and saddle dark gold. Main tail black, sickles black, coverts black, the whole to have a beetle-green sheen. Saddle hackle dark gold, a little lighter gold at tips not objectionable. Wing bows dark gold, same shade as back; coverts or bars black with beetle-green sheen; secondaries forming the bay a flat brown, showing a triangular brown bay; primaries a flat black, with the lower edge flat brown, and all well hidden when the wing is closed and tucked up. Breast and all underbody parts black with patches of golden-brown spangle; solid, shiny black should be striven for in these parts. Undercolour decided blue to blue-grey, with a little buff or light golden-brown in places on breast.

Female plumage: Head and hackle rich gold, the tips of all feathers black, the whole to form a fringe at the cape. Back and wings brown ground ticked or peppered with darker brown or flat black. This may result in a series of black bars across the feathers, which is not objectionable. Tail dull, flat black, a little lighter at the edge of the feathers not a disqualification, but should be discouraged. Breast and all underbody parts red-wheaten or salmon, a level shade all over. Too light a shade for these parts, or too deep a red-wheaten, should not be striven for.

The wheaten

Male plumage: Hackles rich gold. Back and wing bows deep gold. Tail (coverts and sickles) rich beetle green-black. Remainder golden-brown, the colour of a fairly dark bay horse. Undercolour (seen when the feathers are raised) from smoke white to a French or blue-grey, a little light buff fluff at the skin of the breast permissible.

Female plumage: Hackle chestnut with black tips forming a fringe at the base of it. Shoulders and back (upper part) red-wheat; lower part of back to root of tail lighter shade, due to the feathers having a white-wheat edging and red-wheat centre, giving a dappling effect. Wing bows red-wheat, the flights presenting a triangular patch of light brown when closed. Breast white-wheat. Tail dull black with red-wheat edging. Undercolour of back smoke white to blue-grey; of breast pure white.

The white

Male and female plumage: Pure white.

In both sexes and all colours

Beak horn. Eyes rich red with black pupil. Comb, face and wattles red. Ear-lobes white. Legs and feet in all colours green, pale willow to lizard according to variety, toenails horn.

Weights

Male   2.50–2.95 kg ($5\frac{1}{2}$–$6\frac{1}{2}$ lb)
Female   2.00–2.50 kg ($4\frac{1}{2}$–$5\frac{1}{2}$ lb)

Scale of points

Head (lobes 13, comb and wattles 10, other points 10)	33
Plumage	20
Condition	20
Type	15
Legs	12
	100

Serious defects

Want of type. Less than one-third white lobe. Red plumage, legs other than green.

MINORCA

LARGE FOWL

Origin: Mediterranean
Classification: Light: Soft feather
Egg colour: White

The Minorca has been developed in this country as our heaviest light breed, and was at one time famous for its extra-large, white eggs. Crossing with the Langshan and other heavy breeds did not improve the egg production of the breed, and concentration on exaggerated headgear had a similar effect. Those times are passed and wiser counsels now prevail. The result is that a much better, balanced type is aimed for on the show bench with moderate size of lobes and of comb, and a more prominent front.

General characteristics: male

Carriage: Upright and graceful.
Type: Body broad at the shoulders, square and compact. Breast full and rounded. Wings moderate in length, neat fitting close to body. Tail full, sickles long, well arched and carried well back.
Head: Long and broad, so as correctly to carry the comb quite erect. Beak fairly long and stout. Eyes full, bright and expressive. Comb single or rose in large fowl, single only in bantams. The single large, evenly serrated, five serrations preferred, perfectly upright, firmly set on the head, straight in front, free from any twist or thumb mark, reaching well to the back of the head, moderately rough in texture and free from any side sprigs. The rose oblong shape, broad at the base over the eyes, closely fitting, upright, firmly carried, full in front and tapering gradually to the 'leader' at the back, surface evenly covered with small nodules or points, free from hollowness, the 'leader' to follow the curve of the neck but not to touch the hackle. Face fine in quality, as free from feathers or hairs as possible, and not showing any white. Ear-lobes medium in size, almond shaped, smooth, flat, fitting close to the head. The lobe should not exceed 6.88 cm ($2\frac{3}{7}$ in.) deep and 3.75 cm ($1\frac{1}{2}$ in.) at its widest point on the top, tapering as the Valencia almond in shape. No definite size for lobes is fixed in bantams. Wattles, long and rounded at the end.
Neck: Long, nicely arched, with flowing hackle.
Legs and feet: Legs of medium length, and thighs stout. Toes four.

Female

The general characteristics are similar to those of the male, allowing for the natural sexual differences, with the exception of the single comb which drops well down over the side of the face, so as not to obstruct the sight, and the ear-lobes which are 4.44 cm ($1\frac{3}{4}$ in.) deep and 3.13 cm ($1\frac{1}{4}$ in.) wide.

Colour

The black

Male and female plumage: Glossy black with a green sheen.
  In both sexes: Beak dark horn. Eyes dark. Comb, face and wattles blood red. Ear-lobes pure white. Legs black or very dark slate, the latter in adults only.

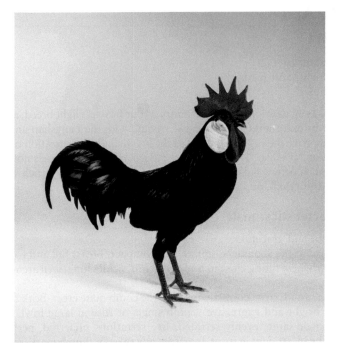

Black Minorca male, bantam

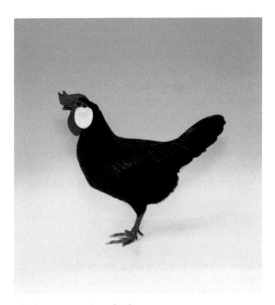

Black Minorca female, bantam

The white

Male and female plumage: Glossy white.

In both sexes: Beak white. Eyes red. Comb, face and wattles blood red. Legs pinky white.

The blue

Male and female plumage: An even medium blue, as free from lacing as possible, the male darker in the hackles, wing bows and back.

In both sexes: Beak, comb, face, ear-lobes and wattles as in the black. Eyes dark brown (darker the better). Legs blue to slate.

Weights

Cock	3.20–3.60 kg (7–8 lb)	Cockerel	2.70–3.60 kg (6–8 lb)
Hen	2.70–3.60 kg (6–8 lb)	Pullet	2.70–3.20 kg (6–7 lb)

Scale of points

The black, the white and the blue

Style, symmetry (type)	10
Size	15
Face	15
Comb	15
Ear-lobes	10
Legs, eyes and beak	8
Colour	10
Condition	10
Breastbone	7
	100

Serious defects

White or blue in face. Feathers on legs. Other than four toes. Wry or squirrel tail. Side sprigs on comb. Plumage other than black, white or blue in the three Standard colours. Purple barring in the blacks. Legs other than black or slate in the blacks and the blues, or white in the whites.

BANTAM

Minorca bantams should be miniatures of their large fowl counterparts and Standard points, colour and defects to be the same for bantams as for large fowl.

Weights

Male	960 g (34 oz)
Female	850 g (30 oz)

Smaller specimens to be favoured, other points being equal.

MODERN GAME

LARGE FOWL

Origin: Great Britain
Classification: Hard feather
Egg colour: Brown

By the introduction of Malay crosses, and with the skill of British fanciers, the Modern Game Fowl was evolved. Black-red, duckwings, brown-reds, piles and birchens were the original recognised varieties, the general characteristics being the same for each, and 13 colours are now standardised.

General characteristics: male

Carriage: Upstanding and active. In the show pen the bird should show plenty of 'lift' as if reaching to its fullest height.
Type: Body short, flat back, wide front and tapering to the tail, shaped like a smoothing iron. Shoulders prominent and carried well up. Wings short and strong. Tail short, fine, closely whipped together, carried slightly above the level of the body, the sickles narrow, well pointed and only slightly curved.
Head: Long, snaky and narrow between the eyes. Beak long, gracefully curved and strong at the base. Eyes prominent. Comb single, small, upright, of fine texture, evenly serrated. Face smooth. Ear-lobes and wattles fine and small to match the comb.
Neck: Long and slightly arched, fitted with 'wiry' feathers, but thin at the junction with the body.
Legs and feet: Legs long and well rounded. Thighs muscular. Shanks free of feathers. Toes four, long, fine and straight, the fourth (or hind) toe straight out and flat on the ground, not downwards against the ball of the foot (or 'duck-footed'), which is most objectionable.
Plumage: Short and hard.

Female

The general characteristics are similar to those of the male, allowing for the natural sexual differences.

Colour

Colour is very important in Modern Game and carries 20 points. Varieties include 13 standardised colours, the blues being included in 1985 and the wheaten in 1993. Legs and beaks vary with the colour varieties, from yellow in piles and whites through willow in black-reds to black in birchens. Toenails to match leg and foot colour. Leg colours are definitely 'tied' to each variety. Thus, whites and piles must always have yellow legs, while shanks are willow in duckwings and black in brown-reds. Eyes similarly vary from bright red to black. Combs and faces vary from bright red to dark purple and black.

The birchen

Male plumage: Hackle, back, saddle, shoulder coverts and wing bows silver-white, the neck hackle with narrow black striping. Remainder rich black, the breast having a narrow silver margin around each feather, giving it a regular laced appearance gradually diminishing to perfect black thighs.
Female plumage: Hackle similar to that of the male. Remainder rich black, the breast very delicately laced as in the male.

In both sexes: Beak very dark horn, black preferred. Eyes black. Comb, face, wattles and ear-lobes mulberry (gypsy-faced) and as dark as possible. Legs and feet black.

The black-red

Male plumage: Cap orange-red. Neck hackle light orange, free from black stripe. Back and saddle rich crimson. Wing bows orange; bars green-black; primaries black; secondaries rich bay on the outer edge, black on the inner and tips, the rich bay alone showing when the wing is closed. Remainder green-black.

Female plumage: Hackle gold, slightly striped with black, running to clear gold on the cap. Breast rich salmon, running to ash on thighs. Tail black, except the top feathers, which should match the body colour. Remainder light partridge-brown, very finely pencilled, and a slight golden tinge pervading the whole, which should be even throughout, free from any ruddiness whatever and with no trace of pencilling on the flight feathers.

In both sexes: Beak dark green. Eyes, comb, face, wattles and ear-lobes bright red. Legs willow.

The brown-red

Male plumage: Hackle, back and wing bows bright lemon, the neck hackle feathers striped down the centre with green-black, not brown. Remainder green-black, the breast feathers edged with pale lemon as low as the top of the thighs.

Female plumage: Neck hackle light lemon to the top of the head, the lower feathers being striped with green-black. Remainder green-black, the breast laced as in the male, the shoulders free from ticking and the back from lacing. (*Note*: There should be only two colours in brown-red Game, namely lemon and black. In the male the lemon should be very rich and bright, and in the female light; the black in both sexes should have a bright green gloss known as beetle green.)

In both sexes: Beak very dark horn, black preferred. Eyes, comb, face, wattles, ear-lobes mulberry (gypsy-faced) and as dark as possible. Legs and feet black.

The gold duckwing

Male plumage: Hackle cream-white, free from striping. Back and saddle pale orange or rich yellow. Wing bows pale orange or rich yellow; bars and primaries black with blue sheen; secondaries pure white on the outer edge, black on inner and tips, the pure white alone showing when the wing is closed. Remainder black with blue sheen.

Female plumage: Hackle silver-white, finely striped with black. Breast pale salmon, diminishing to ash grey on thighs. Tail black, except top feathers, which should match the body colour. Remainder French or steel grey, very lightly pencilled, and even throughout.

In both sexes: Beak dark horn. Eyes ruby red. Comb, face, wattles and ear-lobes red. Legs and feet willow.

The silver duckwing

Male plumage: Hackle, back, saddle, shoulder coverts and wing bows silver-white. Secondaries pure white on the outer edge and black on the inner, with tips of bay, the white alone showing when the wing is closed. Remainder lustrous blue-black.

Female plumage: Hackle silver-white, finely striped with black. Breast pale salmon, diminishing to pale ash grey on thighs. Tail black, except top feathers, which should match the body colour. Remainder light French grey with almost invisible black pencilling.

In both sexes: Beak, etc. as in the golden duckwing.

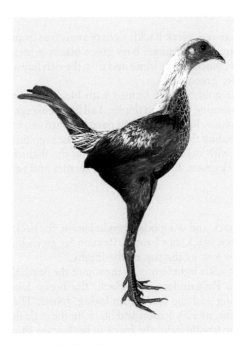

Birchen Modern Game male, bantam

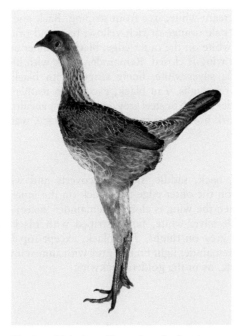

Black-red Modern Game female, bantam

The pile

Male plumage: Hackle one shade of bright orange-yellow. (Dark or washy hackles to be avoided.) Back and saddle rich maroon. Wing bows maroon; bars white and free from splashes; primaries white; secondaries dark chestnut on the outer edge and white on the inner and tips, the dark chestnut alone showing when wings are closed. Remainder pure white.

Female plumage: Hackle white, tinged with gold. Breast rich salmon-red. Remainder pure white.

In both sexes: Beak yellow. Eyes bright cherry-red. Comb, face, wattles and ear-lobes red. Legs and feet rich orange-yellow.

The wheaten

Male plumage: Cap orange-red. Neck hackle light orange, free from black striping. Back and saddle orange to crimson. Wing bows orange; bars green-black; primaries black; secondaries rich bay on outer edge, black on inner and tips, the rich bay alone showing when the wing is closed. Remainder green-black. Altogether showing a brighter top colour than the 'partridge' black-red male.

Female plumage: Hackle golden-orange very lightly striped with black running clear on the cap. Breast light salmon diminishing to fawn or cream on thighs. Body colour pale cinnamon or wheaten. Primaries black with wheaten to outer edge. Tail black except top feathers which, with tail coverts, are darker wheaten.

In both sexes: Beak yellowish-horn. Eyes, comb, face, wattles and ear-lobes red. Legs willow, often showing yellowish soles, a distinguishing mark of the wheaten.

The black

Male and female plumage: Black, free from any other colour, with a purple or green sheen (the latter preferred).

In both sexes: Beak black. Eyes black. Comb, face, wattles and ear-lobes mulberry (gypsy-faced) and as dark as possible. Legs and feet black.

The blue

Male and female plumage: An even, clear, rich medium to pale blue free from lacing but with darker blue top colour in males and hackles of females.

In both sexes: Beak black or blue. Eyes black. Comb, face, wattles and ear-lobes mulberry (gypsy-faced) and as dark as possible. Legs and feet black or blue.

The white

Male and female plumage: Pure white, free from any other colour.

In both sexes: Beak yellow. Eyes, comb, face, wattles and ear-lobes red. Legs and feet yellow.

The blue-red

Male plumage: Cap orange, hackles and saddle gold, free from blue striping. Back and wing bows rich red; bars lustrous blue; outer edge secondaries and edging of lower primaries bay, the bay alone showing when the wing is closed. All other sections an even, clear, rich medium to pale blue except tail, which is a darker shade of blue.

Female plumage: Hackles gold slightly striped with blue. Breast light salmon running to slate blue on thighs. Remainder a rich medium to pale blue; back, shoulders, wing bows, secondaries and top feathers of tail finely and evenly fringed with golden-brown.

In both sexes: Beak horn. Eyes, comb, face, wattles and ear-lobes red. Legs and feet willow.

The silver blue

Male plumage: Cap, hackles, back and wing bows silvery white, hackle feathers striped with blue. Remainder an even, clear, rich, medium to pale blue, breast feathers finely laced with silvery white as far down as top of thighs, with no silver shafting. Tail a darker shade of blue.

Female plumage: Neck hackle silvery white to top of head, lower feathers striped with blue. Remainder an even, clear, rich medium to pale blue, breast laced as in male.

In both sexes: Beak black or blue. Eyes black. Comb, face, wattles and ear-lobes mulberry (gypsy-faced) and as dark as possible. Legs and feet black or blue.

The lemon-blue

Male plumage: Cap, hackles, back and wing bows bright lemon, hackle feathers striped with blue. Remainder an even, clear, rich medium to pale blue, breast feathers finely laced with lemon as far down as top of thighs, with no lemon shafting. Tail a darker shade of blue.

Female plumage: Neck hackle light lemon to top of head, lower feathers striped with blue. Remainder an even, clear, rich medium to pale blue, breast laced as in male.

In both sexes: Beak, etc. as in the blue.

Weights

Male   3.20–4.10 kg (7–9 lb)
Female   2.25–3.20 kg (5–7 lb)

Scale of points

Type and style	30
Colour	20
Head and neck	10
Eyes	10
Tail	10
Legs and feet	10
Condition and shortness of feather	10
	100

Serious defects

Eyes other than Standard colour. Flat shins. Crooked breast. Twisted toes or 'duck' feet. Wry tail. Crooked back.

BANTAM

Modern Game bantams follow the Standard for large fowl. Fine body, 'reachiness' and colour are the main points in bantams. The breed is the favourite of 'die-hard' showmen.

Weights

Male   570–620 g (20–22 oz)
Female   450–510 g (16–18 oz)

MODERN LANGSHAN

LARGE FOWL

Origin: Asia
Classification: Heavy: Rare
Egg colour: Brown

When Major Croad imported his first Langshans in 1872, some poultry experts questioned whether they were significantly different from black Cochins, which at that stage were not as profusely feathered as they have been since about 1900. Some Langshan breeders in the UK decided to emphasise the difference by breeding a taller and tighter feathered type of Langshan. It was this group who retained control of the original Langshan Society, with those favouring the medium feathered type, as first imported, forming a new Croad Langshan Club in 1904. Although the taller birds soon became known as 'Modern Langshans' among poultry keepers in general, the enthusiasts stuck to the names 'Club type' or 'Society type' Langshans for several decades. Modern Langshans gradually declined in popularity through the 1930s, and only just survived to the present day.

General characteristics: male

Carriage: Graceful, upright, alert, strong on the leg with the bearing of an active bird.
Type: Body long and broad but by no means deep. Back horizontal when in normal attitude, and with close compact plumage. Shoulders broad and abundantly furnished saddle. Wings large, closely carried, but neither 'clipped' nor 'pinched in'. Tail full, flowing, spread at base, carried fairly high but not squirrel, furnished with abundant side hangers and two sickles, each feather tapering to a point.
Head: Fine. Beak fairly long and slightly curved. Eyes large. Comb single, straight, upright, fairly small, and evenly serrated with five or six spikes. Face of fine texture. Ear-lobes medium size, pendant and inclined to fold. Wattles medium length, fine texture, neatly rounded.
Neck: Fairly long, broad at base and covered with full hackle.
Legs and feet: Legs rather long, strong and wide apart. Thighs covered with closely fitting feathers, especially around the hocks. Shanks strong but not coarse boned, with an even fringe of feathers (not heavy) on the outer sides. Toes four, long, straight and well spread, the outer (and that alone) slightly feathered.
Plumage: Close and smooth.

Female

With the exception of the tail (not carried high) the general characteristics are similar to those of the male, allowing for the natural sexual differences.

Colour

The black

Male and female plumage: Black with a brilliant beetle-green sheen.
  In both sexes: Beak dark horn to black. Eyes dark brown to black, the darker the better. Comb, face, wattles and ear-lobes brilliant red. Legs and feet dark grey with black scales in front and down the toes, showing pink between the scales (especially down the outer sides of the shanks) and on the skin between the toes. Toenails white. Underfoot pink-white. Skin of the body and thighs white and transparent.

The blue

Male plumage: Hackles, back, tail, sickles, side hangers and wing bows rich deep slate, the darker the better, with brilliant purple sheen. Remainder clear slate blue, each feather distinctly laced (edged) with the same dark shade as the back, the contrast between delicate ground and dark lacing being well defined.

Female plumage: Head and upper part of neck rich dark slate. Remainder clear slate blue, each feather distinctly laced (edged) with dark slate, the lacing being well defined.

In both sexes: Beak, etc. as in the black.

The white

Male and female plumage: Pure white, with brilliant silver gloss.

In both sexes: Beak white with a pink shade near the lower edges. Legs and feet light grey or slate showing pink between the scales and on the skin between the toes. Eyes, comb, face, wattles, ear-lobes, toenails, underfoot and skin as in the black.

Weights

Cock	4.55 kg (10 lb)	Cockerel	3.60 kg (8 lb)
Hen	3.60 kg (8 lb)	Pullet	2.70 kg (6 lb)

Scale of points

Type and carriage	35
Head	15
Legs and feet	10
Size	10
Colour and plumage	20
Condition	10
	100

Serious defects

Yellow skin. Yellow base of beak. Yellow or orange-coloured eyes. Yellow around the eyes. Yellow shanks or underfoot. Legs other than Standard colour. Shanks not feathered. More than four toes. Permanent white in the face or ear-lobes. Comb with side sprigs, or other than single. Wry or squirrel tail. Coloured feathers.

Defects

Absence of pink between toes. Feathering on middle toes. Outer toe not feathered. Too scantily or too heavily feathered shanks or outer toes. Twisted toes. Short shanks. Crooked breast. Twisted or falling comb. General coarseness. Too much fluff. Purple sheen in black; yellow shade in white.

BANTAM

Modern Langshans should follow the large fowl Standard.

Weights

Male	1133 g (40 oz)
Female	910 g (32 oz)

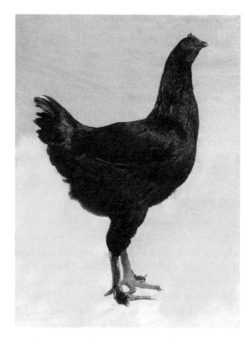

Modern Langshan female

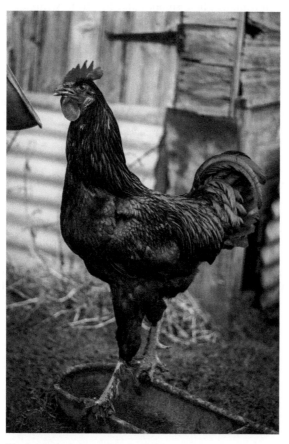

Black Modern Langshan male

NANKIN BANTAM

Origin: Asia
Classification: True Bantam: Rare
Egg colour: Light brown

Nankins, or common yellow bantams, were among the first varieties of bantams introduced into this country. The variety came originally from Java and some parts of India. Once, they were the most widespread of all bantams and are believed to be the progenitors of nearly all buff bantam varieties. The name is thought to have been given from the resemblance of the colour to nankeen cloth. Nankins are excellent layers and the most tameable and engaging of breeds.

General characteristics: male

Carriage: Jaunty and active, with a proud bearing.
Type: Body small and neat, the breast carried well up and forward. Back short and sloping to the tail. Wings large, closely folded and carried very low, almost down to the ground. Tail large and well spread with long well-curved sickles. The whole tail carried high but not squirrel, well furnished with flowing side hangers and coverts.
Head: Small and fine. Beak rather fine and slightly curved. Eyes large and bright. Comb single or rose. The single should be neat, bearing three to six fine spikes. It should be straight and upright and in proportion with the head, carried well away from the head, a flyaway comb being characteristic. The rosecomb should be small and close fitting, finely worked, with a small leader curved gracefully upward. Face smooth, ear-lobes very small, wattles small and well rounded, fine, smooth and free from wrinkles.
Neck: Medium long, well curved and bearing long and abundant hackle.
Legs and feet: Legs short, thighs set well apart, shanks rather short, rounded and fine, free from feathers. Toes four, rather small, straight and well spread.

Female

With the exception of the carriage, which is lower and less arrogant and with the tail carried well spread but slightly lower, the general characteristics are similar to those of the male, allowing for the natural sexual differences.

Colour

Male plumage: Back, neck and saddle hackles a rich orange, wing bows chestnut. Tail main feathers black, sickles and side hangers bronze or copper, shading into black. Remainder of plumage ginger-buff throughout to the skin.
Female plumage: Neck, back, wings, tail and saddle dark ginger-buff. Tail shading into black at the ends. Remainder of plumage light ginger-buff throughout to the skin.

In both sexes: Beak white or horn. Eyes bright orange. Comb, face, ear-lobes and wattles bright red. Legs blue or bluish-white, male often with pinkish stripe on outside of shank. A degree of black on inner web of wings, a smaller amount or none on the female.

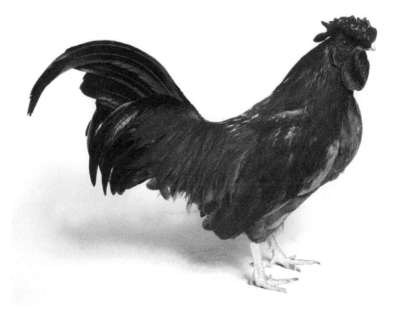

Nankin male

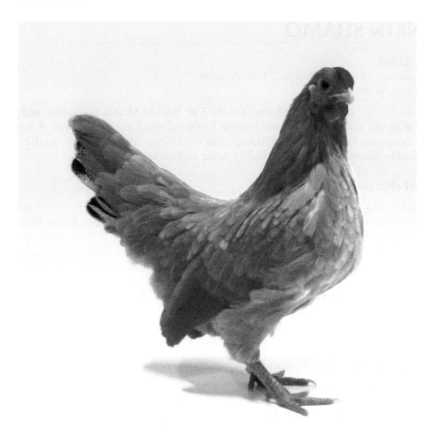

Nankin female

Weights

Male   680–737 g (24–26 oz)
Female   570–620 g (20–22 oz)

Scale of points

Type and carriage   25
Colour   20
Tail   10
Feet and legs   10
Comb   10
Other head points   10
Size   10
Condition   <u> 5</u>
                    <u>100</u>

Serious defects

Wry or squirrel tail. Comb other than rose or single. Comb lopped or twisted or curved down at the rear. Long legs, large feet or twisted toes. White in the ear-lobes or face. Yellow legs. Even colour throughout. White in the base of the tail. All black or buff tails in males, tail lacking black end in females. Visible black in the closed wing. Black striping or flecking on saddle and neck hackle, mealiness in surface or grey undercolour.

NANKIN SHAMO

Origin: Japan
Classification: Asian Hardfeather. True Bantam
Egg colour: White

This is the lightest of the small Shamo breeds. The Nankin Shamo is slimmer and more elegant than the Ko Shamo, is more heavily feathered and has a longer tail. A regional variant exists, the Echigo Nankin Shamo, from the Niigata area. It is very similar to the main Nankin Shamo breed, but is slightly taller and slimmer.

General characteristics: male

Type and carriage: Alert, confident bearing. Upright stance.
Body: Firm and muscular. Body narrowing gradually towards the tail. Rump firm.
Breast: Muscular, with deep keel.
Back: Long. Broadest at the shoulders, sloping down to the tail. Backbone straight.
Wings: Strong and quite long, held downwards and not showing on the back. Shoulders prominent.
Tail: Quite long, well layered, straight and pheasant-like. Held below horizontal. Saddle hackle also quite long, covering the base of the tail.
Head: Medium sized, showing some brow bone. Beak short, strong and curved. Eyes bold and set in oval eyelids. Comb small and compact, triple or walnut. Ear-lobes and wattles small, but with some dewlap.
Neck: Rather long, slightly curved but almost erect. Hackles quite long and thick, but not covering shoulders.
Legs and feet: Legs moderately long. Thighs muscular and rounded. Shanks smooth and round. Toes four, long and straight.

Plumage: Feathers quite long, but narrow and carried close to the body.
Handling: Firm fleshed and muscular.

Female

The general characteristics are similar to those of the male, allowing for the natural sexual differences. Generally of a rather less upright stance.

Colour

Black-red (the 'red' may be any shade from yellow to dark red, with wheaten or partridge females that can be any shade from cream to dark brown, with or without dark markings), duckwing, black, white, splash (any mixture of black, white and shades of red/brown).

In both sexes and all colours: Beak yellow or horn, with darker markings allowed on birds with dark feathers. Legs and feet yellow. Comb, face and wattles bright red. Eyes silver or gold.

Weights

Cock   937 g (2 lb 2 oz)   Cockerel   750 g (1 lb 10 oz)
Hen   750 g (1 lb 10 oz)   Pullet   560 g (1 lb 4 oz)

These are average weights.

Scale of points

Type and carriage	30
Head and neck	20
Condition and plumage quality	20
Legs and feet	10
Eye colour	10
Legs and feet colour	5
Plumage colour	5
	100

Serious defects

Lack of attitude. Any deformity. Comb other than Standard. Poor carriage. Heavy build. Short or rounded tail.

NEW HAMPSHIRE RED

LARGE FOWL

Origin: America
Classification: Heavy: Soft feather
Egg colour: Brown

As if to copy the farmers in the State of Rhode Island who developed the breed carrying its name, those in the neighbouring State of New Hampshire developed and named their breed. The New Hampshire Red was bred by selection from the Rhode Island Red without the introduction of any other breed, taking some thirty years to reach standardisation in 1935. Early maturity, quick feathering and a plump carcase are particular features of the breed. Its body shape and colouring are very different from those of the Rhode Island Red.

General characteristics: male

Carriage: Active and well balanced.

Type: Body of medium length, relatively broad, deep and well rounded. Back of medium length, broad for entire length, gradual concave sweep to tail. Breast deep, full, broad and well rounded, the keel relatively long and extending well to the front at the breast. Wings moderately large, well folded, carried horizontally and close to the body, fronts well covered by breast feathers; primaries and secondaries broad and overlapped in natural order when wing is folded. Tail of medium length, well spread and carried at angle of 45°. Sickles medium length, extending well beyond the main tail; lesser sickles and coverts medium length and broad; main tail feathers broad and overlapping.

Head: Of medium length, fairly deep, inclined to be flat on top rather than round. Beak strong, medium length, regularly curved. Eyes large, full and prominent, moderately high in the head. Comb single, medium size, well developed, set firmly on head, perfectly straight and upright, having five well-defined points, those in front and rear smaller than those in centre; the blade smooth and inclining slightly downward, not following too closely the shape of the neck. Face smooth, full in front of the eyes; skin of fine texture. Wattles moderately large, uniform, free from folds or wrinkles. Ear-lobes elongated oval, smooth and close to head.

Neck: Of medium length, well arched, hackle abundant, flowing well over shoulders. Moderately close feathered.

Legs and feet: Legs well apart, straight when viewed from the front. Lower thighs large, muscular and of medium length. Toes four, medium length, straight and well spread.

Plumage: Feather character to be of broad firm structure, overlapping well and fitting tightly to the body. Fluff moderately full.

Female

The general characteristics are similar to those of the male, allowing for the natural sexual differences. Comb may be slightly tilted at rear. Wattles of medium size, well developed and well rounded. Tail moderately well spread, carried at angle of 35°. Wings rather large, carried nearly horizontal.

Colour

Male plumage: Head and neck hackle brilliant reddish-bay. Breast and front of neck medium chestnut-red. Back brilliant deep chestnut-red. Saddle rich brilliant reddish-bay, slightly darker than neck. Wing fronts medium chestnut-red; bows brilliant chestnut-red; coverts deep chestnut-red; primaries medium chestnut-red, free of peppering desirable, lower web having black stripe adjacent to red shaft, black tips; secondaries upper web black, edged with medium chestnut-red, lower web medium chestnut-red, free of peppering desirable. Tail main feathers black; sickles rich lustrous greenish-black; coverts lustrous greenish-black edged with deep chestnut-red; lesser coverts deep chestnut-red. Body and fluff medium chestnut-red. Lower thighs medium chestnut-red. Undercolour in all sections light salmon, a slight smoky tinge not a defect.

Female plumage: Head medium chestnut-red. Neck medium chestnut-red, each feather edged with brilliant chestnut-red; lower neck feathers distinctly tipped with black; feathers in front of neck medium chestnut-red. Primaries as male, secondaries as male; primary coverts as male. Back, breast, lower thighs, body and fluff medium chestnut-red. Tail main feathers black edged with medium chestnut-red; shaft medium chestnut-red. Undercolour as in male.

In both sexes: Beak reddish-brown. Eyes rich orange-red. Comb, face, wattles and ear-lobes bright red. Legs and toes rich yellow, tinged with reddish-horn. Line of reddish pigment down sides of shanks extending to tips of toes desirable in male.

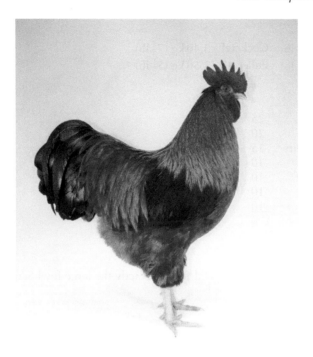

New Hampshire Red male, large

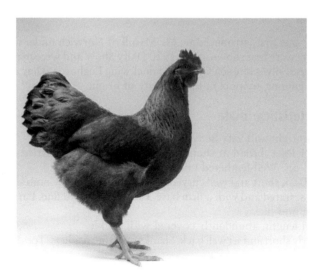

New Hampshire Red female, large

Weights

Cock   3.85 kg (8½ lb)   Cockerel   3.40 kg (7½ lb)
Hen   2.95 kg (6½ lb)   Pullet   2.50 kg (5½ lb)

Scale of points

Type and carriage	25
Colour	20
Dual-purpose quality	15
Head	10
Size and symmetry	10
Legs and feet	10
Condition	10
	100

BANTAM

New Hampshire Red bantams should follow exactly the large fowl Standard.

Weights

Male   980 g (34 oz)
Female   737 g (26 oz)

NORFOLK GREY

LARGE FOWL

Origin: Great Britain
Classification: Heavy: Rare
Egg colour: Brown

The Norfolk Grey was first introduced by Mr Myhill of Norwich under the ugly name of Black Marias. They were first shown at the 1920 Dairy Show and were mainly the result of a cross breed between silver birchen Game and duckwing Leghorns. They appear regularly at shows and are gaining support in their county of origin.

General characteristics: male

Carriage: Fairly upright and very active.
Type: Body rather long, broad at shoulders. Full, round breast carried upwards. Large wings well tucked up. Well-feathered tail.
Head: Skull fine. Beak short and well curved. Eyes large and bold. Comb single, upright, of medium size, well serrated and with a firm base. Face smooth and fine. Ear-lobes small and oval. Wattles long and fine.
Neck: Of medium length, abundantly covered with hackle.
Legs and feet: Fairly short and set well back. Shanks free from feathers. Toes four, well spread.
Plumage: Close.

Female

The general characteristics are similar to those of the male, allowing for the natural sexual differences.

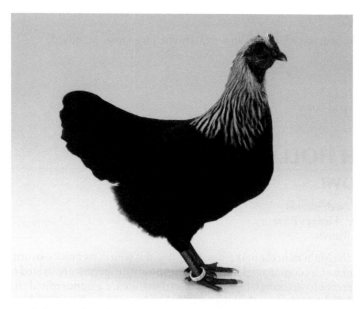

Norfolk Grey female

Colour

Male plumage: Neck, back, saddle, shoulder coverts and wing bars silver-white, the hackles with black striping, free from smuttiness. Remainder a solid black.

Female plumage: Hackle similar to that of the male. Remainder black, the throat very delicately laced with silver (about 5 cm (2 in.) only).

In both sexes: Beak horn. Eyes dark. Comb, face, ear-lobes and wattles red. Legs and feet black or slate black, the former preferred.

Weights

Male   3.20–3.60 kg (7–8 lb)
Female   2.25–2.70 kg (5–6 lb)

Scale of points

	Male	Female
Colour and markings: hackles	20	15
Colour and markings: back and wings	10	15
Colour and markings: breast, thighs and fluff	15	15
Type and size	20	20
Head (comb and lobes 10, eyes 5)	15	15
Legs and feet	5	5
Condition	10	10
Tail	5	5
	100	100

Serious defects

White in lobes. Comb other than single or obstructing the sight. Legs other than black or slate black. Feathers on shanks or feet. Lacing or shaftiness on back, breast or wings of females.

BANTAM

Norfolk Grey bantams should follow exactly the large fowl Standard.

Weights

Male   900 g (32 oz)
Female   680 g (24 oz)

NORTH HOLLAND BLUE

LARGE FOWL

Origin: The Netherlands
Classification: Heavy: Rare
Egg colour: Brown

The blood of the Malines in the make-up of this breed is seen in its quick maturity and rapid growth. To further its commercial importance its utility properties are valued on the show bench in preference to markings. Lightly feathered shanks are a standardised characteristic, and the male is lighter in colour than the female. As a barred breed, the females when mated with unbarred males of breeds with dark downs produce sex-linked offspring, the male chicks having the white head-spot when hatched, which is absent in the female chicks.

General characteristics: male

Carriage: Upright, bold and alert.
Type: Body substantial in build, yet compact. Back broad, flat, horizontal, reasonably long, with slight rise to tail, broad saddle, prominent shoulders. Breast full, rounded and prominent; breastbone long, well fleshed and rounded, neither too shallow nor keel too prominent. Well-rounded sides, good depth of body, with a well-developed abdomen. Wings strong, well developed and close to the body. Tail broad, short, well spread with medium furnishings.
Head: Rounded and of medium length. Beak stout and short. Eyes full, bold, with keen expression, the pupils well formed and large. Face smooth, full fine texture and without heavy eyebrows. Comb single upright, of medium size and fine texture, with five to seven even serrations, following slightly the curve of the neck at the back. Ear-lobes of medium size and silky. Wattles medium in length and size, and fine in texture.
Neck: Somewhat broad, medium in length and not too profusely feathered.
Legs and feet: Legs of medium length, wide apart, well formed and good quality bone with close scales. Thighs well developed and fleshed. Toes four, straight and well spread. Shanks lightly feathered, including outer toe.
Plumage: In general not too profuse. Fine in texture.
Handling: Firm, as befits a table breed. Skin thin and of fine texture. Flesh high-quality table grade.

Female

With the exception of the shanks, which are more heavily feathered, the general characteristics are similar to those of the male, allowing for the natural sexual differences.

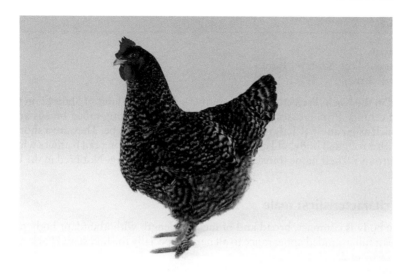

North Holland Blue female

Colour

Male plumage: Lighter blue-grey than female, barred. Undercolour very pale blue-grey, barring immaterial.
Female plumage: Dark grey-blue, slightly barred. Undercolour paler blue-grey, barring immaterial.

In both sexes: Beak white superimposed blue. Eyes orange to red. Comb, wattles face and ear-lobes red. Shanks white, but may be shaded with blue. Skin white.

Weights

Cock   3.85–4.80 kg ($8\frac{1}{2}$–$10\frac{1}{2}$ lb)   Cockerel   3.40–4.30 kg ($7\frac{1}{2}$–$9\frac{1}{2}$ lb)
Hen   3.20–4.10 kg (7–9 lb)   Pullet   2.70–3.60 kg (6–8 lb)

Scale of points

Type and carriage	25
Utility values	25
Colour and markings	20
Head	10
Legs and feet	10
Condition	10
	100

Defects

General coarseness. Superfine bone. Unfeathered shanks. Any points against table, laying or reproductive qualities. Birds may be passed for deformities, crooked breastbone, serious defects and clean shanks devoid of any feathering.

BANTAM

North Holland Blue bantams should follow exactly the large fowl Standard.

Weights

Male   1190 g (42 oz)
Female   1020 g (36 oz)

OHIKI

Origin: Japan
Classification: True Bantam: Rare
Egg colour: Brown

Developed in the Kochi Prefecture on the southern Japanese island of Shikoku in the mid-nineteenth century from crosses (details unknown) between long-tailed breeds and small bantams such as Japanese (Chabo) or others of roughly Pekin type. They are a short-legged bantam with a rounded body, old cocks having extraordinary long tail feathers which drag along the ground. Their name translates: O – tail, hiki – dragging. Not bred in the UK until the 1990s.

General characteristics: male

Type: The body is compact, broad and of medium length with abundant body plumage, which gives a full, rounded appearance to all parts, especially the breast and back. Carriage is nearly horizontal.
Wings: Relatively large and long, carried low so that the tips nearly touch the ground.
Head: Medium size and formation for a bantam of this overall size. Comb is single, no more than medium size, straight and upright, four to six serrations. Ear-lobes of medium size and oval or round. Wattles finely textured, round, of no more than medium size. Eyes large. Beak of medium length and thickness.
Neck: Rather short, with abundant neck hackle feathering which flows over the shoulders and reaches the back.
Saddle and tail: Abundant long and narrow saddle feathers which should reach the ground, and even drag along the ground on exceptional mature cocks. The main tail feathers are long, well spread, and moderately high. They are covered by very long, rather narrow and supple sickles, side hangers and coverts, which flow over the main tail and then down to the ground. This is all that is expected of cockerels, but plumage quality, quantity and length increases with age. The best mature cocks have flexible sickles and side hangers which drag up to 60 cm (2 ft) along the ground. The profile of the neck, back and rise and fall of the tail is said to form an S.
Legs and feet: Thighs short, hidden by the full plumage and low wings. Shanks short to medium in length, strong, smooth, with well-developed pointed spurs on adults. Toes of medium length, straight and well spread.
Plumage: Very abundant and soft.

Female

The general characteristics are similar to those of the male, allowing for the natural sexual differences. Carriage is even more horizontal, the comb is rather small. Females obviously do not have the very long saddle and tail feathers of the male, but their cushion and tail is of full, rounded, elongated oval shape.

Colours

Black-red, duckwing (gold and silver), white (all as in Old English Game).

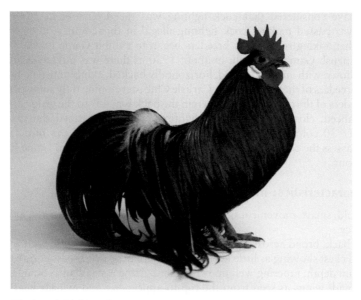

Black-red Ohiki male

Weights

Cock	937 g (33 oz)	Cockerel	750 g (26 oz)
Hen	750 g (26 oz)	Pullet	600 g (21 oz)

Scale of points

Quality, length and number of tail feathers	25
Quality, length and amount of neck and saddle hackles	20
Type, size and carriage	25
Plumage colour	5
Head, including eye and lobe colour	10
Legs and feet	5
Condition	10
	100

Serious defects

Narrow build, long legs, main tail carriage too high or low, much red in lobes, oversized or flopping comb, lack of general abundance of plumage on both sexes and lack of length of saddle and tail feathers on males. Any sign of stiff feathers in tail.

CARLISLE OLD ENGLISH GAME

LARGE FOWL

Origin: Great Britain
Classification: Hard feather
Egg colour: Cream to light brown

When the Romans invaded Britain, Julius Caesar wrote in his commentaries that the Britons kept fowls for pleasure and diversion but not for table purposes. Many well-known authorities have considered that cock fighting was the diversion. In 1849 an Act of Parliament was passed making cock fighting illegal in this country, and, with poultry exhibitions then taking root, many breeders began to exhibit Game Fowls.

The Old English Game Club split in about 1930 as there was already a divergence of birds being shown with larger breasted, horizontally backed, exhibition-type birds tending to win, and breeders of these formed the Carlisle Club, developing only some of the original colours. Breeders of the original type, wherein the back is at 45° to the ground, maintained the well-balanced, close-heeled, athletic fighting fowl, and formed the Oxford Club, retaining over 30 colours. The judge of Oxfords does so with the bird facing away from him to assess the correct balance. It is usually agreed that a good Game Fowl cannot be a bad colour.

General characteristics: male

Carriage: Bold, smart, movement quick and graceful, proud and sprightly, as if ready for any emergency.
Type: Short back, broad across the shoulders, tapering well to the tail, with a full, broad, well-rounded chest showing as little keel as possible. The keel or breast bone to be straight and of medium depth, tapering well up behind and giving a small and compact belly. The whole body with wings as seen from the top to appear flat and as near heart shaped as possible.
Wings: Full and round, inclining to meet under the tail, with strong prominent butts. Feathers to be fairly broad and furnished with hard strong quills. The primaries not to be too long and to be nicely rounded at the ends and to project past the body as little as possible.
Head: Strong, bold, medium length. Beak strong at base, slightly curved. Eyes large, bright, prominent, full of expression. Comb small in both cock and hen. Single, erect and of fine texture. Face of fine texture, to match the comb and wattles. Wattles of fine texture and small. Ear-lobes to match the comb and wattles.
Neck: Long and very strong at the junction with the body. Neck hackle wiry with long feathers, covering the shoulder.
Legs: Thighs short, thick and muscular, shanks of medium length with good round bone, not to be flat on the shins, in-kneed or bow-legged to be considered a serious fault. Spurs low on leg.
Feet: Four toes on each foot, should be clean, even, long and spreading, the back toe standing well backward and flat on the ground.
Tail: In the cock to be carried at a nice angle, neither too low nor too high, and to be straight. Wry and squirrel tail to be considered a serious defect. Feathers to be broad and strong with a pair of good curved sickles of fair length and well furnished with side hangers.
Plumage: Hard, glossy and firm.
Handling: Flesh firm but corky, with plenty of muscle. This is to be considered an important factor.

Female

With the exception of the tail, which is well carried, fairly close and of medium length, the general characteristics are similar to those of the male, allowing for the natural sexual differences.

Colour

The spangle

Male plumage: Neck, hackle and saddle dark red, finely tipped with white. Breast and thighs black, finely and evenly tipped with white. Back and shoulders dark red, finely tipped with white. Wing bows dark red, finely tipped with white with a rich dark blue bar across, finely tipped with white; secondaries deep bay intermixed with white, bay predominating; primaries black intermixed with white. Tail, sickles and side hangers black, tipped with white, straight feathers black intermixed with white.

Female plumage: Neck hackle golden-red, streaked with black, finely tipped with white. Breast and thighs dark salmon, finely and evenly tipped with white. Back and shoulders dark partridge-coloured feathers, finely and evenly tipped with white. Wings secondaries dark partridge intermixed with white, partridge predominating; primaries dark, intermixed with white. Tail black with partridge coverts, finely and evenly tipped with white.

In both sexes: Legs white or yellow, white preferred. Face bright red. Eyes red, both alike.

The black-red (partridge bred)

Male plumage: Neck hackle and saddle orange-red shading to deep orange. Back and shoulders deep crimson. Breast and thighs black. Wing bows deep red, with a rich dark blue bar across; secondaries bay colour on outer web; primaries black. Tail sound black with lustrous green gloss.

Female plumage: (Partridge) neck and hackle golden-red and streaked with black. Breast and thighs shaded salmon. Back and wings partridge colour to be free from rust and shaftiness. Tail black with partridge coverts.

In both sexes: Legs white, yellow or willow. Face bright red. Eyes red, both alike.

The black-red (wheaten bred)

Male plumage: Neck hackle and saddle light golden-red free from streaks. Breast and thighs black. Wing bows bright red; in other respects, including tail, similar to (partridge) black-red.

Female plumage: (Wheaten) neck, hackle golden-red free from striping. Breast and thighs light wheaten. Back and wings wheaten, level on colour, edged with black on primaries. Tail black with a shading of wheaten corresponding with body colour. Clay hens similar to wheaten only darker and harder in colour.

In both sexes: Legs white. Face bright red. Eyes red, both alike.

The brown-red

Male plumage: Neck and saddle lemon or orange, streaked with black. Breast and thighs black laced with brown to top of thighs. Back lemon or orange. Wings, shoulder and wing bows lemon or orange, rest of wing black. Tail black.

Female plumage: Neck lemon or orange, striped with black. Breast and thighs black laced with brown to top of thighs. Body black, tail black.

In both sexes: Legs black. Face gypsy or red, gypsy preferred. Eyes dark, both alike.

The blue-red

Male plumage: Neck, hackle and saddle orange or golden-red. Breast and thighs medium shade of blue. Back and shoulders deep or bright red. Wing bows deep or bright red, with a rich dark blue bar across; secondaries bay colour on the outer web; primaries blue. Tail blue.

Female plumage: Neck golden-red, streaked with blue. Breast and thighs shaded salmon. Back and wings partridge colour, intermixed with blue. Tail blue with partridge coverts.

In both sexes: Legs white or yellow. Face bright red. Eyes red, both alike.

The blue-tailed wheaten hen

Male and female plumage: Similar in all respects to wheatens with the exception of wing, primaries and tail shaded with blue.

In both sexes: Legs white or yellow. Face bright red. Eyes red, both to be alike.

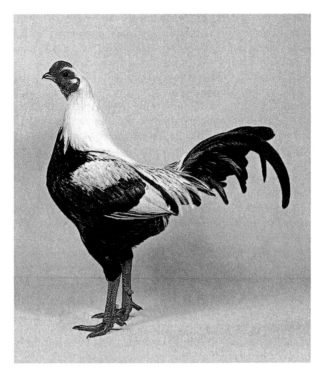

Duckwing Carlisle Old English Game male

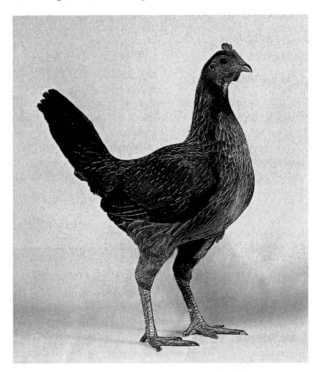

Partridge Carlisle Old English Game female

The birchen grey

Male plumage: Neck, hackle and saddle grey or silver, streaked with black. Breast black laced with grey to top of thighs. Back grey or silver. Wings, shoulders and wing bows grey or silver, rest of wing black. Tail black.

Female plumage: Neck, hackle grey or silver, striped with black. Breast black laced with grey to top of thigh. Body black, tail black.

In both sexes: Legs black. Face gypsy or red, gypsy preferred. Eyes dark, both alike.

The black-breasted grey

Male plumage: Neck, hackle and saddle, grey streaked with black. Back and shoulders grey. Breast, thighs and tail black. Wing bows grey, rest of wing black.

Female plumage: Neck hackle grey striped with black. Breast, thighs, body, wings and tail black.

In both sexes: Legs dark. Face gypsy or red, gypsy preferred. Eyes dark, both alike.

The golden duckwing

Male plumage: Neck hackle creamy white, saddle orange or rich yellow. Breast and thighs black. Back and shoulders orange or rich yellow. Wing bows orange or rich yellow; wing bars steel blue; secondaries white on the outer web; primaries black. Tail black.

Female plumage: Neck hackle silver striped with black. Breast and thighs salmon colour. Back and wings steel grey, free from rust and shaftiness. Tail black, coverts corresponding with body colour.

In both sexes: Legs yellow, white or willow. Face bright red. Eyes red, both alike.

The silver duckwing

Male plumage: Neck and saddle silver-white, free from dark streaks. Breast and thighs black. Back and shoulders silver-white. Wing bows silver-white; wing bars steel blue; secondaries white on outer web; primaries black. Tail black.

Female plumage: As female golden duckwing.

In both sexes: Legs yellow, white or willow. Face bright red. Eyes red, both alike. Pearl eyes permissible with white legs.

The blue duckwing

Male plumage: Neck, hackle, saddle, back, shoulders and wings as for silver duckwing. Breast, thighs and tail blue.

Female plumage: As golden duckwing female but neck silver striped with blue and blue tail.

In both sexes: Legs white. Face bright red. Eyes red, both alike.

The crele

Male plumage: Neck and saddle chequered (barred) orange. Back and shoulders deep chequered orange. Wing bows deep chequered orange with dark grey bar across; secondaries bay colour on the outer web; primaries dark grey. Tail dark grey with light grey bar.

Female plumage: Neck lemon chequered with grey. Breast and thighs chequered salmon. Back and wings chequered blue-grey. Tail dark grey with light grey bar.

In both sexes: Legs white or yellow, white preferred. Face bright red. Eyes red, both alike.

The cuckoo

Male and female plumage: Neck, saddle, back, shoulders, wings and tail bluish-grey in colour, banded across the feathers with darker blue-grey or slate colour, the markings should be as even as possible throughout the plumage.

In both sexes: Legs white or yellow. Face bright red. Eyes red, both alike.

The pile

Male plumage: Neck and saddle orange or chestnut-red. Breast and thighs white. Back and shoulders deep red. Wing bows red with a white bar across; secondaries bay colour on outer web; primaries white. Tail white.

Female plumage: Neck lemon. Breast salmon, lighter towards thighs. Back and wings white. Tail white.

    In both sexes: Legs white or yellow. Face bright red. Eyes red, both alike.

The brassy-backed

Male plumage: Neck, hackle, breast, thighs and tail black. Back, shoulders and saddle brass colour. Wing bows brass with a rich dark blue bar across secondaries; primaries black.

Female plumage: Neck, hackle, breast and thighs black. Back and wings dark brownish. Tail black with light brown coverts.

    In both sexes: Legs black, white or yellow. Face bright red. Eyes red, both alike.

The furness

Male plumage: Neck, hackle and saddle red or gold streaked with black. Back and shoulders red or gold. Breast and thighs sooty black. Wing bows red or gold with a rich dark blue bar across secondaries, bay colour mixed with grey; primaries black.

Female plumage: Neck and hackle gold streaked with black. Breast and thighs deep salmon colour. Back and wings sooty black mixed with a little gold colour, with each feather having a light quill. Tail black.

    In both sexes: Legs white or yellow. Face bright red. Eyes red, both alike.

The blue furness

As for the furness but blue replaces black.

The brassy-backed blue

Male plumage: Neck hackle blue. Back, shoulders and saddle brass colour. Breast and thighs blue. Wing bows brass; primaries and secondaries blue. Tail blue.

Female plumage: Neck hackle, breast and thighs blue. Back and wings light brass or gold. Tail blue with light brass or gold coverts.

    In both sexes: Legs white or yellow. Face bright red. Eyes red, both alike.

The salmon-breasted blue

Male plumage: Neck, hackle and saddle golden, very lightly streaked with blue. Breast deep salmon. Back, shoulders, body, thighs, wings and tail blue.

Female plumage: Neck hackle golden striped with blue. Breast deep salmon. Body, thighs, wings and tail blue.

    In both sexes: Legs white or yellow. Face bright red. Eyes red, both alike.

The crow wing

Male plumage: Neck, hackle, back, shoulders and saddle dark red. Breast and thighs black. Wing bows dark red with a rich dark blue bar across secondaries; primaries black. Tail black with a lustrous green gloss.

Female plumage: Neck hackle black, lightly striped with a bronzy red. Breast and thighs drab black with the upper part of the breast a bronzy red. Wings and back drab black. Tail black.

    In both sexes: Legs white. Face bright red. Eyes red, both alike.

The blue-grey

Male plumage: Neck, hackle, saddle silver streaked with blue. Back and shoulders silver. Breast and thighs blue laced with silver to top of thighs. Wing bows silver; secondaries and primaries blue. Tail blue.

Female plumage: Neck hackle silver striped with blue. Breast and thighs blue, laced with silver to top of thighs. Wings and back blue, free from silver. Tail blue.

In both sexes: Legs dark. Face gypsy or red, gypsy preferred. Eyes dark, both alike.

The lemon-blue

Male plumage: Neck, hackle and saddle lemon streaked with blue. Back and shoulders lemon. Breast blue, laced with lemon to top of thighs. Body and thighs blue. Wing bows lemon; secondaries lemon on outer web; primaries blue. Tail blue.

Female plumage: Neck hackle lemon striped with blue. Breast blue, laced with lemon to top of thighs. Body, thighs, wings and tail blue.

In both sexes: Legs dark. Face bright red. Eyes red, both alike.

The black splashed

Male and female plumage: White splashed with black.

In both sexes: Legs white. Face bright red. Eyes red, both alike.

The blue splashed

As black splashed but blue replaces black.

The self white

Male and female plumage: All over pure white.

In both sexes: Legs white or yellow. Face bright red. Eyes red, both alike.

The self black

Male plumage: Black with brilliant green lustre.

Female plumage: Glossy black.

In both sexes: Legs black, white or yellow. Face red or gypsy. Eyes red, both alike.

The self blue

Male plumage: Neck, hackle and saddle deep rich indigo blue. Breast and thighs soft azure blue. Wing bows deep rich indigo blue; primaries and secondaries azure blue. Tail azure blue.

Female plumage: Hackle and tail dark blue. Breast, back and thighs azure blue.

In both sexes: Legs blue, white or yellow. Face bright red. Eyes red, both alike.

Among other varieties recognised are Hennies, Muffs and Tassels in all colours.

Weights

Male   2.94 kg ($6\frac{1}{2}$ lb)
Female   2.50 kg ($5\frac{1}{2}$ lb)

Scale of points

Shape and carriage	26
Handling and condition	16
Head and eye	10
Legs and feet	15
Colour and plumage	15
Neck	6
Tail	6
Wings	6
	100

Serious defects

Legs too far apart. Cow-hocked. Stork-legged. Roach back.
Flat breasted. Flat or square shins. Squirrel, whip or wry tail.
Duck-footed. Bent toes. Split wing. Rotten plumage.

OXFORD OLD ENGLISH GAME

LARGE FOWL

Origin: Great Britain
Classification: Hard feather
Egg colour: Cream to light brown

When the Romans invaded Britain, Julius Caesar wrote in his commentaries that the Britons kept fowls for pleasure and diversion but not for table purposes. Many well-known authorities have considered that cock fighting was the diversion. In 1849 an Act of Parliament was passed, making cock fighting illegal in this country, and with poultry exhibitions then taking root, many breeders began to exhibit Game Fowls. Over 30 colours of Old English Game have been known.

The Old English Game Club split in about 1930 as there was already a divergence of birds being shown with larger breasted, horizontally backed, exhibition-type birds tending to win. Breeders of these formed the Carlisle Club, developing only some of the original colours. Breeders of the original type maintained the well-balanced, close-heeled, athletic fighting fowl, and formed the Oxford Club, retaining over 30 colours. The judge of Oxfords does so with the bird facing away from him to assess the correct balance. It is usually agreed that a good Game Fowl cannot be a bad colour.

General characteristics: male

Carriage: Proud, defiant, sprightly, active on his feet, ready for any emergency, alert, agile, quick in his movements.
Type: Back short, flat, broad at the shoulders, tapering to the tail. Breast broad, full, prominent, with large pectoral muscles, breast bone not deep or pointed. Wings large, long and powerful with large strong quills, amply protecting the thighs. Tail large, up and spread, main feathers and quills large and strong. Belly small and tight. Thighs short, round and muscular, following the line of the body, or slightly curved.
Head: Small and tapering, skin of face and throat flexible and loose. Beak big, boxing (i.e. the upper mandible shutting tightly and closely over the lower one), crooked or hawk-like, pointed, strong at the setting on. Eyes large, bold, fiery and fearless. Comb, wattles and ear-lobes of fine texture, small and thin in undubbed males and females.

Neck: Large boned, round, strong, and of fair length, neck hackle covering the shoulders.
Legs and feet: Legs strong, clean boned, sinewy, close scaled, not fat and gummy like other fowls, close-heeled, not stiffly upright or too wide apart, and having a good bend or angle at the hock. Spurs are hard and fine and set low on the leg. Toes thin, long, straight and tapering, terminating in long, strong curved nails, hind toe of good length and strength, extending backwards in almost a straight line.
Plumage: Hard sounding, resilient, smooth, glossy and sufficient without much fluff.
Handling: Clever, well balanced, hard yet light fleshed, corky, mellow and warm, with strong contraction of wings and thighs to the body.

Female

With the exception of the tail, which is inclined to fan shape and carried well up, the general characteristics are similar to the male, allowing for the natural sexual differences.

Colour

The black-breasted dark red
Male plumage: Hackle, shoulders and saddle rich dark red (the colour of the shoulders of a black-breasted red). The rest of the plumage black.
Female plumage: Body black or very dark brown, hackle ticked red.
   In both sexes: Fluff (i.e. the down at the roots of the feathers next to the skin) black. Eyes, beak, legs and nails black. Face gypsy or purple.

The black-breasted red
Male plumage: Breast, thighs, belly and tail black. Wing bars steel blue; secondaries (when closed) bay. Hackle and saddle feathers orange-red. Shoulders deep crimson-scarlet.
Female plumage: Hackle golden, lightly striped with black. Breast robin. Belly ash grey. Back, shoulders and wings a good even partridge. Primaries and tail dark.
   In both sexes: The dark-legged birds should have grey fluff; the white- and yellow-legged, white fluff. Face scarlet red. Legs willow, yellow, white, carp or olive.

The shady or streaky-breasted light red
Male plumage: Hackle and back a shade lighter than the black-breasted red male and sometimes red wing bars.

Female plumage: Wheaten, a pale cream colour (like wheat) with clear red hackle. Tail and primaries nearly black. The red wheaten (the colour of red wheat) or light brick-red in body and wings. Hackle dark red. Tail dark.
   In both sexes: Fluff white. Legs white or yellow.

The black-breasted silver duckwing
Male plumage: Resembles the black-breasted red in his black markings and blue wing bars. Rest of the plumage clear, silvery white.
Female plumage: Hackle white, lightly striped black. Body and wings even silvery grey. Breast pale salmon. Primaries and tail nearly black.
   In both sexes: Fluff light grey. Face red, eyes pearl. Legs and beak white. Or eyes red and legs dark.

The black-breasted yellow duckwing
Male plumage: Hackle and saddle yellow-straw. Shoulders deep golden. Wing bars steel blue; secondaries white when closed. Rest of plumage black.

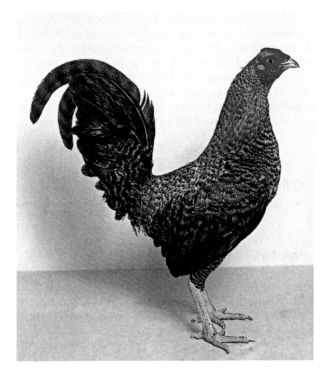

Crele Oxford Old English Game male

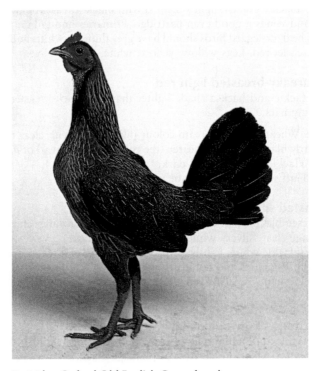

Partridge Oxford Old English Game female

Female plumage: Breast deeper, richer colour and body slightly browner tinge than the silver female.

In both sexes: Fluff light grey. Face red. Legs yellow, willow or dark.

The black-breasted birchen duckwing

Male plumage: Hackle deep rich straw, may be lightly striped. Shoulders maroon; otherwise same as preceding.

Female plumage: Shade darker than yellow duckwing female; hackle more heavily striped with black, and often foxy on the shoulders.

In both sexes: Face slightly darker than in yellow duckwing. Legs yellow or dark.

The black-breasted dark grey

Male plumage: Like the black-breasted red, except hackle, saddle and shoulders a dark, silvery grey, often striped with black.

Female plumage: Nearly black, with grey striped hackle, or body very dark grey.

In both sexes: Fluff black. Beak, eyes and legs black. Face gypsy or purple.

Other greys may have laced, streaked or mottled grey or throstle breasts. Hackle, saddle and shoulders more or less striped with black. Legs and eyes dark; the females dark grey to match. Fluff in both sexes light or dark grey.

Note: Greys all differ from duckwings in having the secondaries, when closed, black, or, if grey, wanting the steel-blue bar across them.

The clear mealy-breasted mealy grey

Male plumage: Nearly white breasted, with hackle and saddle the same, lightly striped. Plumage and most of the tail grey.

Female plumage: Light grey.

In both sexes: Fluff light grey. Eyes and legs dark.

The brown-breasted brown-red

Male plumage: Breast, thighs, belly and closed wing mahogany-brown. Hackle and saddle almost similar. Shoulders crimson. Primaries and tail black or dark bronze-brown.

Female plumage: Dark mottled brown with light shafts to the feathers.

In both sexes: Fluff black. Face deep crimson or purple. Eyes and legs dark.

The streaky-breasted orange-red

Male plumage: Breast streaked, laced or pheasant, black, marked with brown or copper colour. Hackle and saddle brassy or coppery-orange colour. Shoulders crimson, the rest of the wings and the tail black.

Female plumage: Black or nearly black body, with tinsel hackle striped with black, or dark mottled brown and gold striped hackle.

In both sexes: Fluff black or nearly so. Face, eyes and legs dark

The ginger-breasted ginger-red

Male plumage: Breast and thighs deep yellow-ochre, either clear or slightly pencilled or spotted. Hackle and saddle red-golden. Shoulders crimson-red. Tail and flight feathers bronzy.

Female plumage: Golden-yellow throughout, pencilled or spangled, particularly on back and wings, with bronze. Tail pencilled bronze or dark.

In both sexes: Fluff dark. Beak, legs and eyes dark or yellow. Face purple or crimson

The dun-breasted blue dun

Male plumage: Breast, belly, thighs, tail and closed secondaries the colour of a new slate, sometimes the breast marked with the same colour two shades darker. Hackle, saddle and shoulders, and sometimes the tail coverts and the primaries, two shades darker (like a slate colour after being wetted).

Female plumage: Blue-slate colour, with dark hackle like the male, often marked or laced all over with the darker shade.

   In both sexes: Fluff slate blue. Eyes, face and legs dark

The streaky-breasted red dun

Male plumage: Breast slate, streaked with copper-red. Hackle and saddles striped with slate or dark striped. Shoulders crimson. Wing bars and closed secondaries slate, or marked a little with brown. Tail slaty or dark blue.

Female plumage: Body slaty all over, or laced in a darker shade. Hackle golden striped, and sometimes marked with gold on the breast.

   In both sexes: Fluff dark slate. Legs dark or yellow

The yellow, silver and honey dun

These are coloured, respectively, with the following colours; the colour of new honeycomb is intended to describe the honey dun. They may have yellow or dark legs according to body colour, and white legs are permissible in the silver dun, as well as other coloured legs. The females are blue bodied with hackles to match their males. Smoky duns are of a dull smoke colour throughout; legs and eyes should be dark.

The pile

Male plumage: The smock-breasted blood wing pile is marked exactly like the black-breasted light red, except that the black and the blue wing bars are exchanged for a clear creamy white. The breast may be streaked with red in red pile.

Female plumage: White, with salmon breast and golden striped hackle, or streaked all over lightly with red.

In both sexes: Face and eyes red. Legs white, yellow or willow.

Note: Other varieties of piles may be streaky, marbled or robin breasted; and light lemon or custard in top colour, or dun piles having slate-blue markings in place of red. All piles have white fluff.

The spangled

Male and female plumage: These have white tips to their feathers. The more of these spots and the more regularly they are distributed the better. The male should show white ends to the feathers on hackle and saddle. The ground colour may be red, black or brown, or a mixture of all three. Underfluff white.

   In both sexes: Eyes and face red. Legs any colour or mottled to match plumage

The white

Male and female plumage: This variety should be free from any coloured feathers. Fluff pure white.

   In both sexes: Beak and legs white. Face red, eyes pearl; or yellow legs and red eyes

The black

Male and female plumage: This variety should be free from any white or coloured feathers and should possess black fluff.

   In both sexes: Dark beaks, faces and legs and black eyes, though red faces and red eyes are allowed at present

The furness, brassy back and polecat

Male and female plumage: These are blacks with brass colour on their wings or back, and occasionally have yellow legs, which are allowed. The females are chiefly black, but often much streaked with grey-brown on breast and wings. Polecats are streaked with dark tan colour on hackles and saddle in the males. Legs dark.

The cuckoo

Male and female plumage: Cuckoo-breasted cuckoo resembles the Plymouth Rock fowl in markings of a blue-grey barred plumage.

In both sexes: Faces and eyes red. Legs various.

Variations of this colour are yellow cuckoos, also creles, creoles, cirches, mackerels in different provincial dialects, having some mixture of gold or red in the plumage and white fluff, often extremely pretty. Legs white or yellow.

The brown-breasted yellow birchen

Male plumage: Breast reddish-brown. Hackles and saddle straw, striped birchen-brown. Shoulders old gold or birchen. Wing bars and closed secondaries brown. Tail brown or bronze-black.

Female plumage: Yellow-brown, with yellow hackle and robin breast.

In both sexes: Fluff light grey. Beak, legs and eyes yellow

The henny

Male and female plumage: Hencocks should in their plumage resemble hens as closely as possible. They should have their hackle and saddle feathers rounded and the tail coverts hen-like, and not have much sheen on their feathers. This breed often runs large and reachy, which is one of its characteristics. The two centre tail feathers should be straight.

The muff and tassel

Male and female plumage: Both muffs and tassels, or topins, are recognised by the Oxford Club, there being famous strains of both, though now scarce. Tassels vary from a few long feathers (or lark tops) behind the comb to a good-sized bunch. They also occur in some strains of hennies. Muffs of the old breed are stronger, heavier-boned birds than the males bred today, and are rather loose in feather.

Notes

(1) It is desirable that the toenails should match the legs and beak in colour in all Game Fowl.

(2) White- or yellow-legged birds may have white feathers in wings and tail.

(3) The fancier, when he speaks of a brown-red, means the streaky-breasted orange-red; and when talking of a black-red, intends one to infer a black-breasted light red; while black-breasted dark greys are erroneously called 'birchens', although they have no birchen colour in them.

Weights

Male   1.80–2.50 kg (4–5½ lb); it is not considered desirable to breed males over 2.70 kg (6 lb)

Female 0.90–1.36 kg (2–3 lb)

Scale of points

Body (including breast, back and belly)	20
Handling (symmetry, cleverness, hardness of flesh and feathers, condition and constitution)	15
Head (including beak and eyes)	10
Neck	6
Shanks, spurs and feet	10
Plumage and colour	9
Thighs	8
Wings	7
Tail	6
Carriage, action and activity	9
	100

Serious defects

Thin thighs or neck. Flat sided. Deep keel. Pointed, crooked or indented breastbone. Thick insteps or toes. Duck feet. Straight or stork legs. In-knees. Soft flesh. Broken, soft or rotten plumage. Bad carriage or action. Any indication of weakness of constitution.

OLD ENGLISH GAME BANTAM

Origin: Great Britain
Classification: Hard feather
Egg colour: Cream to light brown

This Standard is compiled from that of the Old English Game Bantam Club, and follows the Carlisle ideal. Other Standards exist, but essential differences are slight. Chief variations are in methods of interpretation. Old English Game bantams are of comparatively recent creation. They were evolved largely from the common crossbred bantam of the countryside. Probably there is very little large breed blood in them.

In the large breed it is usually agreed that a good Game bird cannot be a bad colour. This remark does not apply to the bantams, which are show birds only, colour playing a very important part. Nevertheless, the ideal is that the bantam should be a true miniature of the national fighting Game – though this is seldom the case.

General characteristics: male

Head: Small and tapered, skin of face and throat flexible and loose.
Beak: Big, strong at base, slightly curved.
Eyes: Large, bold, fiery and alike in colour.
Comb, wattles and ear-lobes: Of fine texture, small and thin in chickens and hens.
Neck: Large bones, round, strong, and of fair length.
Back: Short, flat, broad at shoulders, tapering to tail.
Breast: Broad, full, prominent, with large pectoral muscles, breast bone not deep or pointed.
Wings: Strong, powerful and carried well up.
Tail: In the cock to be carried at a nice angle, neither too low nor too high, and to be straight. Feathers to be broad and strong with a pair of good curved sickles of fair length and well furnished with side hangers. In the hen well carried, fairly close, of medium length.
Belly: Small and tight.

Thighs: Of medium length, round and muscular, following the line of the body or slightly curved.

Legs: Strong, clean boned, round, sinewy, close scaled, not stiffly upright or wide apart, and having a good bend or angle at the hock.

Feet: Toes thin, long, straight and tapering, terminating in long and strong curved nails, hind toe of good length and strength, extending backwards in almost a straight line.

Spurs: Hard, fine, set low on the leg.

Plumage: Hard, sound, resilient, smooth, glossy and sufficient without much fluff.

Carriage: Proud, defiant, sprightly, active on feet, ready for an emergency, alert, agile and quick in movements.

In-hand: Well balanced, hard, corky, muscular with strong contractions of wings and thighs to the body.

Colour

Colours are very numerous, the most popular being spangles, black-reds (wheaten bred and partridge bred), duckwings, brown-reds, self blacks and blues, furnesses, creles and greys. Most of these main colours follow the usual colour pattern applicable to the variety.

Furnesses are black with brassy hackles, wing shoulders and backs in males; and black with greyish-brown streaked breasts and wings in females. Creles are barred varieties of other colours, distinct from cuckoos, which are plain barred grey. In black-reds, the wheaten bred is brighter in colour and more popular than partridge bred. Off colours are very numerous, but not so popular as in the large breed. Piles and whites are seldom seen. Hennies (hen-feathered males), muffs and tassels (beards and top-knots) are recognised sub-varieties in all colours.

Colour of face, beak, eyes, shanks and toenails varies with the particular colour variety: from red face, red eyes, white legs, toenails and beak in spangles to deep crimson, purple or black faces, black eyes, black legs and feet in brown-reds and similar dark colours. Willow, olive and yellow legs are frequent and permissible in various sub-varieties.

Some of the more popular colour varieties, with the names usually applied to them by showmen, are given below.

The spangle

Male plumage: Neck, hackle and saddle dark red, finely tipped with white. Breast and thighs black, finely and evenly tipped with white. Back and shoulders dark red, finely tipped with white. Wing bows dark red, finely tipped with white with a rich dark blue bar across, finely tipped with white; secondaries deep bay intermixed with white, bay predominating; primaries black intermixed with white. Tail sickles and side hangers tipped with white, straight feathers black intermixed with white.

Female plumage: Neck, hackle golden-red, streaked with black, finely tipped with white. Breast and thighs dark salmon, finely and evenly tipped with white. Back and shoulders partridge-coloured feathers, finely and evenly tipped with white. Wings secondaries partridge, intermixed with white, partridge predominating; primaries dark, intermixed with white. All other feathers partridge colour finely and evenly tipped with white. Tail black with partridge coverts, finely and evenly tipped with white.

In both sexes: Legs white (occasionally yellow). Face bright red. Eyes red, both alike

The black-red (partridge bred)

Male plumage: Neck, hackle and saddle dark rich red shading to deep orange. Breast and thighs black. Back and shoulders deep crimson. Wing bows deep red with a rich dark blue bar across; secondaries bay colour on outer web; primaries black. Tail sound black with lustrous green gloss.

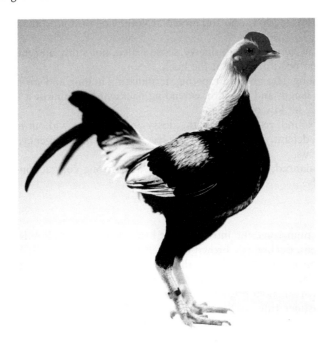

Duckwing Old English Game male, bantam

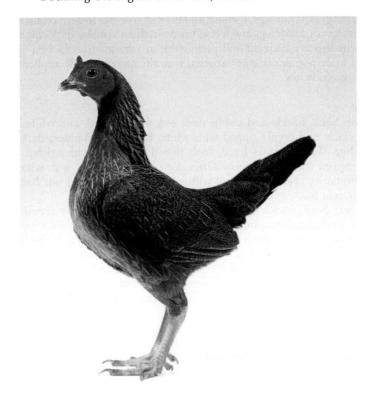

Partridge Old English Game female, bantam

Female plumage: (Partridge) neck golden-red and streaked with black. Breast and thighs shaded salmon. Back and wings partridge colour to be as free from rust and shaftiness as possible. Tail black with partridge coverts.

In both sexes: Legs white, yellow and willow. Face bright red. Eyes red, both alike

The black-red (wheaten bred)

Male plumage: Neck, hackle bright orange, shading off to bright lemon. Back and saddle bright crimson. Breast and thighs black. Wing bows bright red; in other respects, including tail, similar to (partridge) black-red. Tail similar to (partridge) black-red.

Female plumage: (Wheaten) neck hackle white-gold free from streaks. Delicate creamy self colour on remainder. Tail black with a shading of wheaten corresponding with body colour. Clay hens similar to wheaten, only darker or harder in colour.

In both sexes: Legs white. Face bright red. Eyes red, both alike

The golden duckwing

Male plumage: Hackle yellow, saddle straw. Breast and thighs black. Back and shoulders orange or rich yellow (golden). Wing bows orange or rich yellow; wing bars steel blue; secondaries white when closed; primaries black. Tail black.

Female plumage: Neck lightly striped with black. Breast and thighs salmon shading off to ash grey on thighs. Back and wings silvery grey, free from rust and shaftiness. Tail black, coverts corresponding with body colour.

In both sexes: Legs white or yellow. Face bright red. Eyes red or pearl, both alike

The silver duckwing

Male plumage: Neck and saddle white, free from dark streaks. Breast and thighs black. Back and shoulders silver-white. Wing bows silver-white; wing bars steel blue; secondaries white when closed; primaries black. Tail black.

Female plumage: As female golden duckwing.

In both sexes: Legs white or yellow. Face bright red. Eyes red or pearl, both alike

The blue-red

Male plumage: Neck, hackle and saddle orange or golden-red. Breast and thighs medium shade of blue. Back and shoulders deep or bright red. Wing bows deep or bright red, with a rich dark blue bar across; secondaries bay colour on the outer web; primaries blue. Tail blue.

Female plumage: Neck golden-red, streaked with blue. Breast and thighs shaded salmon. Back and wings partridge colour, intermixed with blue. Tail to correspond with body colour.

In both sexes: Legs any self colour. Face bright red. Eyes red, both alike

The blue-tailed wheaten hen

Similar in all respects to wheatens with the exception of wing primaries and tail shaded with blue. Legs any self colour. Face bright red. Eyes red, both to be alike.

The brown-red

Male plumage: Neck and saddle lemon or orange, streaked with black. Breast black laced with brown to top of thighs. Back lemon or orange. Shoulders and wing bows lemon or orange, rest of wing black. Tail black.

Female plumage: Neck, hackle lemon or orange, striped with black. Breast and thighs black laced with brown. Body black, tail black.

In both sexes: Legs dark. Face gypsy or red. Eyes dark, both to be alike

The crele

Male plumage: Neck and saddle chequered (barred) orange. Back and shoulders deep chequered orange. Wing bows deep chequered orange with dark grey bar across; secondaries bay colour on the outer web: primaries dark grey. Tail dark grey.
Female plumage: Neck lemon chequered with grey. Breast and thighs chequered salmon. Back and wings chequered blue-grey. Tail to correspond with body colour.

In both sexes: Legs white or yellow. Face bright red. Eyes red, both to be alike

The cuckoo

Male plumage: Blue-grey barred, variations of this colour are yellow, gold or red in the plumage.
Female plumage: Blue-grey barred all over.

In both sexes: Legs white or yellow. Face bright red. Eyes red, both to be alike

The pile

Male plumage: Neck and saddle orange or chestnut-red. Breast and thighs white. Back and shoulders deep red. Wing bows red with a white bar across; secondaries bay colour on outer web; primaries white. Tail white.
Female plumage: Neck lemon. Breast salmon, lighter towards thighs. Back and wings white. Tail white.

In both sexes: Legs white or yellow (yellow preferred). Face bright red. Eyes red, both to be alike

The furness

Male plumage: Black, with brassy wing bows, wing bays, saddle hangers, brassiness to be allowed in hackles and on back.
Female plumage: Black with salmon breast, brassiness allowed on wings, back, cushion and hackles.

In both sexes: Legs to be any self colour, both alike. Eyes red. Face bright red

The blue furness

Male plumage: Blue, with brassy coloured wing bows, wing bays, saddle hangers, brassiness allowed in neck hackles and on back.
Female plumage: Blue, with salmon breast, brassiness allowed on wings and back, hangers and hackles.

In both sexes: Legs to be any self colour, both alike. Face and eyes red

The brassy-backed black

Male plumage: Black, with brass colour on back, wing bows, hackles and hangers. No bay colour allowed. Clear hackles and hangers allowed.
Female plumage: Polecat. Pale brown to dark brown with black neck hackle, tail and wing flights, brown or brassy streaks allowed in neck hackle. Some speckles and/or lacing allowed on breast and belly.

In both sexes: Legs to be any self colour, both alike. Face and eyes red

The brassy-backed blue

Male plumage: Blue with brass colour on back, wing bows, hackles and hangers. No wing bay colour. Clear hackles and hangers allowed.
Female plumage: Dun. Blue with light to dark brown or honey, or brassiness in neck hackle, cushion, back, wings, breast and belly. Speckling and lacing allowed on breast and belly.

In both sexes: Legs any self colour, both alike. Face and eyes red

The blue duckwing

Male plumage: Cream neck and saddle free from dark streaks. Breast and thighs blue. Back and shoulder silver-white. Wing bay silver-white; wing bars steel blue; secondaries white when closed; primaries blue. Tail blue.

Female plumage: Neck silver lightly striped with black. Breast salmon shading off to blue on thighs. Back and wings silver-grey, free from rust and shaftiness.

In both sexes: Legs white or yellow. Face red. Eyes red or pearl

The lemon-blue

Male plumage: Neck and saddle lemon or orange streaked with blue, breast blue, laced with lemon to top of thighs. Back lemon to orange. Shoulders and wing bows lemon or orange, rest of wings blue. Tail blue.

Female plumage: Neck hackle lemon or orange striped with blue. Breast and thighs blue, laced with brown. Body blue, tail blue.

In both sexes: Legs any self colour. Face gypsy or red. Eyes red or dark, both to be alike

The splashed

Male and female plumage: Mixture of black, white and blue, giving an overall appearance of being light grey.

In both sexes: Legs any self colour. Face red. Eyes red, both to be alike

The blue-grey

Silver where the lemon-blue are lemon. Legs any self colour, both alike. Face red. Eyes red.

The ginger-red

Male plumage: Neck and saddle red-golden. Breast and thighs deep yellow, clear or slightly pencilled or spotted. Back and shoulders crimson-red. Wings and tail bronze or black/dark.

Female plumage: Golden-yellow throughout; pencilled or spangled, particularly on back and wings with bronze. Tail pencilled bronze or black/dark.

In both sexes: Legs dark or yellow or willow. Face dark or red. Eyes dark or red, both to be alike

The self white

All over pure white. Legs white or yellow. Face bright red. Eyes red, both to be alike.

The self black

All over glossy black. Legs any self colour. Face red or dark. Eyes red or dark, both to be alike.

The self blue

Medium shade of blue. Legs any self colour. Face bright red. Eyes red, both alike.

Muffs and tassels

Both muffs and tassels are recognised. Tassels vary from a few long feathers behind the comb to a good-sized bunch.

Weights (suggested)

Male   905–1020 g (32–36 oz)
Female   795–905 g (28–32 oz)

Serious defects

Oversized or coarse. Thin thighs or neck. Flat sided, deep keel. Pointed, crooked or indented breastbone. Thick toes. Duck feet. Straight or stork legs. In-knees. Soft flesh. Broken, soft or rotten plumage. Wry or squirrel tail. Bad carriage or action. Flat shanks. Round or roach back. Unspurred cocks (not cockerels). Incorrect eye colour. Any indication of weakness of constitution.

Scale of points

Head	10
Neck	6
Body	20
Wings	7
Tail	6
Thighs	8
Shanks, spurs and feet	10
Plumage and colour	9
Handling (symmetry, hardness of flesh and feathers, condition and constitution)	15
Carriage and action	9
Total	100

OLD ENGLISH PHEASANT FOWL

LARGE FOWL

Origin: Great Britain
Classification: Light: Rare
Egg colour: White

This breed was given its name of Old English Pheasant Fowl in about 1914, previous to which it had been called the Yorkshire Pheasant, Golden Pheasant and also the Old-fashioned Pheasant. That it is a very old English breed is certain. Some northern breeders retained their strains as Yorkshire Pheasant Fowls until the present tag of 'Old English' was brought officially into use. It has a meaty breast for a light breed, and has always been popular with farmers.

General characteristics: male

Carriage: Alert and active.
Type: Body rather long, deep and round with prominent shoulders. Tail flowing and set well back.
Head: Fine. Beak of medium size. Eyes bright and prominent. Comb rose, moderate in size, not impeding either sight or breathing, fine texture, evenly set, rather square front, the top flat and with plenty of work, tapering to a single leader (or spike) at the back, which should curve gracefully downwards, following the neck line but quite free from it. Face and wattles smooth, free from coarseness or wrinkles. Ear-lobes medium size, oval or almond shaped, smooth.
Neck: Graceful.
Legs and feet: Legs of medium length, well apart, neither coarse nor too fine. Shanks free from feathers. Toes four, well spread.

Female

With the exception of the tail (moderately whipped) the general characteristics are similar to those of the male, allowing for the natural sexual differences.

Colour

The gold

Male plumage: Ground colour bright rich bay. Back rich mahogany-red. Lacing, bars, striping, tipping and tail beetle green-black. Hackles striped and slightly tipped. Saddle a slightly deeper shade than neck. Breast laced. Wing bars (two) marked.
Female plumage: Ground colour bright rich bay. Striping, tipping, spangling and tail beetle green-black. Neck with heavy stripe down centre of each feather. Wing bars crescent spangling; even and well-marked bars a point of great beauty. Tail with slight edging of ground colour carried up from the base along the upper edge of the tail. Remainder each feather tipped with a crescent-shaped spangle. Shafts of all feathers bay.

The silver

Male and female plumage: White with beetle green-black markings.

In both sexes and colours

Beak horn. Eyes fiery red. Comb bright rich red. Face and wattles red. Ear-lobes white. Legs and feet slate blue.

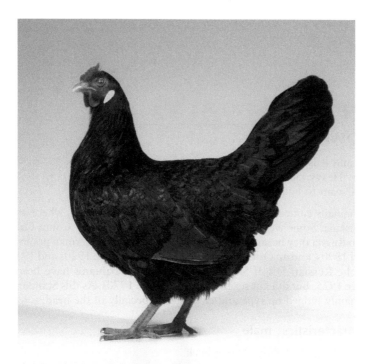

Old English Pheasant Fowl female, large

Weights

Cock   2.70–3.20 kg (6–7 lb)   Cockerel   2.50–2.70 kg (5½–6 lb)
Hen   2.25–2.70 kg (5–6 lb)   Pullet   2.00–2.25 kg (4½–5 lb)

Scale of points

Type (including legs)	20
Head (comb 15, lobes 5, other points 5)	25
Markings	20
Ground colour of body	15
Plumage and flow of feather	10
Size	5
Condition	5
	100

Serious defects

Comb single or over either side. Blushed lobes. Sooty hackles. Definitely black breast in male. Superfine bone. Lack of size. Squirrel tail. Any deformity. Any other defects which would affect health, hardiness, productivity or activity up to 20 points.

BANTAM

Old English Pheasant Fowl bantams should follow exactly the large fowl Standard.

Weights

Male   790 g (28 oz)
Female   680 g (24 oz)

ORLOFF

LARGE FOWL

Origin: Iran and Russia
Classification: Heavy: Soft feather
Egg colour: Cream to light brown

This breed originally came from the Gilan province of northern Iran, where it was known as the Chilianskaia. Some were taken to Moscow and renamed by Count Orloff Techesmensky. From Russia they became known to British, Dutch and German poultry experts in the 1880s and 1890s, and an Orloff Club existed in Britain in the 1920s and 1930s and was reformed as the Russian Orloff Society in 2011. Orloff bantams have been known in Germany since 1925, but did not reach Britain until the 1970s. As this Standard indicates, Orloffs are mainly judged on type and character, especially of the head.

General characteristics: male

Carriage: Upright with slightly sloping back.
Type: Body broad and fairly long. Flat slightly sloping back. Breast rather full and prominent. Closely carried wings of moderate length. Tail of medium size with fairly narrow sickles. Carriage rather low but slightly above horizontal.

Head: Skull wide, of medium size. Beak short, stout and well hooked. Eyes full, and deeply set under well-projecting (beetle) eyebrows, giving a gloomy, vindictive expression. Comb low and flat, shaped somewhat like a raspberry cut through its axis (lengthwise), covered with small protuberances mingled with small, bristle-like feathers, which peculiarity is particularly noticeable in the female. Face muffled, beard and whiskers well developed. Ear-lobes very small, hidden under the muffles. Wattles small, and show only in the male.

Neck: Fairly long and erect, very heavily covered with hackle (boule), the feathers very full at the top but so close at the base of the neck as to appear thin there, and forming a distinct angle with the back.

Legs and feet: Moderately long and stout. Thighs muscular and well apart. Shanks round and finely scaled. Toes four, long and well spread.

Female

With exception of the muffling (which is more developed) and the tail (comparatively long) the general characteristics are similar to those of the male, allowing for the natural sexual differences.

Colour

The black
Male and female plumage: Solid black to the skin from head to tail, with beetle-green sheen.

The black mottled
Male and female plumage: Background colour black with a lustrous beetle-green sheen. White tips to the ends of each feather and to be evenly distributed. Preferably no more than two white flights on each wing, but more not considered a disqualifying fault. Beak should be yellow and legs bright yellow, but black- or horn-coloured mottling or shading not to be a penalized.

Defects: Rust or grey colour in plumage. Uneven white patches in the plumage. Too much white in the hackle and sickles.

The cuckoo
Male and female plumage: As in cuckoo Leghorn.

The mahogany
Male plumage: Beard and whiskers a mixture of black, mahogany and grey, grey preponderating. Neck hackle rich dark orange to mahogany, darkest at the crown and showing very slight black stripes at the base only. Saddle rich mahogany shading to deep orange. Wings rich deep mahogany with a strongly defined green-black sheen.

Female plumage: Muffings as in male. Hackle mahogany, the lower feathers showing black striping. Tail mainly black. Remainder rich dark mahogany uniformly peppered with black, the entire absence of black or heavy and irregular black splashes undesirable.

The spangled
Male plumage: Hackles rich orange to mahogany, with white tips to as many feathers as possible. Back rich mahogany. Wings rich mahogany with black bar showing green or purple sheen, and white flights. Breast solid black with white tips, blotchiness or washiness undesirable. Tail green-black.

Female plumage: Light mahogany with white tips, the spangling to be as uniform as possible.

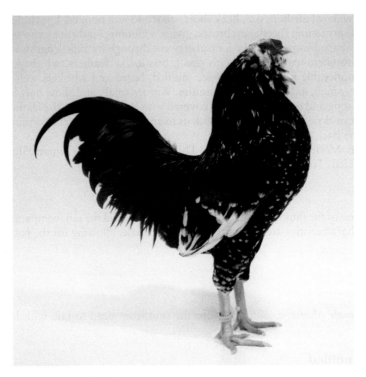

Spangled Orloff male, bantam

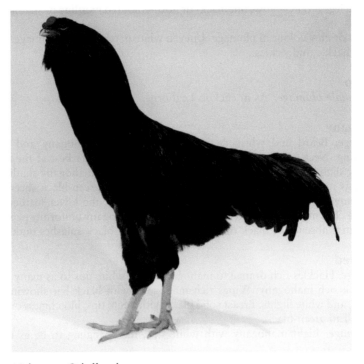

Mahogany Orloff male

The white
Male and female plumage: Lustrous white from head to tail.

In both sexes and all colours
Beak yellow, with a thin rose-tinted skin at base of beak and nostrils. Eyes red or amber. Comb, face, ear-lobes and wattles red. Legs rich yellow.

Weights

Cock	3.6 kg (8 lb)	Cockerel	3.2 kg (7 lb)
Hen	2.70 kg (6 lb)	Pullet	2.25 kg (5 lb)

Scale of points

Comb and other head points, including beard, whiskers and boule	35
Type and carriage	25
Colour	15
Condition	15
Legs	10
	100

Serious defects

The absence of beard, whiskers and boule is considered a serious fault. Legs other than yellow. Comb of any other form than as described. Weak, deformed or diseased specimens.

Disqualifications

In this breed the colour is of secondary importance and is a deciding point only in close competition. The main characteristics of the Orloff are its peculiarities of shape, comb, head and carriage and judges are earnestly requested to bear this in mind when awarding prizes. Slight feathering or down between the toes is not to constitute a disqualification.

BANTAM

Orloff bantams follow the large fowl Standard.

Weights

Cock	1300 g (40 oz)	Cockerel	1200 g (36 oz)
Hen	1000 g (36 oz)	Pullet	900 g (32 oz)

ORPINGTON

LARGE FOWL

Origin: Great Britain
Classification: Heavy: Soft feather
Egg colour: Brown

In the Orpington we have an English breed named after the village in Kent where the originator, William Cook, had his farm. He introduced the black variety in 1886, the white in 1889 and the buff in 1894. Within five years of the original black Orpington being introduced exhibition breeders were crossing Langshan and Cochin and exhibiting the offspring as black Orpingtons, the birds fetching high prices, and attracting many for their immense size. But this crossing at once turned a dual-purpose breed into one solely for show purposes, and it has remained so until today. A late introduction, the Jubilee Orpington, is now rarely seen.

General characteristics: male

Carriage: Bold, upright and graceful; that of an active fowl.

Type: Body deep, broad and cobby. Back nicely curved with a somewhat short, concaved outline. Saddle wide and slightly rising, with full hackle. Breast broad, deep and well rounded, not flat. Wings small, nicely formed and carried in a horizontal position, the ends almost hidden by the saddle hackle. Tail rather short, compact, flowing and high, but by no means a squirrel tail.

Head: Small and neat, fairly full over the eyes. Beak strong and nicely curved. Eyes large and bold. Comb single, small, firmly set on head, evenly serrated and free from side sprigs. In the black variety, comb may be single or rose, the latter small, straight and firm, full of fine work or small spikes, level on top (not hollow in centre), narrowing behind to a distinct peak lying well down to the head (not sticking up). Face smooth. Wattles of medium length, rather oblong and nicely rounded at the bottom. Ear-lobes small and elongated.

Neck: Of medium length, curved, compact and full with full hackle.

Legs and feet: Legs short and strong, the thighs almost hidden by the body feathers, well set apart. Toes four, straight and well spread.

Plumage: Profuse, soft, loose and not fluffy.

Handling: Firm in body.

Female

The general characteristics are similar to those of the male. Her cushion should be wide but almost flat, and slightly rising to the tail, and with no tendency to a ball cushion sufficient to give back a graceful appearance with an outline approaching concave.

Colour

The blue

Male plumage: Hackles, saddle, wing bows, back and tail dark slate blue. Remainder medium slate blue, each feather to show lacing of darker shade as on back.

Female plumage: Medium slate blue, laced with darker shade all through, except head and neck dark slate blue.

In both sexes: Beak black. Eyes black or very dark brown, black preferred. Comb, face, wattles and ear-lobes bright red. Legs and feet black or blue. Toenails white

The black

Male and female plumage: Black with a green sheen.

In both sexes: Beak, etc. as in the blue. Soles of feet white

The buff

Male and female plumage: Clear even buff throughout to the skin.

In both sexes: Beak white or horn. Eyes red orange. Comb, face, ear-lobes and wattles bright red. Legs, feet and toenails white. Skin white

The white

Male and female plumage: Pure snow white.

In both sexes: Beak, legs, feet and skin white. Eyes, face, ear-lobes and wattles red

The jubilee

Male plumage: Ground colour mahogany of a bright shade, and not dark or maroon. Hackles and back mahogany, with black centre stripe, mahogany shaft and white tip. Breast, thighs and fluff mahogany, with black spangle and white tip, the three colours clean and distinct and showing in equal proportions, avoiding a ticked effect on the one hand and a blotchy effect on the other. Wing bows similar to hackles; wing bars black; secondaries mahogany, black and white; primaries similar but more white allowed. Tail sickles white, or black and white, or black, white and mahogany; coverts black edged with mahogany and tipped with white.

Female plumage: Hackle to match that of the cock. Body, thighs and fluff mahogany with spangles and white tips, similar to the breast of the cock. Wings as the body, but with primaries to match those of the cock. Tail as in the cock.

In both sexes: Beak, legs and feet white. Ear-lobes red. Face, comb and wattles red. Eyes red. Toenails and skin white

The spangled

Male plumage: Hackles black with white tips. Back black, slightly ticked with white. Breast, thighs and fluff black with white spangles, the two colours showing in equal proportions, avoiding a ticked effect on the one hand and a blotchy effect on the other. Wing bows similar to back; wing bars black; secondaries and primaries black and white, but more white allowed in the primaries or flights. Tail black and white; the sickles and the coverts black with white tips.

Female plumage: Neck, wings (flights only) and tail, similar to those parts of the cock. Remainder the same as the breast of the cock, the effect to be uniform throughout the bird. (*Note*: In both sexes the black should have a bright glossy beetle-green sheen, and the white should be pure and bright, the two colours distinct and not running into each other.)

In both sexes: Beak black, white or slightly mottled. Eyes red or brown, red preferred. Comb, face, wattles and ear-lobes red. Legs and feet black and white, mottled as evenly as possible. Toenails and skin white

The cuckoo

Male and female plumage: Blue-grey (light shade) ground, each feather barred across with blue-black (dark shade), the markings in keeping with the size of the feather.

In both sexes: Beak white. Eyes red. Comb, face, wattles and ear-lobes red. Legs and feet white. Toenails and skin white

Serious defects

Side spikes on comb. White in ear-lobes. Feathers or fluff on the shanks or feet. Long legs. Any deformity. Yellow skin or yellow on the shanks or feet of any variety. Any yellow or sappiness in the white.

Disqualifications

Trimming or faking.

BANTAMS

Orpington bantams are miniatures of their large fowl counterparts and the Standard for those should be followed.

The jubilee, spangled and cuckoo do not have bantam counterparts standardised.

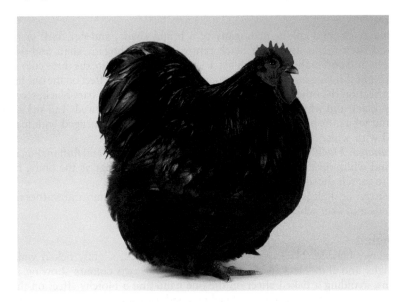

Black Orpington male, bantam

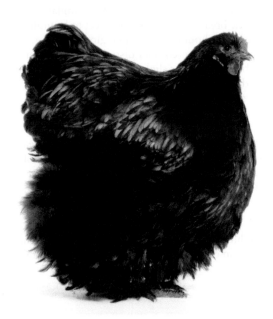

Black Orpington female, large

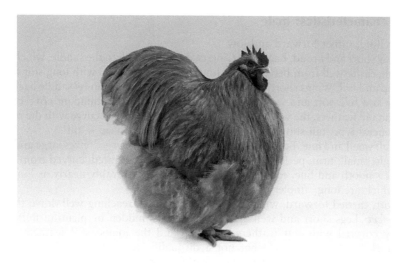

Buff Orpington male, large

Scale of points

	Buff/blue	Black/white	Cuckoo/spangled/jubilee
Type and size	40	40	40
Head	15	20	15
Legs and feet	10	10	10
Colour and plumage	30	25	30
Condition	5	5	5
	100	100	100

Weights and size

Large fowl
Male   4.5 kg (9.9 lb) min.
Female   3.6 kg (7.94 lb) min.

Bantams should be visually 25% of the size of their large fowl counterparts.

BANTAMS

Male   2 kg (4.4 lb)
Female   1.6 kg (3.53 lb)

PEKIN BANTAM

Origin: Asia
Classification: True Bantam
Egg colour: White or cream

This is a genuine bantam breed, very old and having no real relationship to the large breed of Cochins. It was imported from Pekin in the middle of the nineteenth century, hence its name. In recent years new colours have been added to the Standard.

General characteristics: male

Carriage: Bold, rather forward and low.

Type: Body short and broad. Back short, increasing in breadth to the saddle, which should be very full, rising well from between the shoulders and furnished with long soft feathers. Breast deep and full. Wings short, tightly tucked up, the ends hidden by saddle hackle. Tail very short and full, soft and without hard quill feathers, with abundant coverts almost hiding main tail feathers, the whole forming one unbroken duplex curve with the back and saddle. General type: tail should be carried higher than the head – 'tilt'.

Head: Skull small and fine. Beak rather short, stout, slightly curved. Eyes large and bright. Comb single, small, firm, perfectly straight and erect, well serrated, curved from front to back. Face smooth and fine, ear-lobes smooth and fine, preferably nearly as long as the wattles, which are long, ample, smooth and rounded.

Neck: Short, carried forward, with abundant long hackle reaching well down the back.

Legs and feet: Legs short and well apart. Stout thighs hidden by plentiful fluff. Hocks completely covered with soft feathers curling round the joints (stiff feathers forming 'vulture hocks' are objectionable but not a disqualification). Shanks short and thick, abundantly covered with soft outstanding feathers. Toes four, strong and straight, the middle and outer toes plentifully covered with soft feathers to their tips.

Plumage: Very abundant, long and wide, quite soft with very full fluff.

Female

With the exception of the back (rising into a very full and round cushion) the general characteristics are similar to those of the male, allowing for the natural sexual differences.

Colour

The black

Male and female plumage: Rich sound black with lustrous beetle-green sheen throughout, free of white or coloured feathers. (Note: Some light undercolour in adult males is permissible as long as it does not show through.)

The blue

Male and female plumage: A rich pale blue (pigeon blue preferred) free from lacing, but with rich dark blue hackles, back and tail in the male.

The buff

Male and female plumage: Sound buff, of a perfectly even shade throughout, quite sound to roots of feathers, and free from black, white or bronze feathers. The exact shade of buff is not material so long as it is level throughout and free from shaftiness, mealiness or lacing. (*Note*: A pale 'lemon-buff' is usually preferred in the show pen.)

The cuckoo

Male and female plumage: Plumage light French grey, each feather evenly and distinctly banded across several times with dark slate, the markings should be fine and regular and should fuse into each other. The plumage should not be smutty and be free from any white or straw tinge. Cuckoo markings to extend down the feather as far as possible.

The mottled

Male and female plumage: Evenly mottled with white at the tip of each feather on a rich black with beetle-green sheen.

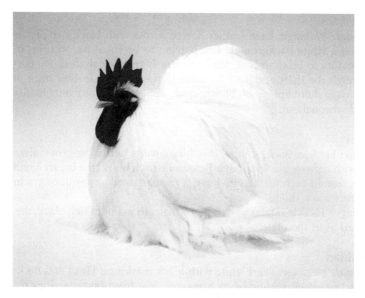

White Pekin Bantam male

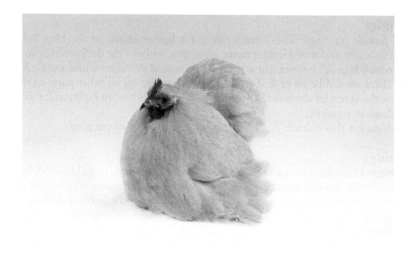

Lavender Pekin Bantam female

The barred

Male and female plumage: Each feather barred across with black bars, having a beetle-green sheen on a white background. The barring to be equal proportions of black and white. The colours to be sharply defined and not blurred or shaded off. Barring should continue through the shaft and into the underfluff, and each feather must finish with a black tip. Plumage should present a bluish, steely appearance free from brassiness and of a uniform shade throughout.

The birchen

Male plumage: Hackle, back, saddle, shoulder coverts and wing bows silver-white, the neck hackle with narrow black striping. Remainder rich black, the breast having a narrow silver margin around each feather, giving it a regular laced appearance gradually diminishing to perfect black thighs.
Female plumage: Hackle similar to that of the male. Remainder rich black, the breast very delicately laced as in the male.

The Columbian

Male and female plumage: Pearl white with black markings. Head and neck white with dense black stripe down middle of each feather, free from black edgings or black tips. Saddle pearl white. Tail feathers and tail coverts glossy green-black, the coverts laced or not with white. Primaries black, or black edged with white; secondaries black on inner edge, white outer. Remainder of plumage entirely white, of pearl grey shade, free from ticking. Undercolour either slate, blue-white or white.

The lavender

Male and female plumage: The lavender is not a lighter shade of the blue Pekin, it is different genetically and is of a lighter more silver tint, without the darker shade associated with the normal blue. The silver tint is more pronounced in the neck and saddle hackle of the male. There should be an even distribution of lavender on all other parts of the body. We look for the lavender shaft in the feathers. The undercolour to be lavender as close to the top colour as possible.
Serious defects for this colour: A dark shaft (quills) denotes dilute Blue.

The partridge

Male plumage: Head dark orange-red, neck hackle bright orange or golden-red, becoming lighter towards the shoulders and preferably shading off as near lemon colour as possible, each feather distinctly striped down the middle with black, and free from shaftiness, black tipping or black fringe. Saddle hackle to resemble neck hackle as nearly as possible. Breast, thighs, underparts, tail, coverts, wing butts and foot feather, hock feather and fluff lustrous green-black, free from grey, rust or white. Back, shoulder coverts and wing bows rich crimson. Primaries black, free from white or grizzle; secondaries black inner web, bay outer, showing a distinct wing bay when closed.
Female plumage: Head and neck hackle light gold or straw, each feather distinctly striped down middle with black. Remainder clear light partridge brown, finely and evenly pencilled all over with concentric rings of dark shade (preferably glossy green-black). The whole of uniform shade and marking, and the ground colour of the soft brown shade frequently described as the colour of a dead oak leaf, with three concentric rings of pencilling or more over as much of the plumage as possible.

The silver partridge

Male plumage: Head silver-white, neck hackle silver-white, each feather distinctly striped with black and free from shaftiness, black tipping or black fringe. Saddle hackle to resemble neck hackle as nearly as possible. Breast, underparts, tail coverts, wing butts and foot feather, hock feather and fluff lustrous green-black, free from grey or white. Back, shoulder coverts and wing bows black. Primaries black, free from grizzle; secondaries black inner web, white outer, showing a distinct wing bay when closed.

Female plumage: Head and neck hackle silver-white, each feather distinctly striped down the middle with black. Remainder silver grey, finely and evenly pencilled all over with concentric rings of dark shade, (preferably glossy green-black). The whole of uniform shade and marking with three concentric rings of pencilling or more, over as much of plumage as possible.

The white

Male and female plumage: Pure snow white, free from cream or yellow tinge, or black splashes or peppering.

In both sexes and all colours

Beak yellow, but in dark colours may be shaded with black or horn. Eyes red, orange or yellow – red preferred. Comb, face, wattles and ear-lobes bright red. Legs and feet yellow. (Dark legs permissible in blacks if the soles of the feet and back of shanks are yellow.)

Weights

Male   680 g (24 oz) max.
Female   570 g (20 oz) max.

Scale of points

Colour and markings	15
Fluff and cushion	15
Leg and foot feather	10
Size and weight	10
Type and carriage	20
Head	10
Length of shank	10
Condition	10
	100

Serious defects

Twisted or drooping comb. Slipped wings. Legs other than yellow (except for blacks). Eyes other than red, orange or yellow. Any deformity.
Split front undesirable, but not a defect.

PLYMOUTH ROCK

LARGE FOWL

Origin: America
Classification: Heavy: Soft feather
Egg colour: Light brown

Specimens of the barred Plymouth Rock were first exhibited in America in 1869, and stock reached here in 1871. The white and black varieties came as sports. About 1890, the buff was exhibited in America and in England. The barred Rock came to us as a dual-purpose breed, but was developed to an exhibition ideal in which body size and frontal development were neglected in order to secure long, narrow, finely barred feathers. With the introduction of sex linkage between the black Leghorn and barred Rock for commercial purposes, utility breeders made use of the Canadian barred Rock, a bird with a roomy body, full breast, lower on the leg but coarser in barring.

General characteristics: male

Carriage: Alert, upright with bold appearance, well balanced and free from stiltiness.
Type: Body large, deep and compact, evenly balanced and symmetrical, broad, the keel bone long and straight. Back broad and of medium length, saddle hackle of good length and abundant. Breast broad and well rounded. Wings of medium size, carried well up, bow and tip covered by breast and saddle feathers, respectively; flights carried horizontally. Tail medium size, rising slightly from the saddle to be carried neatly and not to be fan, squirrel or wry tail, sickles medium length and nicely curved, coverts sufficiently abundant to cover the stiff feathers.
Head: Of medium size, strong and carried well up. Beak short, stout and slightly curved. Eyes large, bright and prominent. Comb single, medium in size, straight and erect with well-defined serrations, smooth and of fine texture, free from side sprigs and thumb marks. Face smooth. Ear-lobes well developed, pendant and of fine texture. Wattles moderately rounded and of equal length, to correspond with size of comb, smooth and of fine texture.
Neck: Of medium length, slightly curved, a full hackle flowing over the shoulders.
Legs and feet: Legs wide apart. Thighs large and of medium length. Shanks medium length, stout, well rounded, smooth and free from feathers. Toes four, strong and perfectly straight, well spread and of medium length.
Fluff: Moderately full, carried closely to the body and of good texture.
Skin: Silky and fine in texture.

Female

The general characteristics are similar to those of the male, allowing for the natural sexual differences, except that comb, ear-lobes and wattles are smaller, the neck is of medium length, carried slightly forward, and the tail is small and compact, carried well back.

Colour

The barred
Male and female plumage: Ground colour white with bluish tinge, barred with black of a beetle-green sheen, the bars to be straight, moderately narrow, of equal breadth and sharply defined, to continue through the shafts of the feathers. Every feather to finish with a black tip. The fluff, or undercolour, to be also barred. The neck and saddle hackles, wing bows and tail to correspond with the rest of the body, presenting a uniformity of colour throughout.

In both sexes: Eyes rich bay. Legs and beak yellow. Face, ear-lobes, wattles and comb red.

The black
Male and female plumage: Black with a beetle-green sheen. Eyes, etc. as in the barred.

The blue
Male and female plumage: One even shade of blue, light to dark, but medium preferred; a clear solid blue, free from mealiness, 'pepper', sandiness or bronze, and quite clear of lacing. Eyes, etc. as in the partridge.

The buff

Male and female plumage: Clear, sound, even golden-buff throughout to the skin. The tail clear buff to harmonise with the body colour, and the undercolour (or fluff) and the quill of the feather also to harmonise with the surface colour. The male of more brilliant lustre than the female. Eyes, etc. as in the barred.

The Columbian

Male plumage: Head pure white. Neck hackle white with a distinct broad black stripe down the centre of each feather, free from white shaft, such stripe to be entirely surrounded by a clearly defined white margin, finishing with a decided white tip, free from black outer edging, black tips and excess of greyness at throat. Saddle hackle pure white. Tail main feathers black with beetle-green sheen; coverts black with beetle-green sheen either laced or not with white. Primaries black or black edged with white; secondaries black on the inner edge and white on the outer edge; remainder pure white, entirely free from ticking. Undercolour white, bluish-white or light slate, not to be visible when feathers are undisturbed.
Female plumage: As for male except tail feathers are black with beetle-green sheen except the top pair, which may or may not be laced with white.

In both sexes: Beak yellow. Eyes rich bay. Face, comb, ear-lobes and wattles red. Legs and feet yellow

The partridge

Male plumage: Head bright red. Neck hackles: web of feather, solid, lustrous, greenish-black, of moderate width, with a narrow edging of a medium shade of rich brilliant red, uniform in width, extending around point of feather; shaft black; plumage on front of neck black, as clear as possible of red. Wing fronts black; bows a medium shade of rich brilliant red; coverts lustrous, greenish-black, forming a well-defined bar of this colour across wing when folded; primaries black, lower edges reddish-bay; secondaries black, outside webs reddish-bay, terminating with greenish-black at the end of each feather, the secondaries when folded forming a reddish-bay wing bay between the wing bars and tips of secondary feathers. Back and saddle a medium shade of rich, brilliant red, with lustrous greenish-black stripe down the middle of each feather, same as in hackle. A slight shafting of rich red is permissible. Tail black; sickles and smaller sickles lustrous greenish-black; coverts lustrous greenish-black, edged with a medium shade of rich brilliant red. Body black; lower feathers slightly tinged with red; fluff black, slightly tinged with red. Breast lustrous black (slight tinge of red allowed). Lower thighs black. Undercolour of all sections slate.
Female plumage: Head deep reddish-bay. Neck reddish-bay, centre portion of feathers black, slightly pencilled, with deep reddish-bay; feathers on front of neck same as breast. Wing shoulders, bows and coverts deep reddish-bay with distinct pencillings of black, outlines of which conform to shape of feathers; primaries black with edging of deep reddish-bay on outer webs; secondaries inner web black, outer web deep reddish-bay with distinct pencillings of black extending around outer edge of feathers. Back deep reddish-bay with distinct pencillings of black, the outlines of which conform to shape of feathers. Tail black, the two top feathers pencilled with deep reddish-bay on upper edge; coverts deep reddish-bay pencilled with black. Body deep reddish-bay pencilled with black; fluff deep reddish-bay. Breast deep reddish-bay with distinct pencillings of black, the outlines of which conform to shape of feathers. Lower thighs deep reddish-bay pencilled with black. Undercolour slate.
Note: Each feather in back, breast, body, wing bows and thighs to have three or more distinct pencillings.

In both sexes: Beak yellow. Eyes reddish-bay. Legs and feet yellow. Comb, face, wattles and ear-lobes bright red

The white
Male and female plumage: Pure snow white, any straw tinge to be avoided.

The silver pencilled
Male plumage: Head silvery white. Neck hackle: web of feather lustrous greenish-black with narrow lacing of silvery white, shafts black. Back, including saddle: web of feather, lustrous greenish-black with narrow lacing of silvery white, a slight shafting of silvery white permissible. Silvery white predominating on surface of upper back, saddle matching with hackle in colour. Tail: main tail, web black. Main and lesser sickles lustrous greenish-black. Coverts lustrous greenish-black with lacing of white. Wing fronts black, bows silvery white. Coverts lustrous greenish-black, forming a distinct bar of this colour across entire wing when folded. Primaries black with narrow edging of white on lower edge of lower webs. Secondaries lower webs, black with lower half white to a point near end of feather, terminating abruptly, leaving ends of feathers black; upper webs black; the secondaries when folded forming a triangular white wing bay between the wing bars and tips of secondary feathers. Breast lustrous greenish-black, slight ticking allowed. Body black. Fluff black, slight tinge of grey permissible. Undercolour slate shading lighter towards base of feathers.
Female plumage: Head silvery grey. Neck hackle black, slightly pencilled with steel grey and laced with silvery white. Front of neck, breast, back, wing bows, wing bars, wing and tail coverts, thighs, body and fluff ground colour steel grey with distinct black pencillings. Main tail black except two top feathers, which have lower web black; upper web, grey pencilled with black. Primaries black with diagonal steel grey pencillings on lower webs. Secondaries lower webs steel grey with black pencillings extending well around tips of feathers; balance of upper webs, black. Undercolour medium slate.
Judging pencilled Plymouth Rocks: Pencilling should be distinct and in sharp contrast to the ground colour, be regular in shape, uniform in width and conform to the contour of the feather. Each feather on the back, breast, body, wing bows and thighs should have three or more pencillings. Pencilling which runs into peppery markings and uneven, broken or barred pencilling constitute defects, as does light shaftiness on feathers of the breast and front of neck. Ground colour to be even throughout.

In both sexes of all colours and varieties

Comb, face, wattles and ear-lobes bright red. Comb to be single, medium size with four to five serrations. Eyes reddish-bay. Beak yellow, horn permissible. Shanks and toes yellow or dusky yellow in the darker coloured varieties, yellow preferred.

Large Plymouth Rocks

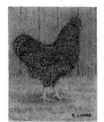
Barred Male

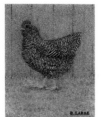
Barred Female

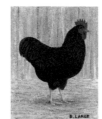
Black Male

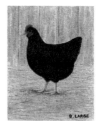
Black Female

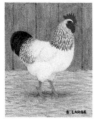
Blue Male

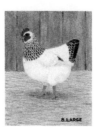
Blue Female

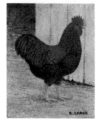
Buff Male

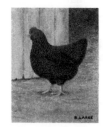
Buff Female

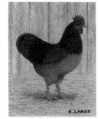
Columbian Male

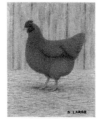
Columbian Female

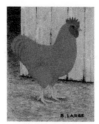
Partridge Male

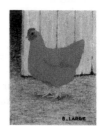
Partridge Female

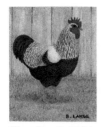
Silver Pencilled Male

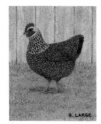
Silver Pencilled Female

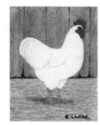
White Male

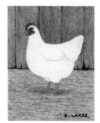
White Female

Artist's impression of large Plymouth Rocks

Weights

Male   3.40 kg (7½ lb) min.
Female   2.95 kg (6½ lb) min.

Scale of points

The barred

Type	30
Barring	20
Colour	15
Size	10
Legs and feet	10
Condition	10
Head	5
	100

The buff

Type (symmetry), shape, size and carriage	30
Colour (general)	20
Quality and texture (general)	15
Condition and fitness	15
Head and comb	10
Eye colour	5
Legs and feet	5
	100

Other varieties

Type	30
Colour	30
Head and eyes	10
Legs and feet	10
Condition	10
Quality and texture	10
	100

Serious defects

The slightest fluff or feather on shanks or feet. Legs other than yellow. White in ear-lobes. In the barred, any feathers of any colour foreign to the variety, black feathers excepted; also lopped or rose comb, decidedly wry tail; crooked back, more than four toes and entire absence of main tail feathers. Other than black feathers in the black. Mealiness, or any black or white in wing or white in tail, spotted hackle, and in the male a spotted saddle and in the female a spotted cushion in the buff. Any coloured feathers in the white. Yellow, straw tinge or sap in white, brown markings, brown undercolour in Columbian.

Disqualifications

Trimming, faking (including unmistakable signs of feathers having been plucked from shanks or feet) and any bodily deformity. Split wing, slipped wing and non-growth of secondaries.

BANTAM

Plymouth Rock bantams are miniatures of their large fowl counterparts and the Standards for large fowl should be used. Colours are buff, barred, partridge, blue, black, white, Columbian and silver-pencilled.

Weights

Male   not to exceed   1.36 kg (3 lb)
Female not to exceed   1.13 kg (2½ lb)

Scale of points

The barred

Type	20
Colour	20
Barring	20
Legs and feet	10
Head	5
Tail	5
Size	10
Condition	10
	100

The buff

Type	20
Carriage and size	10
Colour	20
Quality and texture	15
Head	10
Eye colour	5
Legs and feet	5
Condition	15
	100

The partridge

Type	30
Colour and pencilling	30
Head and eyes	10
Legs and feet	10
Condition	10
Quality and texture	10
	100

Serious defects and disqualifications

As for large fowl.

POLAND

LARGE FOWL

Origin: Poland
Classification: Light: Soft feather
Egg colour: White

The Poland is known for its prominent crest of feathers, which sets it apart from many other breeds. Mentioned in the literature as early as the sixteenth century, the Poland, sometimes in earlier documentation, was associated with the name Paduan or Patavian fowl, although there are illustrations showing the bird without muff or beard. The oldest reference found to date is the stone statue in the Vatican, which bears a very close resemblance to a crested fowl. At the first poultry show in London in 1845, the Poland had classifications for the gold, silver spangled, black and white, and was standardised in the first *Book of Standards* in 1865 in white-crested black, golden and silver varieties. All white-crested varieties are without muffling, while laced and other self varieties have muffs.

General characteristics: male

Carriage: Sprightly and erect.

Type: Back fairly long, flat and tapering to the tail. Breast full and round. Flanks deep, shoulders wide, wings large and closely carried. Tail full, neatly spread and carried rather low, not upright, the sickles and coverts abundant and well curved.

Head: Large, with a decidedly pronounced protuberance on top, and crested. Crest large, full, circular on top and free of any split or parting, high and smooth in front and compact in the centre, falling evenly with long untwisted or reverse-faced feathers far down the nape of the neck, and composed of feathers similar to those of the neck hackle. Beak of medium length, and having large nostrils rising above the curved line of the beak. Eyes large and full. Devoid of comb. Face smooth, without muffling in the white-crested varieties, and completely covered by muffling in the others. Muffling large, full and compact, fitting around to the back of the eyes and almost hiding the face. Ear-lobes very small and round, quite invisible in the muffled varieties. Wattles rather large and long in the white-crested varieties; the others are without wattles.

Neck: Long, with abundant hackle covering the shoulders.

Legs and feet: Legs slender and fairly long, the shanks free of feathers. Toes four, slender and well spread.

Female

With the exception of the crest, which is globular in shape, the general characteristics are similar to those of the male, allowing for the natural sexual differences.

Frizzled

Plumage: The frizzled varieties follow the same Standard as the plain feathered varieties and are standardised in all the same colours in both large fowl and bantam. Feathers must be broad and crisp, curling away from the body towards the head, including the muff in the bearded varieties. The curl should be as close and abundant as possible. The main feathers in the wing and tail are straight and frayed for one-third of their length from the tip.

Colour

The bearded chamois

Male plumage: Rich golden buff ground colour with white markings, crest white at the roots and tips, as free as possible of whole white feathers. Muffling on cheeks and throat laced. Hackle tipped. Back, saddle and wing coverts distinctly laced or spangled at the tips. Breast, thighs, wing bars and secondaries laced. Primaries tipped, tail coverts and sickles laced, the ends of sickles well splashed.

Female plumage: The plumage of the female is one uniform shade of rich golden-buff, every feather laced with white or creamy white except that the primaries are tipped.

In both sexes: Eyes, comb and face red. Ear-lobes blue-white. Beak, legs and feet dark blue and/or horn, soles of feet blue. Skin colour blue

The bearded gold-laced

Male and female plumage: As in the bearded chamois, substituting golden-bay as the ground colour with lustrous black markings and lacing. Undercolour, slate. Eyes, etc. as in the chamois.

The bearded silver laced

Male and female plumage: As in the chamois, substituting silver as the ground colour, with lustrous black markings and lacing. Eyes, etc. as in the chamois. Undercolour slate/silver.

The bearded self white

Male and female plumage: Feathers pure white throughout. Beak, legs and feet blue. Soles and skin blue. Eyes red to dark red.

The bearded self black

Male and female plumage: Rich metallic black throughout. Eyes, etc. as in the chamois.

The bearded self blue

Male and female plumage: An even shade of blue throughout (free from lacing). Undercolour dull blue. Skin colour blue. Legs blue/black. Eyes, etc. as in the chamois.

The non-bearded white-crested black

Male and female plumage: Ground colour lustrous greenish-black, undercolour dull black except the crest, which is pure white with a lustrous greenish-black band at the base of the crest in front.

In both sexes: Eyes, comb, face and wattles red. Ear-lobes white. Beak, legs and feet blue and/or horn, soles of feet white. Skin colour white in all white-crested varieties

The non-bearded white-crested blue

Male and female plumage: An even shade of blue throughout, free from lacing, undercolour dull blue, except the crest, which is snow white with a blue band at the base of the crest in front. Eyes, etc. as in the white-crested black.

The non-bearded white-crested cuckoo

Male and female plumage: Ground colour pale to medium grey patterned with alternating horizontal even bands of grey. The colours reasonably defined but shading into each other. Each feather to have at least three bands and end in a grey tip. Females have fewer, wider and darker bands while males have slightly angled/V-shaped markings in the tail and hackles. Undercolour banded but of a lighter shade of grey. The crest is pure white with a cuckoo band at the base of the crest in front.

In both sexes: Eyes red, wattles bright red. Beak, legs and feet white or blue-white, soles of feet white.

Weights

Male   2.95 kg (6½ lb)
Female   2.25 kg (5 lb)

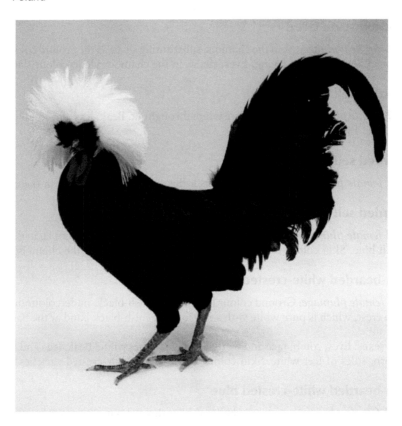

Non-bearded white-crested black Poland male

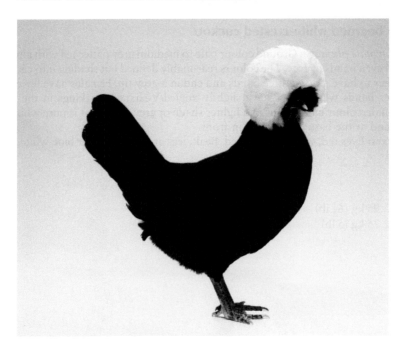

Non-bearded white-crested black Poland female, bantam

Scale of points

The white-crested varieties

Crest	30
Head and wattles	15
Colour/feather quality (to include curl of frizzle feathers)	30
Type	5
Size	10
Condition	10
	100

The other varieties

Crest	30
Head and muffling	15
Colour/feather quality (to include curl of frizzle feathers)	30
Type	5
Size	10
Condition	10
	100

Serious defects

Split or twisted crest. Comb horned. Absence of beard/muffling in laced or self-coloured varieties. Presence of beard/muffling in white-crested varieties. Legs other than blue or slate. Other than four toes on each foot. Any deformity. Absence of black, blue or cuckoo in the front of the crests of the white-crested varieties. In the cuckoo solid black or white feather.

BANTAM

Poland bantams follow the Standards for their large counterparts.

Weights

Male   680–790 g (24–28 oz)
Female   510–680 g (18–24 oz)

Underweight large fowl and overweight bantams will be penalised.

RHODE ISLAND RED

LARGE FOWL

Origin: America
Classification: Heavy: Soft feather
Egg colour: Light brown to brown

No breed made such world progress in so short a time as this American breed. It was developed from Asiatic black-red fowls of Shanghai, Malay and Java types, bred on the farms of Rhode Island Province. Red Javas were known there in 1860, and the original Rhode Island Red had a rose comb, although birds with single combs, probably from brown Leghorn crossings, were bred. They were first exhibited as Rhode Island Reds in 1880 in South Massachusetts. In December 1898, the Rhode Island Red Club of America held its first meeting. In 1904, the single comb variety was admitted to the American

Poultry Association of Perfection, followed in 1906 by the rose combs. The formation of the British Rhode Island Red Club took place in August 1909 and the breed has been one of the most popular in this country for all purposes. Being a gold, males of the breed are utilised extensively in gold–silver sex-linked matings.

General characteristics: male

Carriage: Alert, active and well balanced.

Type: Body deep, broad and long. The keel bone long, straight and extending well forward and back, giving the body an oblong look, rather than square. Back broad, long and horizontal, this being modified by rising curve at hackle and a slightly rising curve at the tail coverts. Saddle feathers of medium length and abundant. Tail of medium length, quite well spread, carried fairly well back, increasing the apparent length of the bird. Sickles of medium length, passing a little beyond the main tail feathers. Lesser sickles and tail coverts of medium length and fairly abundant. Breast broad, deep and carried in a line nearly perpendicular with the base of the beak; it should not be carried further back. Fluff moderately full but with the feathers carried fairly close to the body, not Cochin fluff. Wings of good size, well folded and the flights carried horizontally. With the horizontal back and keel and the breast vertical to the base of the beak, this gives rise to the breed being described as 'brick shaped'.

Head: Of medium size, carried horizontally and slightly forward. Beak medium in length and slightly curved. Eyes full, bright and prominent. Comb single or rose. The single of medium size, fine texture, set firmly in the head, perfectly straight and upright, with five even and well-defined serrations, those in front and rear smaller than the centre ones, of considerable breadth where it is fixed to the head. The rose of medium size, low, set firmly on the head, the top oval in shape, and the surface covered with small points, terminating in a small spike at the rear. The comb to conform to the general curve of the head. Face smooth and of fine texture. Ear-lobes fairly well developed. Wattles medium and equal in length, moderately rounded and of fine texture.

Neck: Of medium length, carried slightly forward, and covered with abundant hackle, flowing over the shoulders but not too loosely feathered.

Legs and feet: Legs well apart. Thighs large, of medium length and well covered with feathers. Shanks of medium length, well rounded and free from feathers. Toes four, of medium length, straight, strong and well spread.

Female

The general characteristics are as those of the males, apart from the sexual differences, e.g. smaller wattles, comb and no sickle feathers, leaving the tail feathers exposed. The tail, however, should not form an apparent angle with the back, nor must it be met by a high rising cushion. It should be quite well spread, carried fairly well back increasing the apparent length of the bird. Neck hackle should be sufficient, but not too coarse in feather. In the mature female the back would be described as broad, while in the pullet it would look somewhat narrower in proportion to the length of her body. The curve from the horizontal back to the hackle or tail should be moderate and gradual.

Colour

Male plumage: The neck red, harmonising with back and breast. Wing primaries the lower web black, with red along outer edging permissible and the upper web red; secondaries the lower web red and the upper black; flight coverts black; wing bows and coverts red. Tail main feathers, including the sickles, black or greenish-black; coverts mainly black, but they may become russet or red as they approach the saddle. The hackle to show a rich brilliant red plumage with no black ticking or lacing. The general surface of the plumage should be a rich brilliant red, except where black is specified. It should be free from shafting, mealy appearance or brassy effect. Absolute evenness of colour is desirable. The bird should be so brilliant in lustre as to have a glossed appearance. The undercolour and quill feather should be red or salmon. With the saddle parted, showing the undercolour at the base of the tail, appearance should be red or salmon, not whitish or smoky. Black or white in the undercolour of any section is undesirable.

Female plumage: Neck hackle to be red, the tips of the lower feather may show black ticking, but not heavy lacing. The tail should be black or greenish-black. However, the upper webs of the two main tail feathers may be edged with red. In all sections of the wing the undercolour and quills of the feathers are as in the males. With the remainder of the plumage the surface should be a rich, dark, even and lustrous red, but not as brilliant a lustre as in the male. It should be free from shafting or mealy appearance.

Note: The 'red' colour nowadays favoured is an extremely deep chocolate-red and, though some breeders disagree with this description, few birds of lighter colour receive prizes.

In both sexes: Other things being equal, the specimen having the richest undercolour shall receive the award. Beak red-horn or yellow. Eyes red. Face, comb, wattles and ear-lobes bright red. Legs and feet yellow or red-horn.

Weights

Cock	3.85 kg (8½ lb)	Cockerel	3.60 kg (8 lb)
Hen	2.95 kg (6½ lb)	Pullet	2.50 kg (5½ lb)

Scale of points

Type (shape 10, size 10, carriage and symmetry 10)	30
Colour (general)	25
Quality and texture (10 + 10)	20
Head and comb (5 + 5)	10
Eye colour	10
Legs	5
	100

Serious defects

Feather or down on shanks or feet, or unmistakable indications of a feather having been plucked from them. Badly lopped comb, side sprig or sprigs on the single comb. Other than four toes. Entire absence of main tail feathers. An ear-lobe showing white (this does not mean pale ear-lobes, but enamelled white). Two absolutely white (so-called wall or fish) eyes. Squirrel or wry tail. A feather entirely white that shows in the outer plumage. Diseased specimens, crooked backs, deformed beaks, shanks and feet other than yellow or red-horn colour. Birds showing any deformity. A pendulous crop shall be cut hard. Coarseness. Toes not straight and well spread. Super-fineness or frizzled, silkie-type defective feather often developed through concentration on lustrous dark plumage. Under all disqualifying causes, the specimen shall have the benefit of the doubt. Robustness is of vital importance.

BANTAM

Rhode Island Red bantams are miniatures of their large fowl counterparts and the Standard for those should be followed.

Weights

Male	790–910 g (28–32 oz)
Female	680–790 g (24–28 oz)

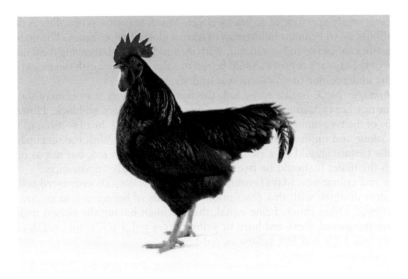

Rhode Island Red male

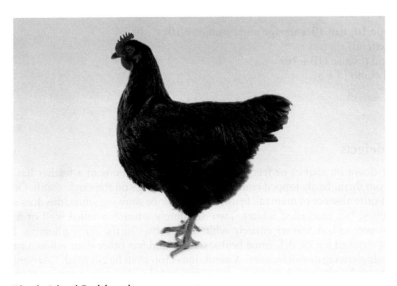

Rhode Island Red female

ROSECOMB BANTAM

Origin: Great Britain
Classification: True Bantam
Egg colour: White or cream

The Rosecomb bantam is a gem of show birds. In former days it achieved probably the highest pitch of artificial perfection ever achieved in exhibition birds.

General characteristics: male

Carriage: Cobby but not dumpy. The back should show one sweeping curve from neck to sickles.
Type: Body short and broad. Back short, shoulders broad and flat. Breast carried well up and forward, with a bold curve from wing bow to wing bow. Wings carried rather low, showing only front half of thighs. Wide flight feathers round ended and broad to ends. Stern flat, broad and thick (not running off to nothing at setting-on of tail), with abundant feather; the saddle hackle long and plentiful and extending from tail to middle of back. Tail carried well back, main feathers broad and overlapping neatly; the sickles being long, circled with a bold sweep, broad from base to rounded ends, main tail feathers not projecting beyond the sickles. Furnishing feathers plentiful, broad from base to end, round ended and uniformly curved with the sickles but hanging somewhat shorter; side hangers broad and long and with the hackles filling the space between stern and wing ends. All feathers broad to ends.
Head: Short and broad. Beak stout and short. Comb rose, neat and long, with square, well-filled front, set firmly, tapering to the setting-on of the spike or leader; top perfectly level and crowded with small round spikes. The leader stout at base, firm, long and perfectly straight, tapering to a fine point. Comb and leader rise slightly from front to rear in one line. Face of fine texture. Ear-lobes absolutely round, with rounded edges, of uniform thickness all over, not hollow or dished, firmly set on the face and kid-like in texture; not smaller than 1.88 cm ($\frac{3}{4}$ in.) or larger than 2.19 cm ($\frac{7}{8}$ in.). Wattles round, neat and fine.
Neck: Rather short, well curved, with wide feathers, the hackle falling gracefully and plentifully over shoulders and wing bows and almost reaching the tail.
Legs and feet: Legs short. Thighs set well apart, stout at top and tapering to hocks. Shanks rather short, round, fine and free of feathers. Toes four, straight and well spread.

Female

With the exception of the ear-lobes, which should not be larger than the now defunct silver threepenny piece (approx. 1.56 cm ($\frac{5}{8}$ in.)), and the wings, which are not carried so low but are tucked up, the general characteristics are similar to those of the male, allowing for the natural sexual differences.

   Note: Standard sizes of ear-lobes are usually considerably exceeded in show specimens.

Colour

The black
Male and female plumage: Black with brilliant green sheen from head to end of tail, the wing bars with extra bright green sheen. Tail feathers and sickles to be rich in green sheen.

   In both sexes: Beak black, eyes hazel to dark (not orange), a dark eye preferred. Legs and feet black

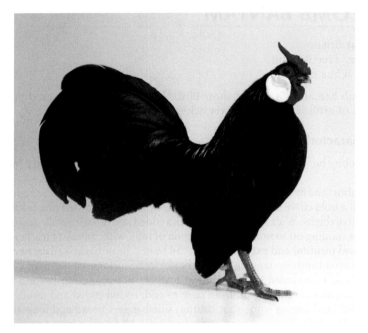

Black Rosecomb bantam, male

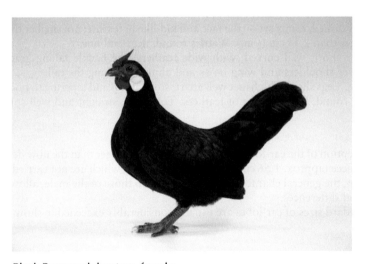

Black Rosecomb bantam, female

The blue

Male and female plumage: Blue of medium shade, free from lacing. The plumage of hackles, back and shoulders in males of a darker shade.

The white

Male and female plumage: Snow white, free from straw tinge.

In both sexes: Beak white, eyes red. Legs and feet white

The black-breasted red

Male plumage: Head lustrous golden-brown. Neck hackle and saddle lustrous golden-brown striped with black. Front of neck black. Breast, body, stern and lower thighs black. Back lustrous golden-red. Shoulders and fronts black. Bows shining golden-red. Coverts greenish-black forming a distinct bar across wing. Primaries black, lower edge of lower web edged with brown. Secondaries black, exposed portion of outer web forming wing bay brown. Main tail black. Sickles, lesser sickles and coverts brilliant greenish-black. Undercolour slate.

Female plumage: Head golden. Neck hackle golden striped with black. Front of neck salmon. Back and cushion surface colour dull black, entire web evenly and finely stippled with golden-brown, free from shafting. Breast salmon, shading lighter at body and blending into body colour. Body and stern ash grey, except where colour blends into wings and back. Shoulders, fronts, bows and coverts same as back. Primaries dull black, lower edge of lower web finely stippled with golden-brown. Lower thighs slaty-brown. Main tail black, two top feathers evenly stippled with golden-brown, shafts black. Coverts same as back. Undercolour slate in all sections.

In both sexes: Legs white. Eyes red

The birchen

Male plumage: Head silvery white. Neck hackle silvery white with slender greenish-black stripe through middle of each feather. Back silvery white. Saddle white with slender greenish-black stripe through middle of each feather. Upper breast black, each feather finely laced with white, from throat down to middle of breast. Lower breast black with some lustre. Shoulders and fronts black. Bows white. Coverts brilliant black forming a distinct bar across wing. Primaries and secondaries black. Body, stern, lower thighs and main tail black. Sickles and lower sickles black with a greenish sheen. Undercolour black.

Female plumage: Head silvery white. Neck hackle silvery white striped with black. Back and cushion black with some lustre. Upper breast black, each feather finely laced with white, from throat down to middle of breast. Lower breast black with some lustre. Body, stern, lower thighs and main tail black. Coverts greenish-black. Shoulders, fronts and bows black. Coverts greenish-black. Primaries and secondaries black. Main tail black, coverts greenish-black.

In both sexes: Legs dark. Face gypsy. Eyes dark

The Columbian

Male plumage: Head white. At least three-quarters of the neck length lustrous greenish-black with a narrow lacing of silvery white. Front of neck white. Breast, body, stern and lower thighs white. Back white, feathers under the hackle black with white edge. Saddle white with lustrous black stripe extending down the middle of each feather. Shoulders, fronts, bows and coverts white. Primaries black with white borders on lower edge of lower web. Secondaries black, upper web laced with white, exposed portion of lower web forming wing bay white. Main tail black, sickles and lesser sickles lustrous greenish-black. Undercolour slaty-blue.

Female plumage: Head white. Neck hackle lustrous greenish-black with a narrow lacing of white, shaft black. Front of neck white. Breast, body, stern and lower thighs white. Wings same as male. Main tail black except two top feathers which should be finely laced with white. Coverts black with narrow lacing of white. Undercolour white.

In both sexes: Legs white. Eyes orange-red

In both sexes and all colours (except birchen face)
Comb, face and wattles brilliant cherry red. Ear-lobes spotlessly white, especially near wattles.

Weights
Male   570–620 g (20–22 oz)
Female   450–510 g (16–18 oz)

Scale of points
Head (comb 20, lobes 15)   35
Tail   15
Colour   12
Type   15
Condition   15
Legs, etc.   <u>8</u>
                                          <u>100</u>

Serious defects
Stiltiness. Narrow chest or back. Hollow-fronted or leafy comb. Coarse bone. Tightly carried wings. Narrow feathers. Blushed lobes. Coloured feathers. White in face. In blacks, grizzled or brown flights, purple sheen or barring, light legs. White tipping in blacks.

RUMPLESS GAME

LARGE FOWL

Origin: Great Britain
Classification: Hard feather: Rare
Egg colour: Brown

As is common with any rumpless breed, the parson's nose or 'caudal appendage' (uropygium) is missing. Foreign breeds like the Barbu d'Anvers has a rumpless version called Barbu du Grubbe. The Barbu d'Uccle has the Barbu d'Everberg as its rumpless version and, even in Japan, there is a Rumpless Yokohama, funny though it may sound, with its long saddle hackle making it feasible. A genetic accident with Old English Game many years ago probably created our own Rumpless Game. The breed, though popular in the bantam form, is not often seen in large fowl.

General characteristics: male

Carriage: Bold and upright.
Type: Body short and small. Back steeply sloping. Breast full and prominent. Wings large and long. Tail completely absent, the whole of the lower back being covered with the saddle feather.

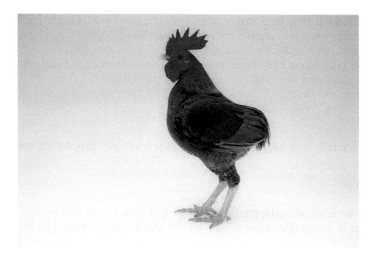

Rumpless Game male, bantam

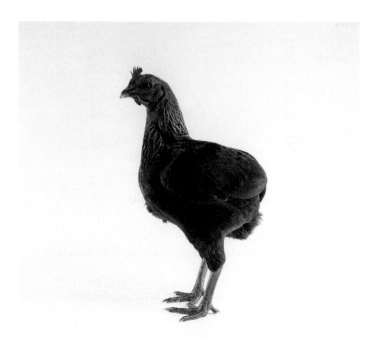

Rumpless Game female

Head: Small and tapering. Beak rather large. Eyes large and bold. Comb single, small and thin, upright. Ear-lobes and wattles fine, small and thin.
Neck: Long and upright; hackle close and wiry.
Legs and feet: Legs strong and of medium length. Thighs short, round and muscular. Toes four, long, straight and tapering.
Plumage: Hard and close.

Female

The general characteristics are similar to those of the male, allowing for the natural sexual differences.

Colour

Plumage colour is of secondary importance in this breed, and almost any recognised 'Game' colour is acceptable. Face, comb, wattles and ear-lobes should be bright red.

Weights

Male   2.25–2.70 kg (5–6 lb)
Female   1.80–2.25 kg (4–5 lb)

Scale of points

Type	25
Carriage and bearing	20
Head	15
Colour	15
Legs and feet	5
Size	15
Condition	5
	100

Disqualifications

Any sign of tail. Other than single comb. Any deformity.

BANTAM

Rumpless Game bantams should follow exactly the large fowl Standard.

Weights

Male   620–740 g (22–26 oz)
Female   510–620 g (18–22 oz)

SATSUMADORI

Origin: Japan
Classification: Asian Hardfeather. Large Fowl
Egg colour: White to light brown

The Satsumadori is a very stylish, flashy Japanese Gamebird developed in Kagoshima (formerly known as Satsuma) on the island of Kyushu. Bred originally for steel spur fighting, this is a powerful, agile bird, with tremendous presence.

General characteristics: male

Type and carriage: General appearance impressive, proud and alert. Stance upright.
Body: Large, firm and well muscled.
Breast: Broad and full with deep keel.
Back: Long, broadest at shoulders, sloping down towards tail and gradually tapering from upper side of thigh. Backbone straight.
Wings: Short, big, strong and bony, carried well down and close to the body, not showing on the back but with prominent shoulders.
Tail: Long, extremely full and luxuriant, carried above horizontal in an unbroken curving fan shape with the spread of feather also extending sideways at a 15° angle to the body. This is a very specific characteristic of the breed.
Head: Deep and broad with wattles and ear-lobes small or absent. Beak strong, broad and curved downwards, but not hooked. Eyes piercing. Comb triple and firm in the male, small or absent in the female.
Neck: Long, strong boned, slightly curved but almost erect. Neck hackle rich and full.
Legs and feet: Thighs long, round and muscular. Legs medium to long – thick and strong with slight bend at hock. Shanks round. Toes four, long and well spread. Hind toe straight and firm on the ground.
Plumage: Feathers narrow and brilliant, rich at neck and tail, otherwise tightly fitting to body. There is also an old type of Satsumadori which is muffed and feather legged, but it is no longer popular.
Handling: Extremely firm fleshed, muscular and well balanced. Strong contraction of wings to body.

Female

The general characteristics are similar to those of the male, allowing for the natural sexual differences.

Colour

Black-red (the red being a brilliant orange-red) with partridge females, silver and gold duckwing, black, white. Beak yellow. Horn colour acceptable in birds with black plumage. Legs and feet yellow. Dark legs acceptable in birds with black plumage. Comb, face, throat, and ear-lobes brilliant red. Eyes silver or gold. Darker eyes acceptable in young birds.

Weights

Male   3–4 kg approx. (6 lb 10 oz–8 lb 12 oz)
Female   2.5–3.5 kg approx. (5 lb 8 oz–7 lb 12 oz)

Scale of points

Type	30
Plumage	25
Head	15
Legs and feet	10
Carriage	10
Condition	10
	100

Serious defects

Poor tail plumage, lack of attitude, 'duck' feet. Any other deformities.

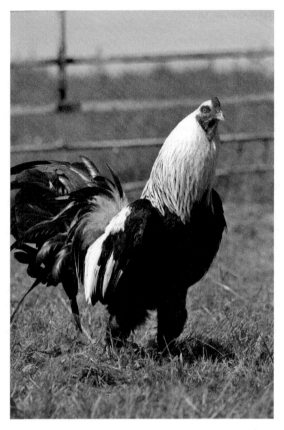

Satsumadori male

SCOTS DUMPY

LARGE FOWL

Origin: Great Britain
Classification: Light: Soft feather
Egg colour: White or cream

This breed has been bred in Scotland for more than a hundred years, and the birds used to be known as Bakies, Crawlers and Creepers. Fowls having identical dumpy characteristics have been shown to exist as early as AD 900. The bird is considered an ideal broody, being an excellent sitter and mother.

General characteristics: male

Carriage: Heavy, with a waddling gait, the extreme shortness of its legs giving the bird the appearance of 'swimming on dry land'. Shortness of leg alone should not constitute the breed's claim to notice. The large, low, heavy body and other points of excellence must be possessed also.
Type: Body long and broad. Back broad and flat. Breast deep. Wings of medium size and neatly carried. Tail full and flowing, the sickles well arched.
Head: Fine. Beak strong and well curved. Eyes large and clear. Comb single, of medium size, upright and straight, free from side sprigs, and the back following the line of the skull, evenly serrated on top. Face smooth. Ear-lobes small and close to the neck. Wattles of medium size.
Neck: Of fair length, in keeping with the size of the body, and covered with flowing hackle.
Legs and feet: Legs very short, the shanks not exceeding 3.75 cm ($1\frac{1}{2}$ in.) Toes four, well spread.

Female

The general characteristics are similar to those of the male, allowing for the natural sexual differences.

Colour

The colours most widely seen are black, cuckoo and white. Other colours seen should only include standardised colours in other breeds.

The black
Male and female plumage: Glossy black with a green sheen. Eyes dark.

The cuckoo
Male and female plumage: Light blue or grey ground, each feather marked across with bands of dark blue or grey. Eyes red.

The white
Male and female plumage: Pure white, free from cream tinge, no black feathers. Eyes red.

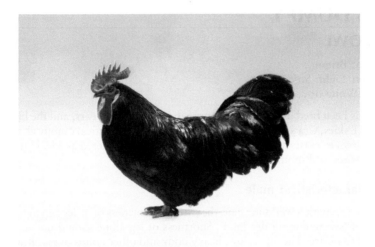

Black Scots Dumpy male

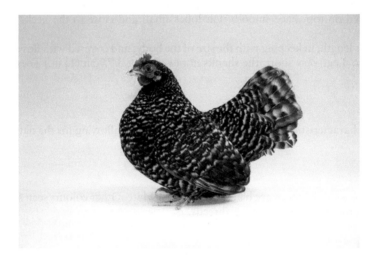

Cuckoo Scots Dumpy female, bantam

The brown-red

Male plumage: Hackle, back and wing bows bright lemon, the neck hackle feathers striped down the centre with green-black. Remainder green-black, the breast feathers edged with pale lemon as low as the top of the thighs.

Female plumage: Neck hackle light lemon to the top of the head, the lower feathers being striped with green-black. Remainder green-black, the breast laced as in the male, the shoulders free from ticking and the back free from lacing.

   In both sexes: Beak very dark horn, black preferred. Legs and feet black or slate. Eyes dark. Comb, face and wattles bright red

The birchen

Male plumage: Hackle, back, saddle, shoulder coverts and wing bows silver-white, the neck hackle with narrow black striping. Remainder rich black, the breast having a narrow silver margin around each feather, giving it a regular laced appearance gradually diminishing to perfect black thighs.

Female plumage: Hackle similar to that of the male. Remainder rich black, the breast very delicately laced as in the male.

   In both sexes: Beak dark horn, black preferred. Eyes dark. Comb, face and wattles bright red

In both sexes and all colours

Comb, face, wattles and ear-lobes bright red. Beak, legs and feet white, except in the black, brown-red and birchen varieties.

Weights

Male   3.20 kg (7 lb)
Female   2.70 kg (6 lb)

Scale of points

Type   45
Size   25
Head   10
Condition   10
Colour   _10_
            100

Serious defects

White ear-lobes. Yellow or feathered shanks or feet. Long legs. Any deformity.

BANTAM

Scots Dumpy bantams should follow the large fowl Standard.

Weights

Male   800 g ($1\frac{3}{4}$ lb)
Female   675 g ($1\frac{1}{2}$ lb)

SCOTS GREY

LARGE FOWL

Origin: Great Britain
Classification: Light: Soft feather
Egg colour: White

A light, non-sitting breed originated in Scotland, it has not been bred extensively outside that country where, even if it is less popular today, it will doubtless be maintained by keen breeders. It has been bred there for over 200 years.

General characteristics: male

Carriage: Erect, active and bold.
Type: Body compact, full of substance and fairly long. Back broad and flat. Breast deep, full and carried upwards. Wings moderately long and well tucked, the bow and tip covered by the neck and saddle hackles. Tail fairly long and well up (but not squirrel fashion) with full sickles.
Head: Long and fine. Beak strong and well curved. Eyes large and bright. Comb single, upright, of medium size, with well-defined serrations, the back following the line of the skull. Face of fine texture. Ear-lobes of medium size. Wattles of medium length with a well-rounded lower edge.
Neck: Finely tapered and with profuse hackle flowing on the back and shoulders.
Legs and feet: Legs long and strong. Thighs wide apart but not quite as prominent as those of Game Fowl. Shanks free from feathers. Toes four, straight and spreading, stout and strong.
Handling: Firm, and somewhat similar to the Game Fowl.

Female

With the exception of the comb, either erect or falling slightly over, the general characteristics are similar to those of the male, allowing for the natural sexual differences.

Colour

Male plumage: Barred. Ground colour of body, thighs and wing feathers steel grey. The barring is black with a metallic lustre, that of the body, thighs and wing feathers straight across, but that of the neck hackle, saddle and tail slightly angled or V shaped. The alternating bars of black are of equal width and proportioned to the size of the feather. The bird should 'read' throughout, i.e. the shade should be the same from head to tail. The plumage should be free from red, black, white or yellow feathers, and the hackle, saddle and tail should be distinctly and evenly barred, while the markings all over should be rather small, even and sharply defined.

Female plumage: Similar to that of the male, except that the markings are not as small, and produce an appearance somewhat resembling a shepherd's tartan.
    In both sexes: Beak white or white streaked with black. Eyes amber. Comb, face, wattles and ear-lobes bright red. Legs and feet white or white mottled with black, but not sooty

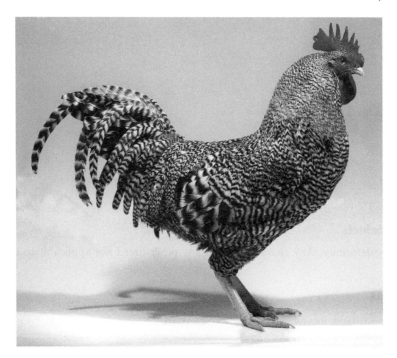

Scots Grey male, large

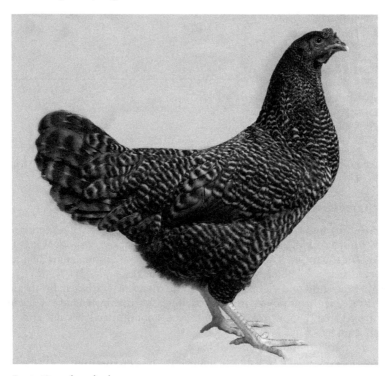

Scots Grey female, large

Weights

Male   3.20 kg (7 lb)
Female 2.25 kg (5 lb)

Scale of points

Colour and markings	30
Size	10
Type	30
Head	10
Condition	10
Legs and feet	10
	100

Serious defects

Any bodily deformity. Any characteristic of any other breed not applicable to the Scots Grey.

BANTAM

Scots Grey bantams follow the large fowl Standard.

Weights

Male   620–680 g (22–24 oz)
Female 510–570 g (18–20 oz)

SEBRIGHT

Origin: Great Britain
Classification: True Bantam
Egg colour: White or cream

This breed is a genuine bantam and one of the oldest British varieties. It has no counterpart in large breeds, but has played a part in the production of other laced fowl, notably Wyandottes. There are two colours, gold and silver.

General characteristics: male

Carriage: Strutting and tremulous, on tip-toe, somewhat resembling a fantail pigeon.
Type: Body compact, with broad and prominent breast. Back very short. Wings large and carried low. Tail square, well spread and carried high. Sebright males are hen feathered, without curved sickles or pointed neck and saddle hackles.
Head: Small. Beak short and slightly curved. Comb rose, square fronted, firmly and evenly set on, top covered with fine points, free from hollows, narrowing behind to a distinct spike or leader, turned slightly upwards. Eyes full. Face smooth. Ear-lobes flat and unfolded. Wattles well rounded.
Neck: Tapering, arched and carried well back.
Legs and feet: Legs short and well apart. Shanks slender and free from feathers. Toes four, straight and well spread.
Plumage: Short and tight, feathers not too wide but never pointed. (Almond-shaped feather is desired.)

Female

The general characteristics are similar to those of the male, allowing for the natural sexual differences. Her neck is upright.

Colour

The gold

Male and female plumage: Uniform golden-bay with glossy green-black lacing and dark undercolour. Each feather evenly and sharply laced all round its edge with a narrow margin of black. Shaftiness is undesirable.

The silver

Male and female *plumage*: Similarly marked on pure, clear silver-white ground colour.

In both sexes and colours

Beak dark horn in golds; dark blue or horn in silvers. Eyes black, or as dark as possible. Comb, face, wattles and ear-lobes mulberry or deep red. Legs and feet slate blue.

Although in males mulberry face is seldom obtainable, the eye should be dark and surrounded with a dark cere.

Weights

Male   620 g (22 oz)
Female   510 g (18 oz)

Scale of points

Lacing	25
Comb	5
Face and lobes	10
Ground colour	15
Tail	10
Type	20
Weight	5
Condition	10
	100

Note: There is at present a decided move to improve type and to discourage the prevailing whip tails and narrow build, particularly in females.

Serious defects

Single comb. Sickle feathers or pointed hackles on the male. Feathers on shanks. Legs other than slate blue. Other than four toes. Any deformity.

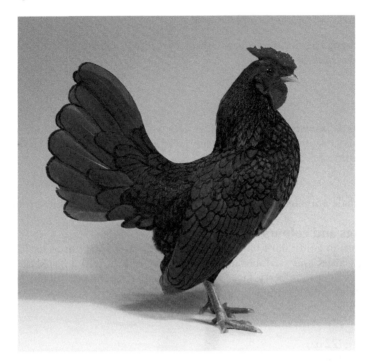

Gold Sebright male

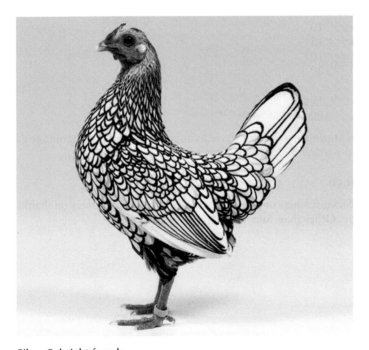

Silver Sebright female

SERAMA

Origin: Malaysia
Classification: True Bantam
Egg colour: Varying from white through to brown

The Malaysian Serama first arrived in the UK in 2004 and The Serama Club of Great Britain was formed in 2005.

The exact origins of the Serama are unclear, but the breed is understood to have been developed at the early part of the 1970s in Kelatan State in Malaysia. The 'Kapan' (a miniature upright pet bantam), various small native game-like birds and the 'Kate' (the native unrefined ancestor of Japanese bantam) were all believed to have been used to create a small lightweight bird with a distinctive outline and character. The breed was given the name 'Serama' after a popular character Sri Rama from the traditional shadow puppet plays. In its native Malaysia today, the Serama is a very popular and highly prized exhibition bird, where they are trained to display themselves on a table before a panel of judges, and are regarded as a 'Living work of art'.

General characteristics: male

Type: Body well muscled with breast carried high, full and well forward. When viewed from above the shape is somewhat elliptical, tapering towards the tail. The back should be short and entirely covered by abundant hackle, covering both the shoulders and secondaries and flowing onto the tail coverts, giving the base of the tail a full appearance.

Carriage and temperament: Assertive and confident yet calm and manageable. Should be easily handled and show no excessive aggression. The bird should pose readily and when viewed from the side should create a vase-like or wide V shape, with the chest, neck and head forming an S shape in pose.

Tail: Tail should be carried high and vertical or within 20° behind vertical, parallel and close to the neck and should be large and full. Main tail feathers should be long and broad and should overlap. The tail should be open and, when viewed from behind, should create an inverted V shape. Sickles should have a slight curve and protrude just above the main tail feathers. Side hangers and tail coverts should be broad, plentiful and curved.

Wings: Fairly large in proportion to the body, they should be held in a vertical position just clearing the ground and leaving the feet partially visible. Shoulders should be set high on the bird. Primaries are long and of medium width, with secondaries moderately long and broad. Slight separation between the primaries and secondaries at the wing tips is acceptable.

Head: Head to be in proportion to the body and carried well back. The single, upright comb is small to medium in size with five regular, pointed serrations as ideal. It should be straight, smooth and free of folds or any deformities and tending towards flyaway type. Wattles are to complement the comb, smaller being preferred and free from folds or wrinkles.

Comb, face and wattles: Bright red, though darker is acceptable in darker coloured birds.

Ear-lobes: Any colour or combination of colours acceptable.

Eyes: Clear and bright, any colour being acceptable.

Legs and feet: The legs are of medium length, straight and set wide apart to allow for full and muscular body. They should be strong and stable. Thighs should be of medium length and well muscled. Shanks to be clean and sturdy, without coarseness. Toes four, straight and well spaced. Any colour legs and feet are acceptable.

Plumage: All feathers should be in good condition with lustrous sheen. Body feathers to be full yet firm, retaining the body's outline.

Colour: Male and female – *any* colour or combination of colours is acceptable and none to be penalised.

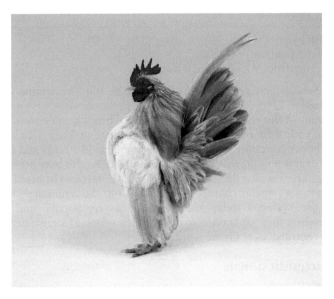

Serama male

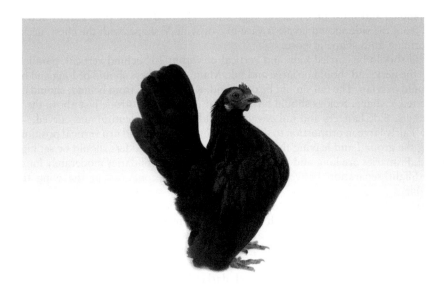

Serama female

Female

The general characteristics are similar to those of the male, allowing for the natural sexual differences.

Weights

Male   up to 500 g
Female   up to 450 g

Scale of points

Type and carriage   55
Temperament   15
Legs and feet   10
Head   10
Condition   <u>10</u>
                   <u>100</u>

Silkied Serama

Silkied feathered Serama are acceptable. The silkied feathered should still retain the typical Serama outline, as in the smooth feathered, but the body feathers should have a silkie, loose feather structure (i.e. feathers should have no central vein). This cannot apply to the primary and secondary wing feathers or the main tail feathers, which would nullify any true Serama type.

All other characteristics should follow the main Standard.

Serious defects

Excessive aggression, nervousness or shyness. Long back. Low tail carriage, decidedly wry tail, squirrel tail. Cow hocks, duck feet, legs too short, course or too fine. Feathering on shanks or feet. Comb other than single. Excessively large comb or wattles. Any general defects. Weight exceeding the upper limit.

SHAMO

Origin: Japan
Classification: Asian Hardfeather. Large Fowl
Egg colour: White to light brown

The Shamo is a Japanese bird of Malayoid type, originally imported to Japan from Thailand in the seventeenth century – the name being a corruption of Siam, the old name for Thailand. In Japan it was developed into a fighting bird of unmatched courage and ferocity. Its feathers are sparse but strong and shiny, and its powerful bone structure and well-muscled body and legs, coupled with its erect posture, make it an impressive and striking bird. Since its importation in the early 1970s the term 'Shamo' has covered all large fowl, but in Japanese classification birds are also divided into Chu Shamo (medium) and O Shamo (large).

General characteristics: male

Type and carriage: General appearance fierce, powerful, proud and alert. Stance very upright.
Body: Large and extremely firm with well-muscled abdomen.
Breast: Broad and full with deep keel.
Back: Long, broadest at shoulders, sloping down towards tail and gradually tapering from upper side of thigh. Backbone straight.
Wings: Short, big, strong and bony, carried well down and close to the body, not showing on the back but with prominent shoulders.
Tail: Carried below horizontal, length to give balance to the bird.
Head: Deep and broad with wattles and ear-lobes small or absent. Beak strong, broad and curved downwards, but not hooked. Eyes deep-set under overhanging brows. Comb triple and firm. Walnut comb rare – but also acceptable.
Neck: Long, strong-boned, slightly curved but almost erect.
Legs and feet: Legs medium to long – thick and strong with slight bend at hock. Thighs long, round and muscular. Shanks thick, strong and round. Toes four, long and well spread. Hind toe straight and firm on the ground.
Plumage: Feathers very short, narrow, hard and brilliant. Scant, and bare showing red skin at throat, keel and point of wing. Neck hackle feathers permitted to curl towards back of neck.
Handling: Extremely firm fleshed, muscular and well balanced. Strong contraction of wings to body.

Female

The general characteristics are similar to those of the male, allowing for the natural sexual differences. Stance very upright, but it is acceptable for a female to be slightly less upright than the male.

Colour

Black-red is the most common colour seen. (The 'red' may be any shade from yellow to dark red, with wheaten or partridge females that can be any shade from cream to dark brown, with or without dark markings.) Ginger, white, black, splash, blue and duckwing are all recognised, and no colour or combination of colours is disqualified.

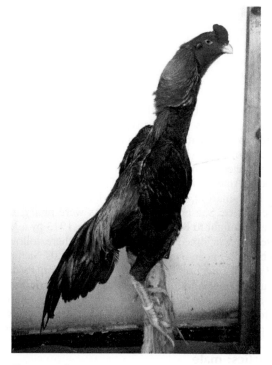

Shamo male

In both sexes and all colours

Beak yellow or horn. Legs and feet yellow. Blackish overcolour acceptable in dark-coloured birds. Comb, face, throat, ear-lobes and any exposed skin brilliant red. Eyes silver or gold. Darker eyes acceptable in young birds.

Weights

Male   3 kg (6 lb 10 oz) min.
Female   2.25 kg (4 lb 14 oz) min.

Chu Shamo – male above 3 kg (6 lb 10 oz) and under 4 kg (8 lb 12 oz); female above 2.25 kg (4 lb 14 oz) and under 3 kg (6 lb 10 oz). O Shamo – male 4 kg (8 lb 12 oz) and above; female 3 kg (6 lb 10 oz) and above

Scale of points

Type and carriage   40
Head   20
Feather/condition   20
Legs and feet   <u> 20</u>
                    100

Serious defects

Lack of attitude. Poor carriage. Overlarge comb. 'Duck' feet.

SICILIAN BUTTERCUP

LARGE FOWL

Origin: Europe
Classification: Light: Rare
Egg colour: White

The distinguishing feature of the breed is the cup-shaped comb. This comb variation has been known for centuries – birds with this type of comb are portrayed on paintings in galleries in Rome and Florence, dating back to the sixteenth century. The first specimens were taken to America from Sicily in the 1830s. Today's stock probably descended from imports and subsequent selection by C.C. Loring of Dedham, Massachusetts, in the 1860s or from eggs imported to America in 1892. In 1907, the breed was widely promoted by the efforts of Mrs James L. Dumaresq, of Easton, Maryland, whose husband had been in the American diplomatic service. She noted 'the chickens were pretty, tame, and abundant layers'. Specimens were brought to Britain in 1910 and in 1913 by a Mrs Colbeck of West Yorkshire. Soon afterwards a breed club was formed; there followed a brief spell of popularity followed by a decline in interest from the late 1920s. Sicilian Flowerbirds were standardised in 1922 as a distinct breed. The Buttercup in bantam form is a recent creation. Obtaining correct plumage markings on females, well-cupped combs on both sexes and a wholly red ear-lobe are the main difficulties in breeding show quality Buttercups. The American Standard for the breed was changed in the late 1920s in favour of a white ear-lobe, hence stock imported to Britain in the 1970s from the USA were white lobed.

General characteristics: male

Carriage: Upright, bold and active.
Type: Body moderately long and deep; broad shoulders and narrow saddle. Full round breast. Broad back sloping downwards to the saddle, which rises in a slightly concave outline to the base of the tail. Long wings, closely tucked. Fairly large tail with long main feathers, carried at an angle of 45°, and fitted with well-curved sickles and abundant coverts.
Head: Skull long and deep. Beak of medium length. Eyes full and keen. Comb beginning at the base of the beak with a single leader and joined to a cup-shaped crown, set firmly on the centre of the skull and surmounted with well-defined and regular points, of medium size and fine texture, and free from decided spikes in the cavity or centre. Ear-lobes almond shaped, flat, smooth and close fitting. Wattles thin and well rounded.
Neck: Rather long, with hackle flowing well over the shoulders.
Legs and feet: Of moderate size and length. Thighs well apart. Shanks slender and free of feathers. Toes four, straight and spreading.

Female

With the exception of the comb (smaller and lower in proportion) the general characteristics are similar to those of the male, allowing for the natural sexual differences.

Colour

The gold
Male plumage: Neck hackle, back, saddle, shoulders and wing bows bright lustrous orange-red. Cape (at base of neck) dark buff marked with distinct black spangles and covered by hackle. Wing bars and bay an even shade of red-bay; primaries black, lower web edged with bay; secondaries red-bay on outer web, black on inner. Breast red-bay. Body light bay. Fluff rich bay shading to light bay on stern, and some feathers on the body fluff with distinct black spangles. Tail black, sickles and coverts green-black, the former showing red-bay at their base and the coverts edged with that colour.
Female plumage: Hackle lustrous golden-buff. Breast and thighs light golden-buff, plain from throat to middle of breast, elsewhere with black spangles. Tail dull black, except the two highest feathers mottled with buff. Wing bows and bars golden-buff with parallel rows of elongated black spangles, each spangle extending slightly diagonally across the web; quill and edge of feathers golden-buff; primaries black edged with buff; secondaries golden-buff regularly barred with black on outer web, black on inner. Back golden-buff regularly spangled with black (the same pattern as the wing bows) and extending over the entire surface, including the saddle and the tail coverts.

The silver
Male and female plumage: Except that the ground is silver-white (free from yellow or straw tinge) instead of red or bay, similar to the golden.

The brown
Male plumage: Neck hackle rich orange-red striped with black, crimson-red in front below wattles. Back and shoulder coverts deep crimson-red or maroon. Saddle rich orange-red with or without a few black stripes. Wing bows deep crimson-red or maroon; coverts steel blue with green reflections forming the bar; primaries brown; secondaries deep bay on outer web, black on inner. Breast and underparts glossy black quite free from brown splashes. Tail green-black, coverts black edged with brown.
Female plumage: Hackle rich golden-yellow, broadly striped with black. Breast salmon-red running into maroon near the wattles and ash grey at the thighs. Body and wings rich brown, very finely and closely pencilled with black, free from any red tinge. Tail black pencilled with brown. (*Note*: The undercolour of both sexes should be slate blue or mouse.)

The white
Male and female plumage: Pure white throughout.

The golden duckwing
Male plumage: Neck and saddle hackles white with cream tinge. Back and saddle maroon-orange shading to cream. Wing butts and bars black; diamond white; bows bright orange to cream. Remainder black.
Female plumage: Hackle white, fairly striped with black or grey. Tail black, except top feathers slightly pencilled with grey. Remainder slate grey, finely pencilled with darker grey or black.

In both sexes and all colours
Beak dark horn lightly shaded with yellow. Eyes red-bay. Comb, face, wattles and ear-lobes bright red (more than one-third white in lobes a serious defect). Legs and feet willow green.

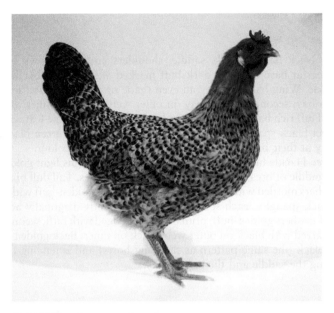

Gold Sicilian Buttercup female

Weights

Male   2.95 kg (6½ lb)
Female   2.50 kg (5½ lb)

Scale of points

Head	30
Colour	25
Type	20
Size	10
Legs and feet	10
Condition	5
	100

Serious defects

Spikes more than 2.5 cm (1 in.) long in cup (or cavity of comb) of male, or any indication of spike in cup (or cavity of comb) of female. Solid white ear-lobes. Shanks other than green. Feathers or stubs on shanks or toes. Any deformity. In golden, solid white in any part of the plumage (except undercolour) or black striping in the male's hackles.

BANTAM

Sicilian Buttercup bantams should follow exactly the large fowl Standard.

Weights

Male   735 g (26 oz)
Female   620 g (22 oz)

SILKIE

LARGE FOWL

Origin: Asia
Classification: Light: Soft feather
Egg colour: Cream

Silkie fowls have been mentioned by authorities for several hundred years. Some think that they originated in India, whilst others favour China and Japan. The Silkie is regarded as a light breed, and as such it must be exhibited. The Silkie's persistent broodiness is a breed characteristic, either pure or crossed.

General characteristics, male

Carriage: Stylish, compact and lively.
Type: Body broad and stout looking. Back short, saddle silky and rising to the tail. Stern broad and abundantly covered with fine fluff, saddle hackles soft, abundant and flowing. Breast broad and full, shoulders stout, square and fairly covered with neck hackle. Wings soft and fluffy at the shoulders with ends of the flights ragged with 'osprey plumage' (i.e. some strands of the flights hang loosely downwards). Tail short and very ragged at the end of the harder feathers of the tail proper. It should not be flowing, but forming a short round curve.
Head: Short and neat, with a good crest which is soft and full and as upright as the comb will permit, having six to twelve soft silky feathers streaming gracefully backwards from the lower back part of the crest to a length of 3.75 cm ($1\frac{1}{2}$ in.). Beak short and broad at the base. Comb almost circular in shape, preferably broader than long with a number of small prominences over it and having a slight indentation or furrow transversely across the middle. Face smooth, wattles concave, nearly semi-circular. Ear-lobes more oval than round. Neck short or medium in length, broad and full at the base with abundant and flowing hackles.
Legs and feet: Free from scaliness. Thighs wide apart and covered with abundant fluff, legs short. Feathers on the legs should be moderate in quantity. Toes five in number, with the fifth toe diverging from the fourth. The middle and outer toes feathered, but these feathers must not be hard.
Plumage: Abundantly silky/fluffy but with an excellent depth and quality of silk.

Female

The saddle broad, with the silkiest of plumage, which should nearly smother the small cushioned tail, the ragged ends alone protruding. The legs are particularly short in the female and the under and thigh fluff should nearly meet the ground. The head crest is short and neat, the eye must not be hidden by the crest, which should stand up and out. Ear-lobes small and roundish. Wattles either absent or very small and oval in shape. Comb small. Other characteristics are as in the male, allowing for the natural sexual differences.

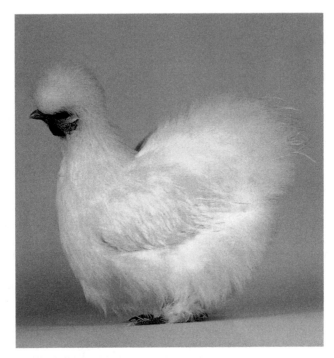

White Silkie female

Colour

The white
Male and female plumage: Pure white.

The black
Male and female plumage: Black all over including the under fluff, with a green sheen in the male. A minimal amount of colour in the hackle is permissible, but not desirable.

The blue
Male and female plumage: An even shade of blue from head to tail.

The gold
Male and female plumage: A bright even shade of gold throughout with darker feathers in the tail of both sexes permissible.

The partridge
Male plumage: Head and crest dark gold. Hackles orange/gold/brown, each feather having a clear black stripe down the centre. Back and shoulders dark gold/partridge brown. Wing bars solid black. Primaries black, free from any white. Secondaries and outer web dark gold, inner web black, the dark gold alone showing when the wing is closed. Tail and sickles black. Leg and foot feather as body. Undercolour slate grey and free from white.
Female plumage: Head and crest dark gold – not black. Neck and breast dark gold striped black. Hackle feathers having a black centre with a lemon or gold edge. Chest lemon or gold and black mingling. Body including wings and cushion subtle black barring on soft partridge brown. Undercolour slate grey and free of white. Leg and foot colour as body. Some black permissible in the tail.

In both sexes and all colours

With the exception of the black the beak should be slatey blue. In the black the beak should be dark slate. Eyes brilliantly black. Comb, face and wattles mulberry, ear-lobes turquoise blue or mulberry, the former being preferable. Legs and feet lead. Nails blue white. Skin mulberry.

The Bearded Silkie

As the Standard silkie but with clearly defined ear muff and beard. The wattles must not be visible.

Weights

Male 1.81 kg (4 lb)
Female 1.36 kg (3 lb)

BANTAM

A counterpart of the large fowl in all respects.

Weights

Male 600 g (22 oz)
Female 500 g (18 oz)

Scale of points

Type	20
Head	30
Legs and feet	10
Colour and plumage	40
	100

Serious defects

Hard feathers. Green beak or tip to beak. Horns protruding from the comb. Ruddy comb, wattles or face. Eye other than black. Incorrect colour in plumage or skin. Plumage not silky. Lack of crest, a Poland-type crest or split crest. The crest must not hang over the eyes. Long pendulous wattles in the male. Green soles to feet. Any deformities, as listed in the Poultry Club's *Book of Standards*, including crooked toes and uneven wattles.

Disqualifications

Single comb. Toes other than five in number. Green legs and/or feet, featherless legs or feet. Vulture hocks.

SPANISH

LARGE FOWL

Origin: Mediterranean
Classification: Light: Rare
Egg colour: White

The white-faced black Spanish is one of our oldest breeds, and was widely kept and admired long before the advent of poultry shows in the latter half of the nineteenth century. Of striking appearance, with its extensive white face, surrounding eyes and ears and extending lower than the wattles, the Spanish was also a good layer of large white eggs. In the last decade, the breed has gained popularity, especially with the reintroduction of the bantam form, although bantam white-faced Spanish were popular around the 1900s.

General characteristics: male

Carriage: Upright, with proud action.
Head: Skull long, broad and deep. Beak long and stout. Eyes full and wide open. Comb single, somewhat small, erect and straight, firm at the base, rather thin at the edge, fitting closely on the neck at the back, of very smooth texture and free from wrinkles, rising well over the eyes but not so as to interfere with the sight, and joining the ear-lobes and wattles. Ear-lobes deep and broad, well rounded at the bottom, extending well below the wattles, meeting in front and going well back on each side of the neck, of fine texture and free from folds or creases. Wattles very long, thin and pendulous.
Neck: Long and fine, with abundant hackle flowing well over the shoulders.
Body: Rather long, fairly broad in front and tapering to the rear. Breast full at the neck and gradually decreasing towards the thighs. Back slanting downwards to the tail, short wings carried closely. Full tail, not carried too high, and with the sickles large and well curved.
Legs and feet: Rather long and slim. Shanks free of feathers. Toes four, slender and straight.

Plumage: Short and close.

Female

With the exception of the comb (which falls gracefully over either side of the face) the general characteristics are similar to those of the male, allowing for the natural sexual differences.

Colour

Male and female plumage: Black with a beetle-green sheen, and free of purple bars.
   In both sexes: Beak dark horn. Eyes black. Comb and wattles bright red. Face and ear-lobes white. Legs and feet pale slate

Weights

Male   3.20 kg (7 lb)
Female   2.70 kg (6 lb)

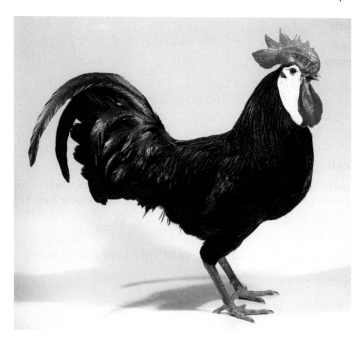

Spanish male

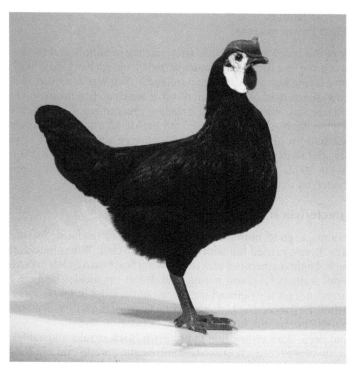

Spanish female

Scale of points

Face and lobes	35
Comb and wattles	15
Type	15
Size	15
Colour	10
Condition	10
	100

Serious defects

Blue, pink or red in face or lobes. Coarse 'cauliflower' face or lobes. Male's comb not erect, side sprigs on comb. Lobes pointed at the bottom. Black or dark legs or feet. Any deformity.

BANTAM

Bantam white-faced Spanish should follow exactly the large fowl Standard.

Weights

Male	1075 g (38 oz)
Female	910 g (32 oz)

SUFFOLK CHEQUER

Origin: Great Britain
Classification: True Bantam
Egg colour: Light brown to cream

The originator of this breed was Trevor Martin, starting in Suffolk and ending in Norfolk, England. He was given by a friend a miniature barred Plymouth Rock male in 1994. Another friend gave him a laying hen, probably not purebred, which was described as brown with a hint of pencilling. When the first eggs from this pair were hatched the male, though poorly barred, had a large tail, which started a breeding programme to produce a breed that resembled a Plymouth Rock with a longer tail as Mr Martin thought that the barred Plymouth Rock had an unfinished look. Although type drifted slightly away from the Plymouth Rock, the birds retained their attractive barring and were first shown in non-Standard classes in 2002. The selection process was based upon Darwinian principles. The breed was accepted by the Poultry Club of Great Britain in 2013.

General characteristics: male

Type: Body compact, good musculature. Back broad and inclined, in side view, to a shallow U shape. Breast carried full with shallow centre cleft. Wings moderate length but carried fairly low. Flight feathers not tucked up. Wing bows usually left uncovered by neck hackle. Main tail feathers long and broad, rounded at tip; sickles medium to long and moderately curved, not greatly outreaching the rest of the tail; side hangers very evident. In side view the whole bird should be U shaped with the top of the tail carried high at an angle of 45–90° from the horizontal, but not squirrel tailed.
Head: Bold and deep. Beak yellow (but faint brown-black streaks allowable), strong and of medium length. Not excessively curved. Comb single, upright and not too large. Well-defined five points with back of comb not held far beyond line of head and top of neck. Texture of comb not fine or smooth but tending to slight 'roughness'. Ear-lobes red with no

indication of white, of smooth texture and only slightly pendulous. Wattles medium size and rounded at the extremities, with texture similar to, but finer than, the comb.

Neck: Sturdy, carried upright but slightly curved when bird is alert, straight and upright when alarmed. Full neck hackle may reach, but not generally cover, the wing bows and shoulders.

Legs and feet: Legs planted firmly and medium width apart. Thighs medium thickness and medium in length. Shanks medium length, rounded, smooth and free from feathers. Toes four, strong and straight and of medium length.

Fluff: Barring to base of feathers but becoming fainter from tip. Moderately full.

Skin: Smooth and fine in texture.

Female

Usually a much darker appearance than the male. General characteristics similar, allowing for the natural sexual differences. Comb, ear-lobes, wattles much smaller than the male. Neck is medium in length, carried in similar fashion to male. The tail is full and pronounced with the main tail feathers carried almost as high as the head.

Colour

Male plumage: Ground colour grey-white. The black bars are fairly well defined but with some faint leakage in the light gaps between. The centres of the black bars have a beetle-green sheen fading away at the edges. The main body feathers have more or less straight black bars, becoming more chevron shaped on neck and saddle hackles, and tail hangers. Barring somewhat straighter on flight feathers.

Female plumage: Much darker than the male, the black bars being relatively wider with even greater leakage into the ground colour (this may be more or less between individuals). The main flight feathers have indistinct barring.

In both sexes: Legs and beak yellow, legs may have a faint red colouration laterally in the male, and front of shank often greyish-brown in the female, with an often more blotched beak. Comb, ear-lobes, face and wattles red. Eyes pale chestnut to amber

General remarks

The body conformation and head should be compact and held boldly with an upright and alert position. When alert, the male should appear U shaped from the side. The female is not so distinctly U shaped.

Defects

Completely black tail or flight feathers. Swollen or deformed rear end of comb in males. Twisted tail feather.

Weights

Male	1200–1500 g (2 lb 13 oz–3 lb 5 oz)	
	not to exceed maximum weight	
Female	1000–1250 g (2 lb 3 oz–2 lb 13 oz)	
	not to exceed maximum weight	

Scale of points

Type (U shape and carriage)	40
Tail size and carriage	10
Barring quality	10
Colour of black bars (beetle-green sheen)	5
Ground colour (lack of black leakage)	5
Legs and feet	10
Head (comb, ear-lobes, wattles, eyes)	10
Condition	10
	100

SULMTALER

LARGE FOWL

Origin: Austria
Classification: Heavy: Rare
Egg colour: Cream to light brown

The origin of the Sulmtaler lies south and south-west of Graz, capital of the Austrian county Stiermarken. Especially in the valleys of Kainach, Lassnitz, Sulm and Saggau (tal = valley), heavy fowls were bred for high-quality fattening, mainly being fed on locally grown maize. From 1865 to 1875, these birds were crossed with Cochin, Houdan and Dorkings and then crossed back again to the local fowls from Stiermarken. By 1900, the Sulmtaler had been developed as a breed in its own right, which then spread into Germany, The Netherlands and England. It is a hardy fowl, fast growing, easy to fatten and a good utility breed.

General characteristics: male

Type: Body full and deep, ratio of deepness to broadness 3:2. Back broad and almost horizontal, medium length with a full saddle and no development of a cushion. Breast very deep, broad, full and well rounded. Wings medium length carried closely. Abdomen broad and full. Thighs strong and well fleshed. Tail full, broad, carried at a 45° angle to the back.
Head: Medium size. Beak strong, slightly short. Eyes round, full and prominent. Comb single, straight, upright, medium size with a tendency to flyaway, evenly serrated but not too deep. Behind the comb is a small tuft of feather or tassel. Ear-lobes are medium size and oblong shape, of fine texture. Wattles are medium length, rounded, of fine texture. Face smooth and fine in texture.
Neck: Medium length, straight, with abundant neck hackle.
Legs and feet: Medium to short in length, clean shanks. Toes four, of medium length, straight and well spread.

Female

Allowing for the natural sexual differences, the hen has a small finely serrated comb, often called in Germany a 'Wickel' or S shape: a comb of which the front part falls to one side and the back to the other side (irregular). The crest at the back of the comb should be half-rounded and should not obscure the vision. The wattles are smaller than those of the male, the body appears heavier with a square, deep and full breast.

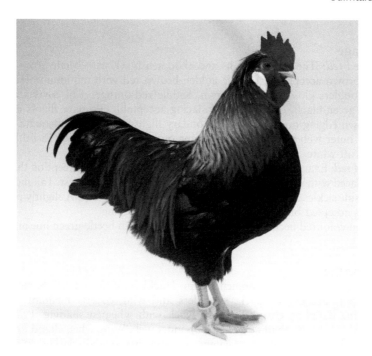

Black-breasted red Sulmtaler male, bantam

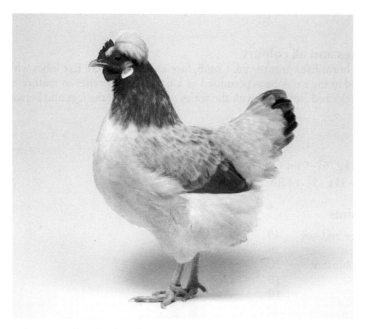

Wheaten Sulmtaler female, bantam

Colour

Male plumage
Black breasted red: The breast, thighs and abdomen black with beetle-green hue. Small amounts of brown acceptable. Hackle golden-brown red with minimum black striping. Back and shoulders glossy reddish-brown. Saddle red-orange. Tail coverts and sickles glossy beetle green-black, minimal brown lacing acceptable. Primary flights matte black with tan brown edging on outer web. Secondary flights must have adequate tan brown colouring on outer web to form triangle shape on wing when closed. Tassel brown-red. Undercolour off-white.

Blue breasted red: Exactly the same as in the black-red males with exception that all black parts are replaced with soft medium blue with slight lacing on the chest. Tail medium blue, with sickles, side sickles and tail coverts being medium to dark blue. A slightly paler hackle in the neck is accepted but not preferred. Minimal peppering.

Faults: Lemon-coloured neck hackle, black, especially with beetle-green hue anywhere on the plumage.

Female plumage
Wheaten: Breast, thighs and abdomen cream. Hackle rich brown-red. Some dull black striping or spots acceptable. Back, shoulders and wing coverts medium red brown-wheaten, giving dappling effect. Tail dull black with wheaten shading. Primaries and secondaries wheaten with shading of black on inner web. Wing when closed forms darker wheaten triangle. Crest is light wheaten. A somewhat overall darker colouration is accepted. Undercolour cream to pale grey.

Blue wheaten: Similar in all respects as in the wheaten females with the exception of wing feathers and tail, where the black is replaced with a soft even medium blue. Minimal peppering.

Faults: Pale-coloured neck hackle; black, especially with beetle-green hue, anywhere on the plumage.

In both sexes and all colours
Beak flesh or horn. Eyes orange-red. Comb, face and wattles red. Ear-lobes white. A small amount of red in the ear-lobe is permitted as a natural occurrence in mature birds over a year in age. Legs and feet white with the scales on the side of the legs and between the toes pinkish-red.

Weights

Male   3–4 kg ($6\frac{1}{2}$–9 lb)
Female   2.5–3 kg ($5\frac{1}{2}$–$6\frac{1}{2}$ lb)

Scale of points

Type, carriage and size	40
Head and crest	20
Colour and plumage	20
Condition	10
Legs	10
	100

Serious defects

Too small, too light, weak, not square enough, coarse bones, long legs, flat breast. Light eyes or fish eyes. Squirrel tailed.

BANTAM

Originated in West Germany, accepted to the Dutch Standard in 1986. Sulmtaler bantams are exact replicas of their large counterparts.

Weights

Male   1000–1200 g (36–43 oz)
Female 800–1000 g (28–36 oz)

SULTAN

LARGE FOWL

Origin: Turkey
Classification: Light: Rare
Egg colour: White

With head crest, beard, vulture hocks, feathered legs, five toes and snow-white plumage, Sultans have always been an ornamental breed. They were originally found strutting around the Sultan of Constantinople's palace garden. All today's Sultans are descended from a crate imported by Miss Elizabeth Watts of Hampstead in January 1854. They have never been numerous, but have a dedicated following.

General characteristics: male

General shape and carriage: Deep, but neat and compact, and very sprightly.
Type: Body rather long and very deep. Breast deep and prominent. Back short and straight. Wings large, long and carried low. Tail long, broad and carried open. Sickles very long and fine. Hangers numerous, long and fine. Coverts abundant and lengthy.
Head: Head medium size. Beak short and curved. Eyes bright. Comb very small, consisting of two spikes only, almost hidden by crest. Face covered with thick muffling. Nostrils horny and large, rising above the curved line of the beak. Crest large, globular and compact. Ear-lobes small and round. Beard very full, joining with the whiskers. Wattles very small, to be hardly perceptible.
Neck: Moderately short, slightly arched and carried well back.
Legs and feet: Thighs short, furnished with heavy vulture hocks to cover the joints. Shanks short, and well covered inside and out with feathers. Toes five in number and of moderate length, completely covered with feather.
Plumage: Long, very abundant and fairly soft.

Female

With the exception of the comb, which is smaller and barely visible, the general characteristics are similar to those of the male, allowing for the natural sexual differences.

Colour

Male and female plumage: Snow white throughout.
   In both sexes: Beak pale blue or white. Eyes red. Comb bright red. Face red. Ear-lobes and wattles bright red. Shanks and toes white or pale blue

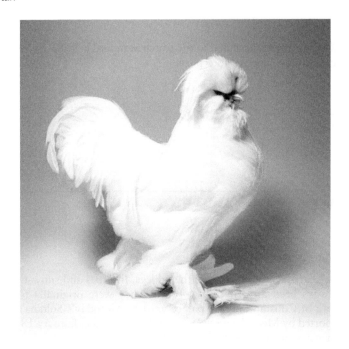

Sultan male

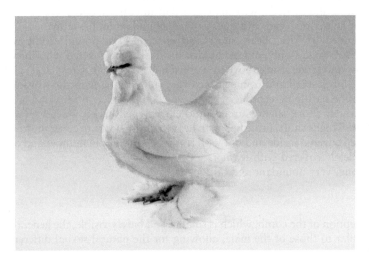

Sultan female

Weights

Male   2.70 kg (6 lb) max.
Female   2.00 kg (4½ lb)

Scale of points

Head and crest	15
Beard and muffling	15
Comb	5
Type and symmetry	12
Colour	15
Leg and foot feathering	15
Size	8
Condition	15
	100

Serious defects

Any deformity. Coloured plumage. Toes other than five in number.

BANTAM

Sultan bantams should follow exactly the large fowl Standard.

Weights

Male   680–790 g (24–28 oz)
Female   510–680 g (18–24 oz)

SUMATRA

LARGE FOWL

Origin: Asia
Classification: Light: Rare
Egg colour: White

The Sumatra, which comes from the island of Sumatra or the Malay Archipelago, was admitted to the American Standard in 1883. With the help of Lewis Wright and Frederick R. Eaton the British Standard was drawn up in 1906 under the name of Black Sumatra. A long, flowing tail, carried horizontally, and a pheasant-like carriage are distinguishing characteristics. Sumatras are prolific layers of white eggs and excellent sitters, especially being used to hatch waterfowl. In the late 1970s, a strain of bantams was recreated.

General characteristics: male

Carriage: Straight and upright in front, pheasant-like, giving a proud and stately appearance.
Type: Body rather long, very firm and muscular, broad, full and rounded breast. Back of medium length, broad at shoulders, very slightly tapering to tail. Saddle hackle very long and flowing. Stern narrower than shoulders, but firm and compact. Strong, long and large wings, carried with fronts lightly raised, the feathers folded very closely together, not carried drooping or over the back. Long drooping tail with a large quantity of sickles and

coverts, which should rise slightly above the stern and then fall streaming behind, nearly to the ground. Sickle and covert feathers not too broad.

Head: Skull small, fine and somewhat rounded. Beak strong, of medium length, slightly curved. Eyes large and very bright, with a quick and fearless expression. Comb pea, low in front, fitting closely, the smaller the better. Face smooth and of fine texture. Ear-lobes as small as possible and fitting very closely.

Neck: Rather long, and covered with very long and flowing hackle.

Legs and feet: Of strictly medium length, thick and strong. Thighs muscular, set well apart. Shanks straight and strong, set well apart, with smooth even scales, not flat or thin. (*Note*: Single spurs are allowed, but multiple spurs are a characteristic of the breed, so are preferred.) Feet broad and flat. Toes four, long, straight, spread well apart, with strong nails, the back toe standing well backward and flat on the ground.

Plumage: Very full and flowing, but not too soft or fluffy.

Female

Main tail feathers are wide and well spread, the top two feathers curved in a convex manner and carried nearly horizontally. Coverts are moderately long, wide and abundant. Otherwise the general characteristics are similar to those of the male, allowing for the natural sexual differences.

Colour

The black

Male and female plumage: Very rich beetle green (green-black) with as much sheen as possible.

The blue

Male plumage: Hackles, saddle, wing bows, back and tail very dark slate blue. Remainder medium slate blue, each feather to show lacing of darker shade as on the back.

Female plumage: Medium slate blue, laced with darker shade throughout, except head and neck, a dark slate blue.

The white

As the black but with plumage snow white throughout. Face as dark as possible.

In both sexes and all colours

Beak black. Eyes very dark brown or black (black preferred). Face, comb, ear-lobes and throat black or gypsy faced (black preferred). Legs and feet dark olive or black (black preferred).

Weights

Male   2.25–2.70 kg (5–6 lb)
Female   1.80 kg (4–5 lb)

Scale of points

Type	20
Head (beak 5, eyes 5, other points 10)	20
Colour	15
Feather, quantity of	15
Condition	15
Legs and feet	10
Neck	5
	100

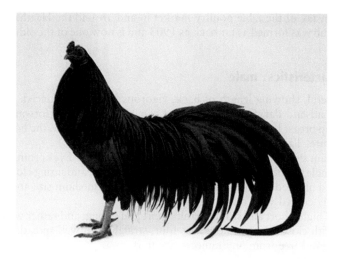

Sumatra

Serious defects

Single or rose comb. Any sign of dubbing. Red colour in comb, face or throat. Any sign of wattles. Other than four toes. Any deformity.

BANTAM

Sumatra bantams should follow exactly the large fowl Standard.

Weights

Male   735 g (26 oz)
Female   625 g (22 oz)

SUSSEX

LARGE FOWL

Origin: Great Britain
Classification: Heavy: Soft feather
Egg colour: Light brown

This is a very old breed, for, although we do not find it included in the first *Book of Standards* of 1865, at the first poultry show of 1845 the classification included Old Sussex or Kent fowls, Surrey fowls and Dorkings. The oldest variety of the Sussex is the speckled. Brahma, Cochin and silver-grey Dorking were used in the make-up of the light. The earlier reds had black breasts, until the red and brown became separate varieties. Old English Game has figured in the make-up of some strains of browns. Buffs appeared about 1920, clearly obtained by sex linkage within the breed. Whites came a few years later, as sports from lights. Silvers are the latest variety. The light is the most widely kept in this country today among Standard as well as commercial breeders. It is one of our most popular breeds for producing table birds. At the time when sex linkage held considerable popularity the light Sussex was one of the most popular breeds of the day, the females being in considerable demand for mating to gold males. At an even earlier stage, the Sussex breed formed the mainstay of the table poultry market in and around the Heathfield area. The Sussex Breed Club was formed as far back as 1903 and is now one of the oldest breed clubs in Britain.

General characteristics: male

Carriage: Graceful, showing length of back, vigorous and well balanced.
Type: Back broad and flat. Breast broad and square, carried well forward, with long, straight and deep breast bone. Shoulders wide. Wings carried close to the body. Skin clear and of fine texture. Tail moderate size, carried at an angle of 45°.
Head: Of medium size and fine quality. Beak short and curved. Eyes prominent, full and bright. Comb single, of medium size, evenly serrated and erect, and fitting close to the head. Face smooth and of good texture. Ear-lobes and wattles of medium size and fine texture.
Neck: Gracefully curved with fairly full hackle.
Legs and feet: Thighs short and stout. Shanks short and strong, and rather wide apart, free from feather, with close-fitting scales. Toes four, straight and well spread.
Plumage: Close and free from any unnecessary fluff.

Female

The general characteristics are similar to those of the male, allowing for the usual sexual differences.

Colour

The brown

Male plumage: Head and neck hackles rich dark mahogany striped with black. Saddle hackle same as neck hackle. Back and wing bows rich dark mahogany. Wing coverts forming the bar blue-black; secondaries and flights black, edged with brown. Breast, tail and thighs black.
Female plumage: Head and neck hackles brown striped with black. Back and wings dark brown, finely peppered with black. Breast and underbody clear pale wheaten-brown. Flights black, edged with brown. Tail black.

The buff

Male and female plumage: Body rich even golden-buff. Head and neck hackles buff, sharply striped with green-black. Wings buff, with black in the flights. Tail and coverts green-black. Dark in undercolour, not penalised at present, but buff is desirable.

The coronation

Best described as a light Sussex with blue in place of black markings. It was bred in 1936 and presented to the King in anticipation of his coronation, the colour emulating the Union flag: red, white and blue.

Male and female plumage: Head and hackles white, striped with even blue, blue centres of each feather to be entirely surrounded by a white margin. Wings white with blue in flights. Tail and coverts blue. Remainder pure white throughout.

The light

Male and female plumage: Head and neck hackles white, striped with black, the black centre of each feather to be entirely surrounded by a white margin. Wings white, with black in flights. Tail and coverts black. Remainder pure white throughout.

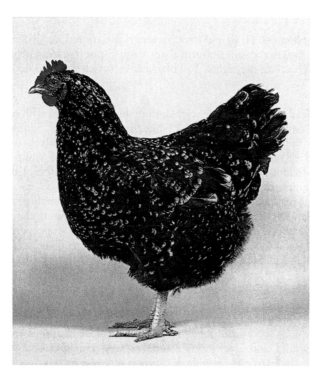

Speckled Sussex female

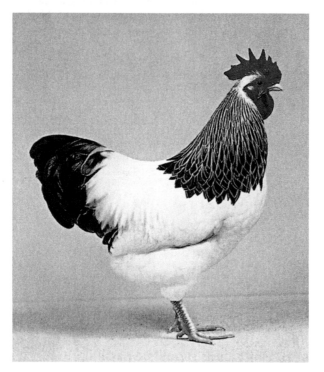

Light Sussex male, bantam

The red
Male and female plumage: Head and neck hackles rich dark red, striped with black. Body and wing bows rich dark red, one uniform shade throughout free from pepperiness. Wings rich dark red with black in the flights. Tail black; coverts rich dark red. Undercolour slate.

The speckled
Male plumage: Head and neck hackles rich dark mahogany, striped with black and tipped with white. Wing bows speckled; primaries white, brown and black. Saddle hackle similar to neck hackle. Tail main feathers black and white, sickles black with white tips. Remainder rich dark mahogany, each feather tipped with a small white spot, a narrow glossy black bar dividing the white from the remainder of the feather. Undercolour slate and red with a minimum of white.
Female plumage: Head, neck and body ground colour rich dark mahogany, each feather tipped with a small white spot, a narrow glossy black bar dividing the white from the remainder of the feathers, the mahogany part of feather free from pepperiness, neither of the colours to run into each other, and to show the three colours distinctly; undercolour as for male. Tail black and brown with white tip. Flights black, brown and white.

The silver
Male plumage: Head, neck and saddle hackles white striped with black, the black centre of each feather to be entirely surrounded by a white margin. Wing bows and back silvery white; coverts forming bar black; flights and secondaries black tinged with grey. Breast black with white shafts, and silver lacing round feathers. Thighs dark grey showing faint lacing. Tail black. Undercolour grey-black shading to white at skin.
Female plumage: Head and neck hackles as in the male. Back and wing bows greyish, each feather showing white shaft with fine silver lacing surrounding it; flights and secondaries greyish-black. Tail black. Breast and thighs lighter shade of greyish-black with white shafts and silver lacing to correspond with the top colour. Undercolour as in the male.

The white
Male and female plumage: Pure white throughout and to the skin.

In both sexes and all colours
Beak white or horn generally, dark or horn with the brown and dark shading to white with the silver. Eyes: brown – brown or red; buff, red and speckled – red; light, silver and white – orange. Face, comb, ear-lobes and wattles red. Shanks and feet white. Flesh and skin white.

Weights

Male   4.10 kg (9 lb) min.
Female   3.20 kg (7 lb) min.

Scale of points

Type, size and weight	40
Plumage and markings	35
Head	15
Legs and feet	10
	100

Serious defects (for which birds should be passed)

Other than four toes. Wry tail or any other deformity. Feather on shanks and toes. Rosecomb.

BANTAM

Sussex bantams conform to the large fowl Standard.

Weights

Male   1530 g (54 oz) max.
Female   1133 g (40 oz) max.

Scale of points

Type, size and weight   35
Hackle, tail and wing   20
Body colour   15
Head and eye   15
Feet and legs   _15_
                        100

TAIWAN

Origin: Taiwan
Classification: Asian Hardfeather. Large Fowl
Egg colour: White or light brown

The Taiwan is a very large bird of Malayoid type. The breed is sometimes called Taiwan Shamo, but as this is not a Japanese breed that name is incorrect. The breed's origins are in the island of Taiwan (formerly Formosa).

It is of a similar type to the Shamo, but generally bigger and heavier with longer legs.

There is a tendency in Europe to call any unidentifiable big Asian Game breed 'Taiwan', and these birds are often clumsy and of poor carriage. Birds of similar type have been called 'Saipan' in USA, also 'Chinese Shamo'.

The true breed is an impressive, strong, agile, upright bird.

General characteristics: male

Type and carriage: General appearance large, powerful, alert and agile, balanced and full of aggressive spirit.
Body: Large, firm and well muscled.
Breast: Broad and full with deep keel.
Back: Long, broadest at shoulders, sloping down towards tail and gradually tapering from upper side of thigh. Backbone straight.
Wings: Short, big, strong and bony, carried close to the body, not showing on the back.
Tail: Carried horizontally or below, length to give balance to the bird.
Head: Strong, deep and broad with wattles and ear-lobes small or absent. Beak powerful, broad and curved downwards, but not hooked. Eyes deep-set under overhanging brows. Comb triple or walnut, set low on a broad base.
Neck: Long, strong boned and slightly curved.
Legs and feet: Legs long, thick and strong with slight bend at hock. Thighs long, round and muscular, shanks shorter than thighs. Toes four, long and well spread. Hind toe straight and firm on the ground.
Plumage: Feathers short, narrow and hard, often showing red skin at throat, keel and point of wing.

Handling: Extremely firm fleshed, muscular and well balanced. Strong contraction of wings to body.

Female

The general characteristics are similar to those of the male, allowing for the natural sexual differences.

Colour

Black-red (wheaten) is the most common colour, but no colour or combination of colours is disqualified.

In both sexes and all colours
Beak yellow or horn. Legs and feet yellow, or yellow with blackish over-colour in dark-coloured birds. Comb, face, throat, ear-lobes and any exposed skin brilliant red. Eyes pearl to gold. Darker eyes acceptable in young birds.

Weights

Male   5–7 kg approx. (11–15 lb plus)
Female   4–5.5 kg approx. (9–12 lb plus)

Scale of points

Type and carriage	40
Head	20
Feather/condition	20
Legs and feet	20
	100

Serious defects

Lack of attitude. Lack of size. Overlarge comb. 'Duck' feet.

THAI GAME

Origin: Thailand
Classification: Asian Hardfeather. Large Fowl
Egg colour: White or light brown

Thai Game is a large game breed of Malayoid type, kept and fought in its country of origin – Thailand. The Standard is intended to preserve this original type. Their general appearance is very Shamo-like, the major differences being lighter build, a less exaggeratedly upright stance, less prominent shoulders and a characteristically full tail carried slightly above horizontal.

General characteristics: male

Type and carriage: General appearance agile, alert and full of aggressive spirit.
Body: Firm and well muscled.
Breast: Broad and full with deep keel.
Back: Long, broadest at shoulders, sloping down towards tail and gradually tapering from upper side of thigh. Backbone straight.

Wings: Short, strong and bony, carried close to the body, not showing on the back.

Tail: Characteristically full with strong sickles, rising above the horizontal to form a graceful curve. Length to give balance to the bird.

Head: Strong, deep and broad with wattles and ear-lobes small or absent. Beak powerful, broad and curved downwards, but not hooked. Eyes deep-set under overhanging brows. Comb triple or walnut, set low on a broad base.

Neck: Long, strong boned and slightly curved.

Legs and feet: Legs medium to long, thick and strong with slight bend at hock. Thighs long, round and muscular. Shanks strong and round. Toes four, long and well spread. Hind toe straight and firm on the ground.

Plumage: Feathers short, narrow and hard, often showing red skin at throat, keel and point of wing.

Handling: Extremely firm fleshed, muscular and well balanced. Strong contraction of wings to body.

Female

The general characteristics are similar to those of the male, allowing for the natural sexual differences.

Colour

No colour or combination of colours is disqualified.

In both sexes and all colours

Beak yellow or horn. Legs and feet pale preferred, but any colour acceptable. Comb, face, throat, ear-lobes and any exposed skin brilliant red. Eyes pearl to gold. Darker eyes acceptable in young birds.

Weights

Male   3.5 kg approx. (7 lb 12 oz)
Female   2.5 kg approx. (5 lb 8 oz)

Scale of points

Type and carriage   40
Head   20
Feather/condition   20
Legs and feet   <u>20</u>
                    100

Serious defects

Lack of attitude. Overlarge comb. 'Duck' feet.

THÜRINGIAN

Origin: Germany
Classification: Light: Rare
Egg colour: White

The first recorded mention of these fowls in the Thüringen state of Germany was in 1793. They were known as Thüringer Pausbäckchen until they were standardised under their present German name of Thüringer Barthuhn on 8 March 1907. They have been seen at British poultry shows since about 2000 but initially only in the chamois and silver spangled colour varieties, with other colours appearing later. They are gaining in popularity in Britain, however maintaining the small size of the bantams remains a priority.

General characteristics: male

Type: Body full and strong. Breast broad and full. Abdomen well developed, full and broad. Back moderately long and broad, tapering towards tail with a full saddle, carried nearly horizontally, sloping slightly down with rise to base of tail. Wings long and broad, carried well up. Tail full and well spread, with rather long, well-curved sickles. Tail is carried about 45° above the horizontal. Carriage is lively and active.

Head: Medium size, well rounded and broad. Beak short and broad, well curved. Eyes large. Comb single, upright, no more than medium sized, finely and evenly serrated with five or six points, well-rounded behind, curved down but clear of head. Ear-lobes small, completely covered by full beard. Wattles absent or very small, not visible because of beard. Beard long feathered, full and undivided right up around the face and cheeks. This is an important point, as Thüringian Beardeds do not have the tri-lobed formation seen on some other bearded breeds.

Neck: Medium length, somewhat curved and richly feathered, especially to the rear.

Legs and feet: Thighs short and strong with full but not fluffy feather. Shanks medium length, smooth and free of feather. Toes four, well spaced.

Female

The general characteristics are as for the male, allowing for the natural sexual differences, except that the neck hackle is particularly full at the rear, forming the characteristic ruffle. This becomes more pronounced in older hens. The comb is small and upright.

Colour

The black

Male and female plumage: Glossy black with a beetle-green sheen. Undercolour dark slate grey to black.

In both sexes: Legs and beak dark grey to black. Eyes dark brown.

Colour defects: Dull plumage, purple stripes, strong blue sheen, red feathers.

The silver spangled

Male plumage: Ground colour silver-white with black underfluff. Head, neck and saddle silver-white tipped with black. Shoulders silver-white. Primaries black with silver and white tips. Secondaries inner web silver mottled black, outer web silver so that a purely silver wing edge can be seen when closed. Breast silver-white with black spangles at the ends of the feathers. Beard, abdomen and tail green-black. Slight white edging of sickles is permitted.

Female plumage: Ground colour, underfluff and wing markings as on male. Head, beard and abdomen black. Neck, breast, back and tail all silver-white with black spangles towards the end.

In both sexes: Legs slate blue. Eyes orange to reddish-brown.

Colour defects: Yellow tinge. Too much white in the tail, incorrect markings.

The gold spangled

Male and female plumage: As for silver spangled, except that the ground colour is gold-brown to gold-red. Light golden-brown flecking allowed in sickles. Small white feather tips permitted in primaries.

In both sexes: Legs slate blue. Eyes brown to orange.

Colour defects: Too light or too dark base colour or irregular shading. Too much brown in the tail, strong mottling in hackle feathers of the hen.

The chamois spangled

Male and female plumage: As for silver spangled, except that the ground colour is buff, the cock a little more intense in colour than the female. The spotted pattern is creamy white. Buff is allowed in the sickles. Creamy white beard.

In both sexes: Legs slate blue. Eyes orange to reddish-brown.

Colour defects: Too light, brownish or strong non-Standard base colour. Incorrect marking, which should be as in silver spangled.

The white

Male and female plumage: Pure white.

In both sexes: Legs blue but white/flesh permitted. Eyes orange.

Colour defects: Strong yellow tinge. Different coloured feathers.

The cuckoo

Male and female plumage: Each feather has barring of black and light blue slightly arched transversely, the dark part of the feathers being wider than the light. The markings are not strongly defined, the barring being blurred. Male and female have no difference in width of barring.

In both sexes: Legs flesh but grey permitted. Eyes orange.

Colour defects: Strongly blurred markings, brown tinge, too much white in sickles.

The blue laced

Male and female plumage: Pure grey-blue base colour with each feather with a darker black-blue edge. Head, neck and hackles of the cock dark blue. Undercolour dark slate blue.

In both sexes: Legs dark slate grey. Eyes brown.

Colour defects: Brownish or sooty base colour. Missing or blurred lacing.

The partridge

Male plumage: Head dark gold, hackles dark gold with wide black feather shafts. Back, shoulders and wing coverts red-gold. Primaries black with narrow brown outer edge. Secondaries black on feather ends, outer web brown forming the wing triangle. Black colour has green sheen. Beard, chest, legs and abdomen black. Tail black with green sheen.

Female plumage: Head dark gold colour, hackles dark gold with wide black feather shafts. Body grey-brown plumage with a clearly prominent and highly uniform black shaft line, light brown highlights, light brown quills. Primaries black with mottled brown rim. Secondaries brown inside web black, outside brown with black flecking. Beard rust, rusty red breast becoming grey towards the belly. Legs and abdomen grey-brown, tail dark brown.

In both sexes: Legs slate blue. Eyes reddish-brown to orange.

Colour defects: Brown or buff flecking, too dark top colour, chest or leg markings (leakage). In the hen, bright primary colour, too weak partridge markings.

Weights

Male $\quad$ 2–2.5 kg (4$\frac{1}{2}$–5$\frac{1}{2}$ lb)
Female $\quad$ 1.5–2 kg (3$\frac{1}{2}$–4$\frac{1}{2}$ lb)

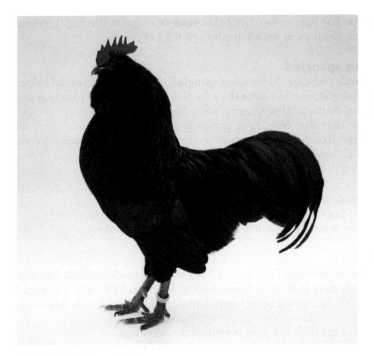

Black Thüringian male, bantam

Scale of points

Type	25
Colour and markings	20
Head	10
Beard	15
Legs and feet	10
Size	10
Condition	10
	100

Serious defects

Uneven, folded or twisted comb, or side sprigs. Narrow, divided or underdeveloped beard. Visible wattles. Squirrel or low tail carriage. Lack of furnishings in male or lack of fullness in neck feather of female. Incorrect plumage colour or colour of legs or feet, as specified.

BANTAM

Thüringian bantams should follow exactly the large fowl Standard.

Weights

Male   700–800 g (25–28 oz)
Female 600–700 g (21–25 oz)

TRANSYLVANIAN NAKED NECK

LARGE FOWL

Origin: Europe
Classification: Heavy: Rare
Egg colour: Light brown

Transylvania has been part of Romania since 1918, but was once part of the Ottoman Turkish Empire, and then part of the Austro-Hungarian Empire. Naked Neck chickens have been recorded in many parts of Europe and the Middle East, so it is difficult to be sure about their origin. Exhibition Naked Necks, bred to a Standard with completely bare necks, have always been most popular in Austria and Germany: there were 110 Naked Necks at the 1907 Leipzig Show. Karl Huth exhibited the first recorded Naked Neck bantams at the 1898 German National Show. They have never been more than a rare novelty in the UK.

They are active foragers and productive birds, and their bare necks and reduced plumage are not a problem, especially in warm climates. Indeed, the speed with which cockerels can be hand plucked and ready for cooking has no doubt ensured their popularity among smallholders. There are now several naked-necked broiler hybrids, a good example of how even the most unexpected old breed can be useful in today's poultry industry.

General characteristics: male

Carriage: Alert, upright and bold.
Type: Body large, deep and compact, well balanced and symmetrical. Back broad and of medium length, saddle hackle long and abundant. Breast broad and well rounded. Wings of medium size, carried well up. Tail medium size carried at an angle of 45°, sickles large and well curved.
Head: Medium size. Beak short, stout and slightly curved. Eyes large, bright and prominent. Comb single, medium in size, straight and erect, with well-formed spikes. Face smooth. Ear-lobes and wattles of medium size, fine in texture and smooth: the head to carry an oval cap of feathers surrounding the base of the comb, even in shape, with a small tassel at the back.
Neck: Of medium length, slightly curved, completely without feathering, stubs or fluff: the skin of the neck to be smooth and fine in texture, free from wrinkles or roughness. (A small tassel of feathers at the bottom of the neck above the breast feathers is permitted, but not desirable.)
Legs and feet: Legs of medium length, strong and stout. Shanks round and free of feathers. Toes four, strong, straight and well spread.

Female

The general characteristics are similar to those of the male, allowing for the natural sexual differences.

Colour

The black
Male and female plumage: Dense black with a rich green sheen.

The white
Male and female plumage: Snow white throughout.

The cuckoo
Male and female plumage: Colour as in Cochin.

The buff
Male and female plumage: Colour as in buff Rocks.

The red
Male and female plumage: Colour as in Rhode Island Reds.

The blue
Male and female plumage: Colour as in blue Minorca.

In both sexes and all colours
Eyes orange. Face, comb, ear-lobes, wattles and neck bright red. Buff, cuckoo, red and white varieties have a white or light horn beak and white legs and feet. Blacks and blues have a dark horn or black beak and the legs and feet are black or slate blue.

Weights
Male   3.20–3.60 kg (7–8 lb)
Female   2.50–2.70 kg (5½–6½ lb)

Scale of points
Type and carriage	20
Head and neck	35
Legs and feet	10
Colour and markings	15
Size	10
Condition	10
	100

Serious defects
Any noticeable feather, fluff or stubs on the neck. Absence of cap of feathers on the head. Feathered legs. Other than four toes. Any deformity.

BANTAM
Bantam Naked Necks are to be replicas of their large fowl counterparts.

Weights
Male   910 g (32 oz)
Female   680 g (24 oz)

TUZO

Origin: USA and Europe from Oriental bloodlines
Classification: Asian Hardfeather. True Bantam
Egg colour: White or light brown

The Tuzo is a hard feather true bantam developed in the USA and Europe from Oriental bloodlines. (Standardised in Germany in 1983.)

General characteristics: male

Type and carriage: Small and elegant with upright stance.
Body: Extremely firm and muscular. Broad at front, becoming narrower towards the saddle.
Breast: Broad and well rounded, thrust forward a little.
Back: Short and straight. Held at a steep angle. Saddle feathers short and narrow.
Wings: Short and broad, fitting close to the body but with prominent shoulders. Showing bare red skin at point of wing.
Tail: Well developed. Carried horizontally or a little below and only moderately curved.
Head: Broad and rounded with a short, strong, well-curved beak. Well-developed brows and protruding cheeks. Small triple comb. Wattles and lobes (if any) insignificant. In old birds there is a definite dewlap.
Neck: Medium length, well curved, held upright. Neck hackle short, not covering shoulders.
Legs and feet: Thighs strong with slight bend at hock. Shanks medium length, strong and straight. Toes four, straight.
Plumage: Very narrow, short, hard and brilliant.
Handling: Extremely firm fleshed, muscular and well balanced.

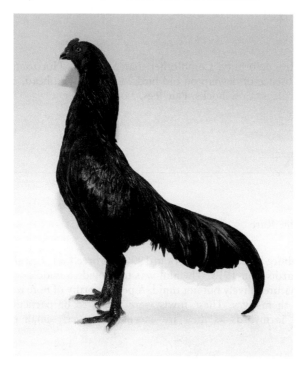

Black Tuzo male

Female

The general characteristics are similar to those of the male, allowing for the natural sexual differences. Generally of a rather less upright stance.

Colour

Male and female: Plumage black with green sheen. Blue and white are also accepted. In the white, the colour should be pure white throughout. In the blue, the body colour should be a medium slate blue with or without darker lacing, and with darker slate-blue head and neck in females; hackle, saddle, wingbow and tail in males.

Beak dark horn to black. Legs and feet dark olive to black, with light soles. Comb, face, ear-lobes and wattles bright red in males, face may be darker in females. Eyes pearl to yellow (darker allowed in young birds).

Weights

Male   1–1.5 kg (2 lb 4 oz–3 lb 7 oz)
Female   1 kg approx. (2 lb 4 oz)

Scale of points

Type and carriage   40
Plumage quality   10
Colour   10
Head   20
Legs and feet   10
Condition   <u>10</u>
                    100

Serious defects

Lack of attitude. Any deformity. Comb other than Standard. Horizontal carriage. Wattles too big. Absence of dewlap on old birds. Long pointed head. Pointed beak. Short legs. Cow hocks. Pale legs. Loose feather.

VORWERK

LARGE FOWL

Origin: Germany
Classification: Light: Rare
Egg colour: Cream

Originated in Hamburg by Oskar Vorwerk in 1900, the breed was first shown at Hanover in 1912 and standardised in 1913. The aim was to provide a middle-weight economical utility fowl, good natured, lively but not timid. A point worthy of note is the compatibility of males amongst themselves. These fowls were found to be particularly suitable for smallholdings and farmyards as they are excellent foragers, small eaters and quick maturing.

General characteristics: male

Carriage: Very powerful, compact utility shape, carriage low rather than high, not too much bone, markings the same in both sexes, lively but not timid.
Type: Body of considerable size, as broad and deep as possible like a rounded rectangle. Back broad, slightly sloping with a full saddle. Breast broad, deep and well rounded. Wings closely carried. Tail moderately tight, held at a lowish angle with well-rounded sickles of moderate length.
Head: Medium size and moderately broad. Face covered with small feathers. Comb single, of medium size at the most, with four to six serrations. Wattles of medium length, well rounded. Lobes of barely average size. Eyes alert.

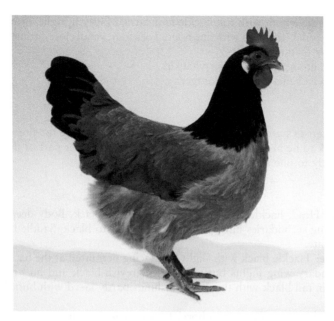

Vorwerk female, large

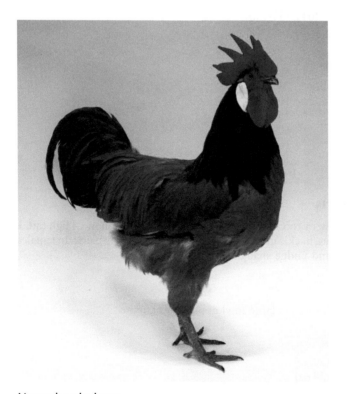

Vorwerk male, large

Neck: Of moderate length with full hackle and carried fairly upright, proudly.
Legs and feet: Moderate length with fine bone. Toes four, small close-fitting scales. Thighs fleshy and tightly feathered.
Plumage: Close fitting, glossy, velvety hackle.
Handling: Firm as befits an active forager.

Female

General characteristics are similar to those of the male, allowing for the natural sexual differences. Back to be broad with almost no cushion. The latter part of the small comb may bend slightly to one side.

Colour

Male plumage: Head, hackle and tail should be velvety black. Body deep buff, under-colour grey. Wing secondaries buff; primaries dark grey to black. Saddle buff with light striping. Legs slate.
Female plumage: Hackle black with slight buff lacing permitted at the back of the head. Body and secondary wing flights buff; primaries greyish-black and buff mixed. Visible parts of the main tail black with the tail furnishings partly laced with buff. Undercolour grey.

In both sexes: Beak greyish-blue to horn. Eyes orange or orange-red. Comb, face and wattles red. Lobes white. Legs and feet slate

Weights

Male   2.50–3.20 kg ($5\frac{1}{2}$–7 lb)
Female   2.00–2.50 kg ($4\frac{1}{2}$–$5\frac{1}{2}$ lb)

Scale of points

Type/utility quality	25
Head	10
Colour	25
Legs and feet	10
Size	15
Condition	15
	100

Serious defects

Body too narrow or too light. Carriage too high. Coarse bone. High tail. Lobes too red. Pale legs. In males, hackle unduly buff or grey, saddle nearly black. In females, lack of black in neck or tail and undue spangling in body feathers.

BANTAM

The same Standard as in large fowl applies to bantams.

Weights

Male   910 g (32 oz)
Female   680 g (24 oz)

WELSUMMER

LARGE FOWL

Origin: The Netherlands
Classification: Light: Soft feather
Egg colour: Deep red-brown

Named after the village of Welsum, this Dutch breed has in its make-up such breeds as the partridge Cochin, partridge Wyandotte and partridge Leghorn, and still later the Barnevelder and the Rhode Island Red. In 1928, stock was imported into this country from The Netherlands, in particular for its large brown egg, which remains its special feature, some products being mottled with brown spots. It has distinctive markings and colour, and comes into the light-breed category, although it has good body size. It enters the medium class in the country of its origin. Judges and breeders work to a Standard that values indications of productiveness, so that laying merits can be combined with beauty.

General characteristics: male

Carriage: Upright, alert and active.
Type: Body well built on good constitutional lines. Back broad and long. Breast full, well rounded and broad. Wings moderately long, carried closely to the sides. Tail fairly large and full, carried high, but not squirrel. Abdomen long, deep and wide.
Head: Symmetrical, well balanced, of fine quality without coarseness, excesses or exaggeration. Skull refined, especially at back. Beak strong, short and deep. Eyes keen in expression, bold, full, highly placed in skull and standing out prominently when viewed from front or back; pupils large and free from defective shape. Comb single, of medium size, firm, upright, free from any twists or excess around nostrils, clear of nostrils, and of fine, silky texture, five to seven broad and even serrations, the back following closely but not touching the line of the skull and neck. Face smooth, open and of silky texture, free from wrinkles or surfeit of flesh and without overhanging eyebrows. Ear-lobes small and almond shaped. Wattles of medium size, fine and silky texture and close together.
Neck: Fairly long, slender at top but finishing with abundant hackle.
Legs and feet: Thighs to show clear of body without loss of breast. Shanks of medium length, medium bone and well set apart, free from feathers and with soft, pliable sinews, free from coarseness. Toes four, long, straight and well spread out, back toe to follow in straight line, free from feathers between toes.
Plumage: Tight, silky and waxy, free from excess or coarseness, silky at abdomen and free from bagginess at thighs.
Handling: Compact, firm and neat bone throughout.

Female

The general characteristics are similar to those of the male, allowing for the natural sexual differences.

Handling: Pelvic bones fine and pliable; abdomen pliable; flesh and skin of fine texture and free from coarseness; plumage sleek; abdomen capacious, but well supported by long breastbone and not drooping; general handling of a fit, keen and active layer.

Colour

Male plumage: Head and neck rich golden-brown. Hackles rich golden-brown as uniform as possible, free from black striping, yet underparts (out of sight) may show a little striping at present. Back, shoulder coverts and wing bows bright red-brown. Wing coverts black with green sheen forming a broad bar across (a little brown peppering at present permissible); primaries (out of sight when wing is closed) inner web black, outer web brown; secondaries outer web brown, inner web black with brown peppering. Tail (main) black with a beetle-green sheen; coverts upper black, lower black edged with brown. Breast black with red mottling. Abdominal and thigh fluff black and red mottled.

Female plumage: Head golden-brown. Hackle golden-brown or copper, the lower feathers with black striping and golden shaft. Breast rich chestnut-red going well down to the lower parts. Back and wing bows reddish-brown, each feather stippled or peppered with black specks (i.e. partridge marking), shaft of feather showing lighter and very distinct. Wing bars chestnut-brown; primaries inner web black, outer brown; secondaries outer web brown, coarsely stippled with black, inner web black, slightly peppered with brown. Abdomen and thighs brown with grey shading. Tail black, outer feathers pencilled with brown.

The silver duckwing

Male plumage: Head, neck and hackles white. Breast black with white mottling. Back shoulder coverts and wing bows white. Wing primaries flight feathers (out of sight as wings closed) inner web black, outer web white; secondaries outer web white, inner web black, with white peppering; coverts black with green sheen forming a broad bar across primaries. Tail main black with beetle-green sheen; coverts upper black, lower black, edged with white. Abdominal and thigh fluff black with white mottling.

Female plumage: Head and skull silvery white. Hackle silvery white and lower feathers with black striping and white shaft. Breast salmon-red or robin red. Back and wing bows silvery grey, each feather stippled or peppered with black specks (i.e. partridge marking), shaft of feather showing light and very distinct. Wing bars silvery grey; primaries inner web black, outer web white; secondaries outer web white, coarsely stippled with black, inner web black slightly peppered with white. Abdomen and thighs silvery grey. Tail black, outer feathers pencilled with white.

In both sexes and colours

Beak yellow or horn. Eyes red. Comb, face, ear-lobes and wattles bright red. Legs and feet yellow. Undercolour dark slate grey.

Weights

Cock 3.20 kg (7 lb) Cockerel 2.70 kg (6 lb)
Hen 2.70 kg (6 lb) Pullet 2.00–2.25 kg ($4\frac{1}{2}$–5 lb)

These weights should be taken as minimum Standards.

Scale of points

General type	20
Handling, size and indications of productiveness	30
Head	10
Legs and feet	10
Colour	20
Condition	10
	100

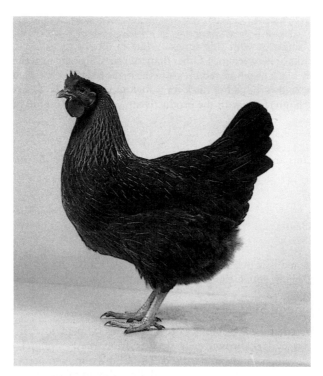

Welsummer female, large

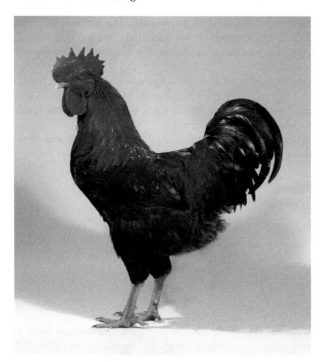

Welsummer male, large

Serious defects

Comb other than single or with side sprigs. White in lobe. Excessive white in plumage. Feather on legs, hocks or between toes. Other than four toes. Striping in neck hackle or saddle of male. Absolutely black or whole red breast in the male. Salmon breast in the female. Legs other than yellow. Badly crooked or duck toes. Any body deformity. Coarseness, beefiness and anything which interferes with the productiveness and general utility of the breed.

BANTAM

Welsummer bantams are to be miniatures of the large fowl and so the Standard for large applies.

Weights

Male   1020 g (36 oz)
Female   790 g (28 oz)

At present, more realistic maximum weights are male 1360 g (48 oz) and female 1133 g (40 oz). All things being equal, the smaller bird is the preferred.

The Welsummer egg Standard

The brown egg preceded the Welsummer breed. Various farmers' fowl around the village of Welsum laid large dark brown eggs. It was from these mongrel flocks that the Welsummer was developed and standardised. The Club's aim is to perpetuate the laying qualities and brown egg capabilities of the breed. Eggs should follow the weight Standards laid out by the Poultry Club in the unified Egg Standard.

Colour: A rich deep red-brown, as dark as possible. The pigment to be evenly distributed over the whole surface. Some products are speckled, mottled and occasionally blotched.
Shape: Egg shaped: the top, containing the air space, domed, the bottom less so and more pointed, with ample girth.
Size: Exhibition eggs should be of good size. Eggs should follow the weight Standards laid out by the Poultry Club in the unified Egg Standard.
Shell texture: Matt, smooth and free from ridges, pimples or porosity. Glossy eggs can be produced but the matt egg is the preferred.
Appearance and bloom: Exhibition eggs should be fresh, clean, with new laid bloom and with minimal nest marks and scratches.

Scale of points

Colour	25
Shape	25
Size	20
Shell texture	20
Appearance and bloom	10
	100

Serious defects

Pale colour. Poor shape: spherical, narrow or equally domed at both ends. Small size. Uneven shell texture: ridges, calcareous pimples or roughness at either end. Very glossy or thin and porous shell. Excessive nest marks or scratches. Dirty or stained. Anything interfering with hatchability. Staleness. When more than one egg forms a single exhibit they should match and be similar in all respects: failure to do so constitutes a serious defect.

WYANDOTTE

LARGE FOWL

Origin: America
Classification: Heavy: Soft feather
Egg colour: Brown

The first variety of the Wyandotte family was the silver laced, originated in America, where it was standardised in 1883. The variety was introduced into England at the time, and our breeders immediately perfected the lacings and open ground colouring. Partridge Cochin and gold spangled Hamburgh males were crossed with the silver females to produce the gold laced variety. The white Wyandotte came as a sport from the silver laced; the buff followed by crossing buff Cochin with the silver laced. In 1896, the partridge variety was introduced from America, the result of blending partridge Cochin and Indian Game blood with that of the gold laced, the variety being perfected for markings in England. It was once called the gold pencilled, and the silver pencilled soon followed from partridge Wyandotte and dark Brahma crossings. Columbians were the result of crossing the white Wyandotte with the barred Rock, and it was the crossing of the gold laced and the white varieties which produced the buff laced and the blue laced, first seen here in 1897. Blacks, blues and barred have been made in different ways in this country. The latest variety to be introduced is the red, created in Lancashire, from the gold laced variety, with selective matings with white Wyandotte, Barnevelder and Rhode Island Red. It is clear that, while the family of the Wyandotte is large, every variety is a made one from various blendings of breeds.

General characteristics: male

Carriage: Graceful, well balanced, alert and active, but docile.
Type: Body short and deep with well-rounded sides. Back broad and short with full and broad saddle rising with a concave sweep to the tail. Breast full, broad and round with a straight keel bone. Wings of medium size, nicely folded to the side. Tail medium size but full and spread at the base, the main feathers carried rather upright, the sickles of medium length.
Head: Short and broad. Beak stout and well curved. Eyes intelligent and prominent. Comb rose, firmly and evenly set on head, medium in height and width, low, and square at front, gradually tapering towards the back and terminating in a well-defined spike (or leader), which should follow the curve of the neck without any upward tendency. The top should be oval and covered with small and rounded points; the side outline being convex to conform to the shape of the skull. Face smooth and fine in texture. Ear-lobes oblong, wattles medium length, fine in texture.
Neck: Of medium length and well arched with full hackle.
Legs and feet: Thighs of medium length, well covered with soft feathers; the fluff fairly close and silky. Shanks medium in length, strong, well rounded, good quality, and free of feather or fluff. Toes four, straight and well spread.
Plumage: Fairly close and silky, not too abundant or fluffy.

Female

The general characteristics are similar to those of the male, allowing for the natural sexual differences.

Colour

The barred
Male and female plumage: Equal width of black (with beetle-green sheen) and white bars, clear-cut and horizontal, carried to the skin and finished with a black tip. It is important that there is a sharpness in the barring and that there should be an overall flow making a distinct pattern over the body. Undercolour barred to the skin with as many bars as possible. Any black or white feathers in wings or body is a disqualification.
Colour defects: Irregular and broken barring, V-shaped barring with the exception of the neck and saddle hackles of the male due to the natural shape of the barbs. Brassiness in any part of the plumage.

The black
Male plumage: Black with beetle-green sheen, undercolour as dark (black) as possible but some white or grey undercolour is permissible as long as it does not show through.
Female plumage: Black with beetle-green sheen, undercolour as dark (black) as possible.

The blue
Male and female plumage: One even shade of blue, light to dark, but medium preferred; a clear solid blue, free from mealiness, 'pepper', sandiness or bronze, and quite clear of lacing; a 'self colour' in fact.

The lavender
Male and female plumage: The lavender is not a lighter shade of the blue Wyandotte. It is different genetically and is of a lighter more silver tint without the darker shade associated with the normal blue. The silver tint is more pronounced on the neck and saddle hackles of the male. All other parts to be an even shade of lavender. Feathers to have a lavender shaft, the undercolour to be lavender as close to the top colour as possible.

The buff
Male and female plumage: Clear, sound buff throughout to skin, allowing greater lustre on the hackles and wing bows of the male. With these exceptions the colour should be perfectly uniform, but washiness or a red tinge, mealiness or 'pepper' to be avoided.

The chocolate
Male plumage: To be a distinct two-tone chocolate. The breast and thighs to be an even shade of chocolate brown. The undercolour to be as dark a shade of chocolate as possible.
Female plumage: All parts to be an even shade of chocolate, including the undercolour, which is a uniform shade of chocolate.

The Columbian
Male and female plumage: Pearl-white with black markings. Primaries (wing) black or black edged with white; secondaries black inner web and white outer. The male's neck hackle broadly striped with intense black down the centre of each feather, such stripe entirely surrounded by a clearly defined white margin and finishing with a decided white point (free from black outer edging or black tips). Saddle hackle white. Tail glossy green-black, coverts either laced or not with white. The female's hackle bright intense black, each feather entirely surrounded by a well-defined white margin. Tail feathers black, except the top pair, which may or may not be laced with white. Remainder (in both sexes) white, entirely free of ticking, with slate or blue-white undercolour.

The partridge

Male plumage: Head dark orange. Hackles bright orange-yellow, shading to bright lemon-yellow, free from washiness, each feather having a clearly defined glossy black stripe down the middle, not running out at the tip, and free from light shaft. Back and shoulders bright red of a scarlet shade, free from maroon or purple tint. Wing bars solid, glossy black; primaries solid black, free from white; secondaries rich bay outer web and black inner and end of feather, the rich bay alone showing when the wing is closed. Undercolour black or dark grey, free from white. Breast and fluff metallic black, free from red or grey ticking. Tail (including sickles and tail coverts) metallic black, free from white at roots.

Female plumage: Head and hackle rich golden-yellow, the larger feathers finely and clearly pencilled. Breast, back, cushion and wings soft light partridge brown, quite even and free from red or yellow tinge, each feather plentifully and distinctly pencilled with black, the pencilling to follow the form of the feather, and to be even and uniform throughout. Fine, sharply defined pencilling with three or more distinct lines of black is preferred to coarse, broad marking, especially in females, in which the pencilling is generally better defined than in pullets. Pencilling that runs into the brown, peppery markings and uneven, broken or barred pencilling constitute defects. Light shafts to feathers on the breast must be penalised. Fluff brown (same shade as body), as clearly pencilled as possible. Primaries (wing) black; secondaries brown (same shade as body), pencilled with black on outer web, black on inner web, showing pencilling when the wing is closed. Tail black, with or without brown markings, with clearly pencilled feathers up to the point of the tail.

The blue partridge

Male and female plumage: Similar to that of the partridge, with the exception that the black of the partridge is replaced by grey-blue. The grey-blue colour should be bright and as even as possible in all areas. It is permissible for the blue partridge to be a little lighter in ground colour in the female and a little lighter in the red, orange and lemon areas in the male than the partridge.

The silver pencilled

Male and female plumage: Except that the ground is silver-white in the male and steel grey in the female, instead of red, brown, etc. (of various shades), the silver pencilled is similar to the partridge.

The blue silver pencilled

Male and female plumage: Similar to that of the silver pencilled, with the exception that the black of the silver pencilled is replaced by grey-blue. The grey-blue colour should be bright and as even as possible in all areas.

The red

Male and female plumage: Surface rich, bright, glossy red. Neck hackle of medium shade to match body colour, with a black stripe down the centre of each feather at the lower part. Tail and coverts green-black. Wing primaries inner half black, outer half red; secondaries inner half dark slate or black, outer half to match body. Undercolour dark or slate, clearly defined.

The white

Male and female plumage: Pure white, free from yellow or straw tinge.

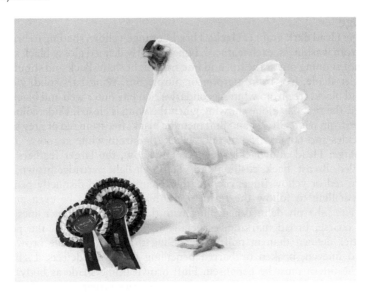

White Wyandotte female, large

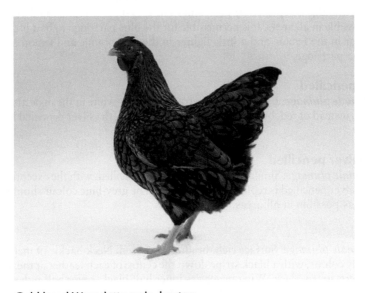

Gold laced Wyandotte male, bantam

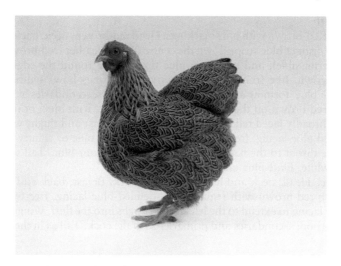

Partridge Wyandotte female, bantam

The silver laced

Male plumage: Silvery white with black markings. Head silvery white. Neck, hackles and saddle silvery white with distinct black stripe through the centre of each feather (white at centre of black stripe is permissible), free from ticks. Back and shoulders silvery white, free from yellow or straw colour. Wing bows silvery white; coverts evenly laced, forming at least two well-defined bars; secondaries black on inner and wide white stripe on outer web, the edge laced with black; primaries black on inner web and broadly laced white on outer edge. Breast and thighs the web white with well-defined black lacing, free from double or white outer lacing, lacing regular from throat to back of thighs, showing green lustre. Undercolour dark slate. True tail feathers, sickles and coverts black with green lustre. Fluff black or dark slate.

Female plumage: Head, neck and hackle as in the cock. Breast, back and thighs undercolour dark slate, web white with regular, well-defined black lacing, free from double or outer lacing and showing green lustre. Wings same as back on the broad portion; secondaries and primaries as in the cock. Tail black showing green lustre, the coverts black with a white centre to each feather. Fluff as in the cock.

The gold laced

Male plumage: Rich golden-bay with black markings. Head golden-bay; neck, hackles and saddle golden-bay with distinct black stripe down the centre of each feather (golden-bay at centre of black stripe is permissible), free from ticks, black outer edging or black tips. Back and shoulders golden-bay, free from black, or from deep maroon. Wing bows rich golden-bay; coverts evenly laced, forming at least two well-defined bars; secondaries black on inner and wide golden stripe on outer web, the edge laced with black; primaries black on inner web, and broadly laced gold on outer edge. Breast and thighs the web golden-bay with well-defined black lacing, free from double or bay outer lacing, the markings regular from throat to back of thighs, showing green lustre. Undercolour black or dark slate. Tail black, with green lustre. Fluff black or dark slate.

Female plumage: Head, neck and hackle as in the cock. Breast, back and thighs undercolour dark slate, web golden-bay with regular, well-defined black lacing, free from double or outer lacing and showing green lustre. Wings same as back on the broad portion; secondaries and primaries as in the cock. Tail as in the cock. Fluff as in the cock.

The blue laced

Male plumage: Red-brown with blue markings. Head red-brown; neck, hackles and saddle red-brown with distinct blue stripe down the centre of each feather (red-brown at centre of blue stripe is permissible), and free from blue tips or blue round the edging. Back and shoulders red-brown, free from blue, or smutty blue. Wings bows red-brown; coverts evenly laced with blue, forming at least two well-defined bars; secondaries blue on the inner web, and wide red-brown on the outer web, the edge laced with blue; primaries blue on inner web, and broadly laced red-brown on outer edge. Breast and thighs web red-brown with well-defined blue lacing, free from double or outer or blue or smutty marking, and regular from the throat to the back of the thighs. Undercolour blue. Tail solid blue, free from black or white. Fluff blue powdered with gold.

Female plumage: Head, neck and hackle as in the cock. Breast, back and thighs undercolour blue, web red-brown with regular, well-defined blue lacing, free from double or outer lacing, the lacing to extend to the back of the thighs into the fluff. Wings same as back on the broad portion; secondaries and primaries as in the cock. Tail as in the cock. Fluff as in the cock.

The buff laced

Male plumage: Rich buff with white markings. Head buff; neck, hackles and saddle buff with distinct white stripe down the centre of each feather (buff at centre of white stripe is permissible), free from ticks, white outer edging, or white tips. Back and shoulders rich buff, free from white. Wing bows rich buff; coverts evenly laced with white, forming at least two well-defined bars; secondaries white on the inner web, and wide rich buff strip on the outer web, the edge laced with white; primaries white on the inner web, and broadly laced buff on outer edge. Breast and thighs web rich buff with well-defined pure white lacing, free from double or buff outer lacing, the markings regular from throat to back of thighs. Undercolour pure white. Tail pure white. Fluff pure white.

Female plumage: Head, neck and hackle as in the cock. Breast, back and thighs undercolour pure white, web rich buff with regular white lacing, and the lacing on the cushion may continue into the tail coverts. Wings same as back on the broad portion; secondaries and primaries as in the cock. Tail as in the cock. Fluff as in the cock.

In both sexes and all colours

Beak, legs and feet yellow or horn, which may dilute to straw in adults or laying pullets. Yellow preferred. Eyes bright bay, orange or red. Bright bay preferred.

Note: In all colours and sexes, regularity of lacing to count above any breadth of lacing. Brightness and uniformity of ground colour to be considered of more value than any particular shade.

Scale of points for all laced colours

Lacing (including striping)	35
Colour	25
Type	20
Head	10
Condition	10
	100

Birds to be passed over for serious defects as in all colours, and points to be deducted for lack of presentation.

Weights

Cock   not less than 4.08 kg (9 lb)   Cockerel   not less than 3.62 kg (8 lb)
Hen   not less than 3.17 kg (7 lb)   Pullet   not less than 2.72 kg (6 lb)

Scale of points

The black

Colour (surface 25, undercolour 10)	35
Type	25
Head	10
Size and condition	15
Legs	15
	100

The blue and the lavender

Type	25
Colour	25
Head	15
Legs	15
Size	10
Condition	10
	100

Serious defects: These include black legs devoid of yellow.

The buff

Type (back 8, body 10, wings 8, tail 9)	35
Colour	35
Head	10
Legs	5
Condition	15
	100

The Columbian

Type	35
Body colour	15
Hackle/tail	20
Head	10
Legs	5
Condition	15
	100

Serious defects (which should be heavily penalised): These include badly crooked breastbone, coarseness. Inactivity. Excess of feather. Overhanging eyebrows. Crooked toes. Brown undercolour. Green eyes.

The partridge, blue partridge, blue silver pencilled and silver pencilled male

Type	22
Head, beak, neck (comb 7, eyes 5, lobes and wattles 4)	16
Legs and feet	6
Colour and markings (colour of hackles 8, striping of hackles 8, top colour 8, breast 7, flights 5, tail 4, undercolour 4, fluff 4)	48
Size and condition	8
	100

The partridge, blue partridge, blue silver pencilled and silver pencilled female

Type	22
Head, beak, neck (comb 6, eyes 5, lobes 4)	15
Legs and feet	10
Colour and markings (ground colour 15, formation – breadth and form of black or blue marks – of pencilling 11, clearness of pencilling 10, fluff 5, hackle 4)	45
Size and condition	8
	100

Serious defects: These include slipped wings, wall eyes or eyes that do not match.

The red

Type	35
Colour	35
Head	10
Legs	5
Condition	15
	100

The barred

Type	30
Colour/markings	30
Head	10
Legs	10
Condition	20
	100

Serious defects: These include shanks other than yellow (allowance made for adult birds and heavy laying females). Coarseness, superfine bone. Any points against egg production, reproduction or stamina values. Absence of any dark undercolour, and any deformity for which a bird may be passed.

The white

Type	25
Colour	25
Head	15
Legs and feet	10
Size	15
Condition	10
	100

Serious defects (for which a bird may be passed): These include feathers other than white in colour. Coarseness and 'Orpington' type.

Serious defects in all colours

Any feathers on shanks or toes. Permanent white or yellow in ear-lobe covering more than one-third of its surface. Comb other than rose, or falling over one side, or so large as to obstruct the sight. Shanks other than yellow, except in mature birds, which may shade to light straw. Any deformity.

BANTAM

Wyandotte bantams are miniatures of the large fowl and the Standards in every respect are the same, with the exception of weights and some scales of points. White laced buffs, violet laced, blue laced, buff and cuckoo are also seen in bantams.

Colour

In both sexes: Beak bright yellow, except in marked and laced varieties, in which it may be horn, shaded with yellow. (*Note*: Yellow beaks are unobtainable in black males with dark undercolour, and beak colour in these should be black, shaded with yellow.) Eyes bright bay in all colours. Comb, face, wattles and ear-lobes bright red. Legs and feet bright yellow

Weights

Male   not to exceed 1.70 kg ($3\frac{3}{4}$ lb)
Female   not to exceed 1.36 kg (3 lb)

Scale of points

The white
Colour	25
Type	25
Head	5
Comb	10
Lobes	5
Eyes	5
Leg colour	5
Size	10
Condition	10
	100

The black
Colour	20
Undercolour	15
Type	20
Head	5
Comb and lobes	10
Leg colour	10
Size	12
Condition	8
	100

The Columbian
Comb	10
Eyes	5
Lobes and wattles	5
Hackle and tail	15
Body colour	15
Legs	5
Type and symmetry	35
Condition	10
	100

Serious defects

Feathers on shanks or toes. Permanent white or yellow in ear-lobes, covering more than one-third of the surface. Comb other than rose or flopping or obstructing the sight. Shanks other than yellow. Any deformity. Slipped wings (which should be penalised strongly). Eyes not matching or other than bright bay. Conspicuous peppering on ground colour of laced varieties. Any form of double lacing in laced varieties.

YAKIDO

Origin: Japan
Classification: Asian Hardfeather. True Bantam
Egg colour: White or light brown

The Yakido is a small Shamo variety that was created around 1850 (the Tokugawa period) in the Mie province. The breed is of Shamo type, but comes below the Chu Shamo in weight, and is shown as a bantam. It was bred originally as a sparring partner for the bigger birds.

General characteristics: male

Type and carriage: General appearance fierce, proud and alert. Stance very upright.
Body: Muscular and powerful for size of bird.
Breast: Broad and full with deep keel.
Back: Long, broadest at shoulders, sloping down towards tail and gradually tapering from upper side of thigh. Backbone straight.
Wings: Long and muscular, carried well down and close to the body, not showing on the back but with prominent shoulders.
Tail: Long with narrow sickles, held horizontally or below.
Head: Medium size and not over-long, wattles and ear-lobes small or absent. Beak strong, broad and curved downwards, but not hooked. Eyes deep-set under fine but overhanging brows. Comb triple and firm.
Neck: Medium length, strong boned and muscular, slightly curved but almost erect.
Legs and feet: Legs strong boned, medium to long, with slight bend at hock. Thighs long, round and muscular. Shanks strong and round. Toes four, long and well spread. Hind toe straight and firm on the ground, spurs straight.
Plumage: Feathers very tight and hard, showing bare red skin at throat, keel and point of wing. Neck hackle not extending to shoulders.
Handling: Extremely firm fleshed, muscular and well balanced. Strong contraction of wings to body.

Female

The general characteristics are similar to those of the male, allowing for the natural sexual differences. Stance very upright, but it is acceptable for a female to be slightly less upright than the male.

Colour

The only Standard colour is black with beetle-green gloss. Some reddish feather in hackle and/or saddle is acceptable, but pure black is preferred. Beak yellow, with some black pigmentation acceptable. In hens an all-black beak is acceptable. Legs and feet yellow. It is acceptable to have some black pigmentation and for hens to have black legs with yellow sole. Comb, face, throat, ear-lobes and any exposed skin brilliant red. Eyes silver is preferred, gold is acceptable.

Weights

Male   2.6 kg (6 lb) or below (stag av. weight 2.1 kg (5 lb))
Female 2.1 kg (5 lb) or below (pullet av. weight 1.65 kg (3 lb 8 oz))

Scale of points

Type and carriage	40
Head	20
Plumage quality	10
Colour	10
Legs and feet	10
Condition	10
	100

Serious defects

Lack of attitude. Poor carriage. Overlarge comb.
Poor leg colour. 'Duck' feet.

YAMATO GUNKEI

Origin: Japan
Classification: Asian Hardfeather. Large Fowl
Egg colour: White or tinted

The Yamato is the largest of the small Shamo breeds, and could be considered an intermediate size (with the Chibi Shamo being its bantam equivalent). In Britain it is exhibited as large fowl.

It is an ancient ornamental breed, and the aim is to be as thick-set, exaggerated and full of character as possible within the weight limits. The main feature is a very heavily wrinkled face, which gets more and more grotesque with age.

General characteristics: male

Type and carriage: Upright stance. Solid, powerful appearance. Full of character.
Body: Extremely powerful and muscular.
Breast: Broad, deep, well rounded and muscular.
Back: Medium length and broad. Widest at the shoulders, giving the appearance of a wide gap between the wings, and gradually narrowing from above the thighs. Backbone straight, sloping down towards the tail. Saddle feathers should be sparse, narrow and short.
Wings: Short, muscular and strong with prominent shoulders held away from the body, but with primaries tightly folded into the body. Wing tips should stop at the base of the saddle hackle and should not be carried over the back. Primary and secondary feathers should be broad and in well-ordered layers. Birds of the best type are usually found to have split wing. In the Yamato this should never be judged a fault.
Tail: Very short, and carried low. Main tail slightly fanned with sickles and tail coverts very short and curved forming a 'prawn' tail, with feather tips pointing down and inwards.

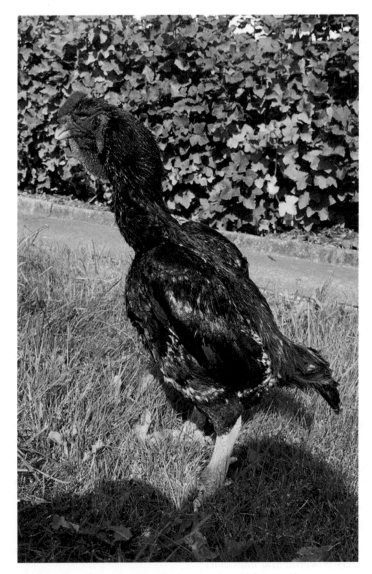

Black-red Yamato Gunkei male

Head: Large, broad and flattened at the top, wider at the front than the back. Prominent eyebrows to suggest ferocity. Beak thick, short, well curved and deep from top to bottom. Comb triple or walnut, firmly set to the head. Eyes large, penetrating and deep-set under heavy overhanging eyebrows. Wattles small. Ear-lobes thick and firm. Throat skin thick and very wrinkled with a dewlap of bare red skin.

Neck: Long, strong, thick and almost erect. The bare skin of the dewlap extends well down the front of the neck. Neck hackle feathers are very short and narrow, hardly reaching the base of the neck.

Legs and feet: Thighs of medium length, well muscled and rounded. Legs well apart, accentuated by the general sparse plumage of body and legs. Shanks straight, thick and strong. Toes four, short, straight, powerful and well spread.

Plumage: Very hard and sparse. Bare red skin showing at keel, vent and point of wing. The shoulder coverts show clearly on the back giving the characteristic 'five hills' – this is seen across the back, looking from the head to the tail by: one shoulder/shoulder coverts/back/ shoulder coverts/other wing.

Handling: Extremely firm fleshed and muscular.

Female

The general characteristics are similar to those of the male, allowing for the natural sexual differences. However, the female is rarely as exaggerated, and the short tail, carried well down, is straight and spread horizontally.

Colour

Black-red (the red may be any shade from yellow to dark red, with wheaten or partridge females that can be any shade from cream to dark brown with or without dark markings), duckwing, black, white, blue, ginger, splash, spangle and cuckoo are all recognised.

In both sexes and all colours

Beak yellow or horn, with dark markings acceptable. Legs and feet yellow, dusky markings acceptable in dark-coloured birds. Comb, face, ear-lobes, wattles and any exposed skin red. Eyes silver or gold. Darker eyes acceptable in young birds.

Weights

Cock	2 kg (4 lb 4 oz)	Cockerel	1.5 kg (3 lb 7 oz)
Hen	1.7 kg (4 lb)	Pullet	1.3 kg (3 lb)

Scale of points

Type and carriage	30
Head and neck	20
Condition and plumage quality	20
Legs and feet	10
Eye colour	10
Legs and feet colour	5
Plumage colour	5
	100

Serious defects

Poor carriage. Overlarge comb. 'Duck' feet. Long tail.

YOKOHAMA

LARGE FOWL

Origin: Japan and Europe
Classification: Light: Rare
Egg colour: White or light brown

The earliest recorded long-tailed fowls were found in China and sent home by Japanese diplomatic representatives. This was sometime between AD 600 and 800 in our calendar. Not all accounts agree about dates and details of events so long ago. The original type birds were called Shokoku in Japan, and from them were developed several other Japanese long-tailed breeds, which are summarised at the end of this Standard. Several of these Japanese long-tailed breeds were exported to Europe, the first recorded by M. Girard, a French missionary, in 1864. These and later shipments were consigned from the port of Yoko-hama, which became the name by which all long-tailed fowls were called by Europeans who were not able, or did not bother, to discover the true breed names and details from Japanese experts. A leading German fancier, Hugo du Roi, bred and promoted the red lobed and, somewhat gamey, red saddled white Yokohama (circa 1880), but it is not clear if he made them himself by crossing various imports or actually imported birds of this colour and type. This variety is unknown in Japan now, but might have existed then. In an effort to bring some order to their assortment of imported types, German fanciers restricted the name Yokohama to the red saddled whites, and invented a new name, Phoenix, for the white lobed, single combed type. British fanciers formed a Yokohama Club about 1904 and decided to use that name for all types; which is why we now have one very long and complex Standard for what really should be several breeds. Yokohama bantams were made by various German fanciers by crossing large Yokohamas with assorted bantams of appropriate colours.

General characteristics: male

Type: Body fairly long and deep, full round breast, long back tapering to tail, long wings carried rather low but close to the body. Tail as long and flowing as possible, with a great abundance of side hangers – the whole tail carried low and forming a graceful curve. Saddle hackles extremely abundant, long and narrow and covering the wing tips. The saddle hackles are long enough to drag on the ground on good old cocks. Carriage is stylish and pheasant-like.
Head: Skull small, slightly long and tapering. Beak strong and curved. Eyes bright. Comb single, pea or walnut (single comb not permitted on red saddled variety). Single comb: small and upright. Pea comb: small, neat and straight. Walnut: medium sized. Face of fine texture. Ear-lobes small, oval, closely fitting. Wattles are medium sized and rounded (small or absent on red saddled variety).
Neck: Long and furnished with flowing hackle, which should completely encircle the neck.
Legs and feet: Legs of medium length (longer legs allowed on red saddled variety), the shanks fine and free of feather. Toes four, well spread.

Female

The back long, tapering to the tail and furnished with long tail covert feathers. Tail very long and carried horizontally with the two top feathers gracefully curved, and the side coverts sickle-like. The remaining general characteristics are similar to those of the male, allowing for the natural sexual differences.

Colour

The black-red

Male plumage: Head bay. Neck and saddle hackles reddish-bay with or without black centre striping. Breast, thighs and tail black with a beetle-green lustre. Back reddish-bay. Wing bows deep bay, bars black with blue sheen; primaries black; secondaries outer web bay, inner web black.
Female plumage: Head brown. Neck hackle golden-orange with or without black centre striping. Breast salmon, a lighter shade below. Thighs grey-brown. Back and shoulders brown, each feather with a light shaft. Tail coverts brown. Tail black, the two uppermost feathers spotted or grizzled with light brown. Wing primaries black; secondaries outer web brown, inner web black.

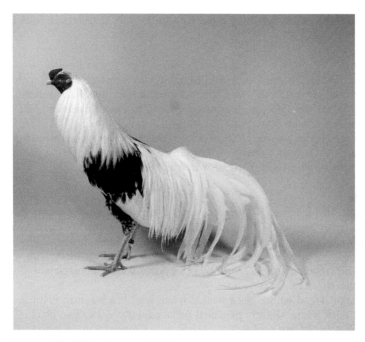

Red saddled Yokohama male, large

The silver duckwing
Male plumage: Head silver-white. Neck and saddle hackles silver-white with or without black centre striping. Breast, thighs and tail black with beetle-green lustre. Back silver-white. Wing bows silver-white, bars black with blue sheen; primaries black; secondaries outer web silver-white, inner web black.
Female plumage: Head light grey. Neck hackle light grey with black centre striping. Breast salmon, a lighter shade below. Thighs grey. Back and shoulders grey, each feather with a light shaft. Tail coverts grey. Tail black, the two uppermost feathers spotted or grizzled with grey. Wing primaries black; secondaries outer web mottled grey, inner web black.

The gold duckwing
Male plumage: Head light yellow or straw. Neck and saddle hackles light yellow or straw with or without black centre striping. Breast, thighs and tail black with beetle-green lustre. Back orange-bay. Wing bows orange-bay, bars black with blue sheen; primaries black; secondaries outer web light yellow or straw, inner web black.
Female plumage: Similar to silver duckwing female except for slight brownish tinge over back and wings, and the breast is a deeper, richer shade of salmon.

The white
Male and female plumage: Snow white, free from straw tinge.

The black
Male and female plumage: Dense black with a rich green sheen.

Black-tailed buff
Male and female plumage: All plumage except for wings and tail a rich lustrous buff with pale slatey-buff undercolour. Wing primaries black, edged with buff; secondaries outer

web buff, inner web black, heavily fringed with buff. Main tail black; sickles and coverts black edged with buff.

The blue-red

Male plumage: Head bay. Neck and saddle hackles orange or golden-red with or without blue centre striping. Breast, thighs and tail medium shade of blue. Back and shoulders deep or bright red. Wing bows deep or bright red, bars dark blue; primaries blue; secondaries outer web bay, inner web blue.

Female plumage: Head brown. Neck hackle golden-red with blue centre striping. Breast and thighs salmon. Back and shoulders brown with fine blue peppering. Wing primaries blue; secondaries outer web mottled brown, inner web blue.

The spangled

Male plumage: Head white. Neck hackle white, the lower feathers near the shoulders having black centre striping. Breast and thighs black, each feather tipped with a white crescent. Back white. Saddle hackle white near the wings, then with some light black centre striping, this striping heavier near the tail. Wing bows white, bars black with white lacing; primaries black; secondaries white with black on inner web. Tail black with distinct white lacing on lower coverts.

Female plumage: Head white. Neck hackle white with black centre striping. Breast and thighs white. Back white, slightly pencilled or laced with black. Tail black.

In both sexes of the above colours

Beak horn (yellow or white allowed with white plumage). Eyes red-brown. Comb, face and wattles red. Ear-lobes white or red (only red on walnut combed whites, as these are related to the red saddled). Legs and feet yellow, willow, slate blue or white.

The red saddled

Male and female plumage: White and red. Breast and thighs red in the male and red-buff in the female, with well-defined white, kite-shaped spangles at the end of each feather. The male's back and wing bows bright red, the former shading into the saddle. Remainder white.

In both sexes: Beak yellow. Eyes red. Comb, face, wattles and lobes red. Legs and feet yellow

The above colours and markings are ideal, but general type, quality and length of tail and hackles are more important than colour on Yokohamas.

Weights

Large male	1.8–2.7 kg (4–6 lb)
Large female	1.1–1.8 kg (2½–4 lb)
Bantam male	570–680 g (20–24 oz)
Bantam female	450–570 g (16–20 oz)

Breeders and judges should give preference to large Yokohamas and small Yokohama bantams to maintain the difference between them.

Scale of points

Quality and length of tail and number of feathers	25
Quality and length of neck and saddle hackles	20
Type and carriage	20
Head	10
Size	10
Colour	5
Condition	5
Legs and feet	5
	100

Serious defects

Broken tail feathers. Short saddle hackles. Too high tail carriage. White marbling in face. Yellow or straw-coloured feathers in the white. Any deformity.

LONG-TAILED BREEDS STANDARDISED IN JAPAN

Kurokashiwa

Another long-tailed long-crower. Single comb. Red ear-lobes. Colour black.

Minohiki

(Mino = saddle feather, Hiki = dragging). In Japan they were mainly bred in Aichi and Shizuoka Prefectures on the main Japanese island of Honshu. Very long saddle hackle. Medium length tail. Triple, walnut or 'chalice' comb. Red ear-lobes. Red-brown eyes. Colours: black-red, silver duckwing, gold duckwing, white, ginger and 'five coloured' (the same colour and pattern as Koeyoshi long-crower).

Onagadori

Developed in the Kochi area of Shikoku in the mid-seventeenth century, which is still the only area where they are bred in Japan. Tail over 1.5 m long, with a 12 m tail having been recorded. They are recognised as a living National Treasure of Japan. The tail feathers of males grow very quickly, and under ideal conditions continue to grow without moulting, sixteen to eighteen of them for the life of the bird. Also extremely long saddle hackle feathers. Single comb. White ear-lobes. Red-brown eyes. Colours: black-red, silver duckwing, gold duckwing, white, ginger.

Shôkokur

Believed to be the original long-tailed breed as mentioned in the introduction. Single comb. Red ear-lobes. Red-brown eyes. Very long tail and saddle hackles. Colours: silver duckwing, gold duckwing, white.

Tôtenkô

These look identical to normal black-red Yokohamas as described in the Standard above, but are a long-crowing breed. They are widely bred in Japan today. Single comb. White ear-lobes. Red-brown eyes. Colour: black-red.

Japanese long-crowers

Koeyoshi

Large and heavy, fairly upright stance, with Shamo-type head – heavy eyebrows, triple comb and pale eyes, red face, yellow legs and strong bone. Plumage colour goshiki ('five coloured', which looks like streaked duckwing in the male, and dull light brown ground colour with black lacing in the female).

Kurokashiwa

Pheasant-like body and long tail held low, single comb, red face sometimes with black markings (hens sometimes have all-black faces), orange-red eyes and dark legs. Plumage colour pure black with green sheen. In Britain this breed is included in the Yokohama Standard.

Tomaru

Compact body with sweeping tail held above horizontal. Single comb, red face sometimes with black markings (hens sometimes have all-black faces), orange-red eyes and dark legs. Plumage colour black with green sheen.

Tôtenkô

Pheasant-like body and long tail held low, single comb, red face with white ear-lobes, orange-red eyes, olive legs. Plumage colour black-red. In Britain this breed is included in the Yokohama Standard.

Turkish long-crower

Denizli

Male average weight 3 kg. Compact body, high to squirrel tail carriage, single or rose comb, red face, dark eyes, slate legs. Plumage colours: variations on birchen/duckwing and brown/black-red, also black.

Russian long-crower

Jurlower (Yurlov Golosysti)

Average weight male 4–5 kg, female 3–4 kg. Solid build. Back slightly roached. Comb single, small, straight and upright or a unique type of rose comb, thick and high giving the effect of a helmet, and with a short straight leader. Red face, white smutty legs. Plumage colour: variations of brown/black-red, and birchen with variable lacing.

German long-crower

Bergische Kraher

Considered to be an Old National Breed and has had a German Standard since 1885. Also known as Mountain Long Crower. Light breed, back slightly roached, single comb, white ear-lobes, dark eyes, slate legs. Plumage colour black with variable gold lacing.

There are several other long-crowing breeds throughout the world, including the white Berat from Yugoslavia/Albania, the Indonesian Ayam Pelung and the 'Musician Fowl of Brazil', but no examples in the UK up to 2007.

Turkeys

The turkey dates back to the Aztec period, when it was kept for its meat and decorative feathering. Explorers introduced the birds to Europe in the early sixteenth century. William Strickland is reputed to have brought the turkey to England from Spain in 1524. Over the centuries it has also been displayed for its exotic features.

Classes for turkeys were offered at the first English Poultry Show in 1845 and a Standard for turkeys appeared in the first English *Book of Standards* in 1865. The Standards published here relate solely to the traditional varieties of turkey, which are naturally bred and not related in any way to the modern-day, commercial, broad-breasted or dimple-breasted types, which are not considered appropriate for the show pen.

GENERAL STANDARD: HEAVY BREEDS

General characteristics: Male and female

Carriage: Stately and moderately upright.
Type: Body long, deep and well rounded. Back curving with good slope to tail. Breast broad, full, long and straight. Wings strong and large. Tail long in proportion to body.
Head: Long, broad and carunculated. Beak strong, curved and well set. Eyes bright, bold and clear.
Snood: The fleshy protuberance above the beak of a male turkey. This is a muscle that elongates to as much as 15.24 cm (6 in.) down over the beak when displaying. It can be retracted to form a short erect cone above the beak when not displaying. The snood will vary in colour from pale pink to very deep pink on all varieties, according to activity and behaviour.
Throat – wattle: Large and pendant.
Caruncles: The fleshy round prominences on the head and neck, which are larger on the front of the neck, below the throat wattle. They can change from bright red through to bluish white.
Neck: Long, curving backward towards saddle.
Beard or tassel: A cluster of black, hair-like growth attached to the centre of the upper part of the breast in all adult males. The beard can grow to around 15.24 cm (6 in.) in length. Females have a beard but generally no more than 1 cm in length, which is usually hidden by breast feathers.
Legs and feet: Thighs long and stout. Fluff – the feathers between the legs and base of the vent, which are soft and short. Shanks large, strong, well rounded and of medium length. Toes four, straight and strong and well spread.

GENERAL STANDARD: LIGHT BREEDS

The general characteristics are the same as for the Heavy breeds with the following exceptions.

British Poultry Standards, Seventh Edition. Edited by J. Ian H. Allonby and Philippe B. Wilson.
© 2019 Poultry Club of Great Britain. Published 2019 by John Wiley & Sons Ltd.

General characteristics: Male and female

Carriage: Active and upright.
Legs and feet: Shanks large, strong and fairly long.

JUDGING – SCALE OF POINTS FOR ALL COLOURS

Type and size	35
Head	15
Legs and feet	15
Colour	25
Condition	10
	100

SERIOUS DEFECTS

Crooked or other deformity of the breast bone. Wry tail. Feathers other than the colour stipulated for the variety. Any birds exceeding the weights laid down in the Standard. Any abnormality.

DISQUALIFICATIONS

Double-breasted varieties.

TURKEY EGGS
Shape

Turkey eggs should be shown in their own classes. Turkey eggs should have a greater length than width and be much roomier in the top than the bottom, which should be more curved.

Size

Turkey egg weights vary between heavy and light varieties:

Heavy breeds would be expected to lay heavier eggs: 85.0–98.0 g (3.0–3 $\frac{1}{2}$ oz)
Light breeds: 73.0–87.0 g (2$\frac{1}{2}$–3$\frac{1}{2}$ oz)
A pullet's egg can be 6.0 g lighter.

Colour

The turkey lays a speckled egg. The speckles range from a deep brown to reddish-chestnut. Blotches or mottling of colour should be considered a fault.

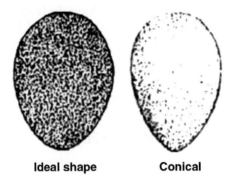

Ideal shape   **Conical**

BLUE

Origin: North America
Classification: Light

The breed has been developed on the lines of the Slate turkey. However, the feathers of the Blue are an even colour throughout. The female is usually slighter lighter in shade than the male. This has been a very popular exhibition bird in the past but fewer are seen than at the beginning of the twentieth century.

Male

Head: Red, changeable to bluish-white.
Eyes: Dark to black.
Beak: Slate blue.
Throat – wattle: Red, changeable to bluish-white.
Plumage: A light or dark shade of sound and even blue, free from black or brown feathers.
Legs and feet: Slate blue.

Female

Similar to the male.

Standard weights

| Mature stag | 10–12.7 kg (22–28 lb) | Young stag | 8–11.2 kg (18–25 lb) |
| Mature hen | 5.4–8.1 kg (12–18 lb) | Young hen | 3.6–6.3 kg (8–14 lb) |

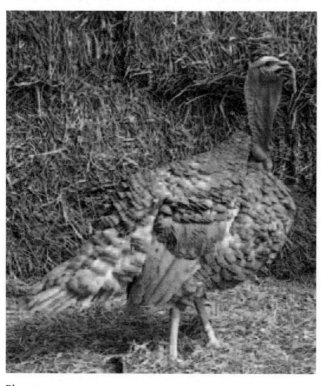

Blue stag

Defects

Presence of any other colour feather.

Day-old poults

Poults are a yellowish-white with an extremely pale tinge of blue.

BOURBON RED

Origin: North America
Classification: Heavy

The Bourbon Red turkey is named after Bourbon County in Kentucky's Bluegrass Region, where it originated in the late 1800s. It was admitted to the American Standard of Perfection in 1909.

Male

Head: Red, changeable to bluish white.
Beak: Light horn at tip, darker at base.
Eyes: Dark brown.
Throat – wattle: Red, changeable to bluish white.

Plumage

Neck: A rich, dark, chestnut-mahogany.
Back: Rich, dark, chestnut-mahogany, each feather from point of shoulders to base of main tail having a very narrow edging of black.
Tail: Main tail – pure white, with an indistinct bar of soft red crossing each main tail feather near the tip. Coverts – deep brownish-red.

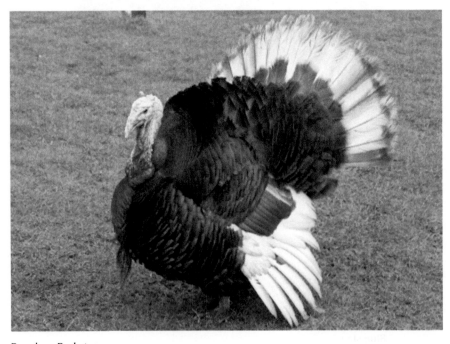

Bourbon Red stag

Wings: Fronts, bows and coverts – rich, dark, chestnut-mahogany, each feather having a very narrow edging of black. Primaries and secondaries – pure white.

Breast: Rich, dark, chestnut-mahogany, feathers having a very narrow edging of lustrous black.

Body and fluff: Body – deep, brownish-red, each feather edged with a very fine line of black. Fluff – a lighter shade of brownish-red.

Legs and feet: Lower thighs – dark, chestnut-mahogany. Shanks and toes – reddish-pink in adults; deep reddish-horn in young. Undercolour of all sections: red, shading to a light salmon at base.

Female

Similar to that of the male, except there is no black edging in any section. On the breast, each feather has a narrow thread-like edging of white.

Standard weights

Mature stag	14.9 kg (33 lb)	Young stag	10.4 kg (23 lb)
Mature hen	8.1 kg (18 lb)	Young hen	6.3 kg (14 lb)

Defects

More than one-third any colour other than white showing in either primaries, secondaries or main tail feathers. Entire absence of black edging in plumage of stags on breast, wing fronts and saddle. Entire absence of white edging on feathers in upper breast and neck sections of hens.

Day-old poults

Head is a light reddish-brown with a darker brown mark on the back of the head. The neck and back is a light yellowish-brown with three dark brown stripes running from the shoulders, with the middle stripe being the broadest of the three. The wings go from dark brown at the front through to cream at the tips. Throat, breast and thighs are a pale yellowish-white. As feathering appears the growing poult takes on a pale beige colouring with white markings, these disappear as the adult feathers emerge.

BRONZE

Origin: Europe
Classification: Heavy

The bronze turkey is the closest in colouring to the Eastern Wild. It is the most popular variety of turkey there is and a good Bronze is difficult to beat at exhibitions. The Bronze was further developed in England and reintroduced to the Americas, where it became extremely popular. They are often confused with the broad breasted (meat birds). There are far fewer pure standard Bronzes than broad-breasted Bronzes. In the *British Poultry Standards*, third edition (1978), the Mammoth Bronze and Cambridge Bronze were Standardised under the name Bronze.

Male

Head: Red, changeable to bluish-white.
Eyes: Iris a dark hazel; pupil blue-black.
Beak: Horn.
Throat – wattle: Bright rich red.

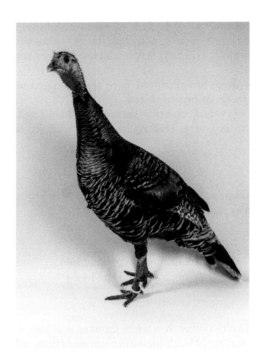

Bronze hen

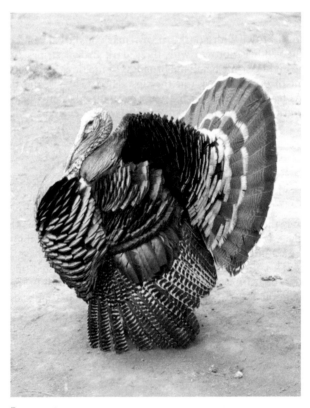

Bronze stag

Plumage

Plumage of both sexes a good metallic bronze throughout.

Neck: Copperish-bronze.

Back: From neck to middle of back – a rich copperish-bronze, each feather terminating in a narrow black band, extending across end. From middle of back to tail coverts – black, each feather having a broad, copperish-bronze band extending across it near the end, the feathers ending in a distinct black band, gradually narrowing as the tail coverts approached.

Tail: Main tail and coverts – dull black, each feather evenly and distinctly marked transversely with a parallel line of brown; each feather having a bronze band extending across the feather, bordered on each side by a distinct band of intense black; the feather terminating in a wide edging of white.

Wings: Shoulder and wing bow coverts – rich copperish-bronze, ending in a narrow band of black; coverts rich bronze, forming a broad band across wings when folded, feathers terminating in a black band, separating them from the secondaries. Primaries, each feather alternately crossed with distinct parallel black and white bars of equal width; flight coverts barred similar to primaries; secondaries dull black, alternately crossed with distinct parallel black and white bars, the black bar taking on a bronze cast on the shorter top secondaries and the white bar becoming less distinct.

Breast: Exposed surface of feathers rich bronze, unexposed parts black. Each feather on lower part of breast approaching body terminating in a narrow black band extending across the end.

Body and fluff: Body black, each feather with a wide bronze band extending across it at the end, a narrow band of black bordering the bronze and terminating in a narrow edging of pure white. Fluff, a dull black.

Legs and feet: Thighs dull black with slight edgings of greyish white. Shanks and toes dull black but changing to horn with maturity.

Toenails: Horn.

Female

As male but with faint white lacing on the breast.

Standard weights

Mature stag	13.6–18.14 kg (30–40 lb)	Young stag	11.33–15.87 kg (25–35 lb)
Mature hen	8.16–11.79 kg (18–26 lb)	Young hen	6.35–9.97 kg (14–22 lb)

Defects

Wings showing one or more primary or secondary feathers completely black or white or brown, or absence of white bars more than one-half of the length of primaries.

Disqualifications

Double-breasted varieties.

Day-old poults

The head is light brown with dark brown blotches and streaks. The neck and back have a broader dark streak down the centre with narrower streaks on either side. The wings have two dark streaks in the centre and a dark spot near the tip. The underneath of the poult is a yellowish-white on the surface and pale grey beneath. The legs and feet are mainly flesh coloured with some smoky pigmentation below.

BUFF

Origin: America
Classification: Light

The Buff is named for the rich cinnamon colour of its body feathers. The breed was recognised by the American Poultry Association in 1874 but very few now exist in America and there is no longer a Standard for it there. The breed was extremely popular in Britain at the turn of the last century with its own Buff Turkey Club in the early 1900s.

Male

Head: Red, changeable to bluish-white.
Eyes: Iris dark hazel; pupil blue-black.
Beak: Light horn.
Throat – wattle: Brighter rich red.
Plumage: A deep cinnamon-buff colour.
Tail: Deep cinnamon-buff throughout edged with a paler band at the tip.
Wings: Secondaries very pale buff. Primaries white.
Legs and feet: Pink and flesh colour.
Toenails: Light horn.

Female

Similar to the male.

Standard weights

Mature stag   10–12.7 kg (22–28 lb)   Young stag   7.25–10.4 kg (16–23 lb)
Mature hen   5.4–8.1 kg (8–14 lb)   Young hen   3.6–6.3 kg (8–14 lb)

Defects

Any black on feathering. More than one-third any colour other than buff showing in either primaries, secondaries or main tail feathers.

Day-old poults

A pale creamy brown throughout.

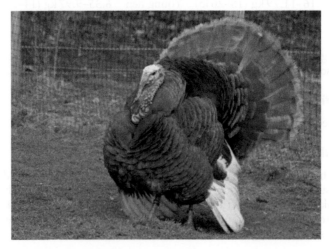

Buff stag

CRIMSON DAWN/BLACK-WINGED BRONZE

Origin: Europe
Classification: Heavy

The last Standard published was in the fifth edition, although referenced in the sixth edition 'All characteristics the same as the Bronze except for the wings'. These are rarely seen.

Wings: Shoulder and wing bow coverts – rich copperish-bronze. Some white permitted. Primaries – solid black. Secondaries – black with white tips.

Disqualifications

Double-breasted varieties.

CROLLWITZER (PIED)

Origin: Europe
Classification: White

The Pied turkey has been in existence in Europe since the 1700s. It is very ornamental and a popular exhibition bird. The Pied is more suited as an egg producer than a meat bird.

Male

Head: Red, changeable to bluish-white.
Eyes: Light brown.
Beak: Light horn.
Throat – wattle: Red, changeable to bluish-white.

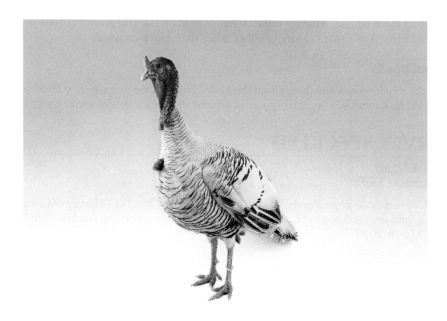

Crollwitzer (Pied) stag

Plumage

Neck: White with every feather ending in a fine black edge.

Back: White with metallic black over saddle, fringed with white.

Tail: Main tail pure white with a wide black band across each feather near the end, terminating in pure white at the tip. Coverts and lesser coverts white with wide band of metallic black extending across the feather near the end, terminating in a wide edge of white.

Wings: Fronts and bows white with narrow edge of black across each feather. Coverts white with narrow edge of black on end of each feather forming a black band when wing is folded. Primaries dull black. Secondaries white with exposed portion of each feather having a black strip running about 10 cm (4 in.) in length on each feather; becoming shorter on top secondaries to form a distinct spot on each feather.

Breast: Exposed portion of each feather pure white ending in a band of black to form a contrast of black and white giving the effect of scales of a fish.

Body and fluff: Body white with each feather ending in a black band terminating in white. Fluff white.

Legs and feet: Thighs white with very light black edging. Shanks and toes – in mature birds, deep pink; in young birds, pinkish-white.

Toenails: Light horn.

Female

Similar to male.

Standard weights

Mature stag	9–10 kg (20–22 lb)	Young stag	7.2 kg (16 lb)
Mature hen	5.4 kg (12 lb)	Young hen	4.5 kg (10 lb)

Defects

Absence of black edging. Absence of black bands in main tail and greater coverts in both stags and hens. Any other coloured feather other than black or white.

Day-old poults

Poults are a yellowish-white throughout the body. Through the down pure white feathers grow and black markings begin to appear at around six to eight weeks, sometimes sooner.

HARVEY SPECKLED

Origin: England

Classification: Light

A speckled turkey developed in the late twentieth century by Mr. D.C. Harvey of Cornwall, England. Initially bred as a light commercial bird. Standard passed by Poultry Club Great Britain March 2016

Male

Head: Red, changeable to bluish-white.

Eyes: Iris dark hazel; pupil black.

Beak: Light horn.

Throat – wattle: Red changeable to bluish-white.

Plumage: Overall colour is creamy white with distinct cinnamon speckles.

Tail: Creamy white.

Wings: Flights and secondaries creamy white.

Body and fluff: Creamy white everywhere with some light cinnamon stippling.
Legs and feet: Salmon pink with touch of horn, ageing to predominantly horn.
Toenails: Horn.

Female

Same as male but less heavily speckled.

Standard weights

| Mature stag | 10–12.7 kg (22–28 lb) | Young stag | 7.25–10 kg (16–23 lb) |
| Mature hen | 5.4–8.1 kg (12–18 lb) | Young hen | 3.6–6.3 kg (8–14 lb) |

Defects

Any colour other than cinnamon. Speckles running into each other, areas of solid colour or barring of solid colour.

Day-old poults

Creamy white.

NARRAGANSETT

Origin: North America
Classification: Heavy

The Narragansett turkey is named after the Narragansett Bay region in Rhode Island, USA. It is believed the Narragansett was originally founded through Black turkeys from England being taken to America and breeding with the Eastern Wild turkey. The breed was admitted to the American Standards of Perfection in 1874.

Male

Head: Red, changeable to bluish-white.
Beak: Horn.
Eyes: Brown.
Throat – wattle: Red, changeable to bluish-white.

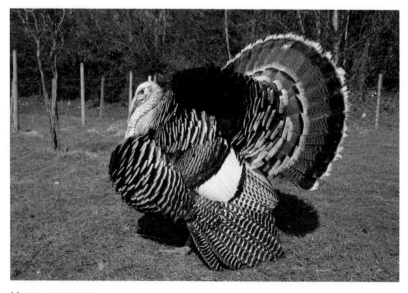

Narragansett stag

Plumage

Neck: Unexposed part of the feather black, the exposed surface of each feather steel grey approaching white; finishing in a narrow black band across the feather. The band increasing in width as the back is approached.

Back: Rich, metallic black free from any bronze cast. Saddle – black, each feather ending in a broad, steel-grey band going to white, the light band increasing in width as the tail coverts are approached.

Tail: Main tail – dull black, each feather regularly pencilled with parallel lines of tan, ending in a broad band of metallic black, free from bronze cast, edged with steel grey going to white. Coverts and lesser coverts – dull black, each feather regularly pencilled with parallel lines of tan, having a wide band of metallic black – free from bronze cast – extending across it near the end, terminating in a wide edging of light steel grey approaching white.

Wings: Shoulder and wing bow coverts – light steel grey ending in a narrow black band. Coverts – a light steel grey, forming a broad steel-grey band across the wings when folded, feathers terminating in a distinct black band, forming a glossy, ribbon-like mark, which separates them from secondaries. Primaries – each feather, throughout its entire length, alternately crossed with distinct, parallel black and white bars of equal width. Flight coverts – barred similar to primaries. Secondaries – alternately crossed with distinct parallel black and white bars, the black bar taking on a light steel-grey cast on the shorter top secondaries, the white bar becoming less distinct.

Breast: Unexposed part of each feather black, ending in a broad, light steel-grey band which becomes darker the closer you get to the underbody; each feather ending with a distinct black band, narrow at the throat and becoming wider on the lower breast.

Body and fluff: Body dull black, feathers ending with a distinct band of white. Fluff black, terminating in white.

Legs and feet: Lower thighs intense black edged with light steel grey. Shanks and toes – in mature specimens, deep salmon; in young specimens, dark approaching salmon.

Female

The female is smaller and finer in bone structure than the male. Plumage is similar in all sections to the male except that feathers on the back should end with a distinct white edging of medium width, the black edging terminating at cape and breast gradually changing to a white edging, which widens as it approaches the rear.

Standard weights

Mature stag	14.9 kg (33 lb)	Young stag	10.4 kg (23 lb)
Mature hen	8.1 kg (18 lb)	Young hen	6.3 kg (14 lb)

Defects

Wings showing one or more primary or secondary feathers completely black or brown, or absence of white or grey bars more than one-half of the length of primaries; white or grey bars showing on main tail feathers beyond greater main tail coverts, except the terminating wide edging of white. Entire absence of black bands on greater tail coverts. Edging of brown in secondary feathers.

Day-old poults

The head is yellowish-grey, mottled with dark brown with three dark streaks, the middle being widest, running from the top of the head down the neck. The upper parts of the body are light greyish-brown mottled with very dark brown and the three dark streaks continue along the back to the tail. The underparts of the body are yellowish-white to almost white on the surface. Undercolour of body down throughout is a light grey. The shank, legs and feet are the same as the Bronze. Although the breasts of Narragansett poults are paler than in the Bronze it is very difficult to segregate the two varieties accurately until they are around six weeks old.

NEBRASKAN

Origin: America
Classification: Heavy

A pied colour mutation produced by a non-sex-linked recessive gene, which appeared in 1947 in a closed flock of broad-breasted Bronze. Thirteen poults were hatched in the first year and these formed the basis of a new true-breeding variety named Nebraskan by the originator R.H. Jandebeur of North Platte, Nebraska. Believed to be no longer in the UK.

Male

Head: Red, changeable to bluish-white.
Eyes: Bluish-pearl.
Beak: Horn.
Throat – wattle: Red, changeable to bluish-white.

Plumage
Neck: White with surface flecking.
Back: White with flecking. The saddle has the most abundant flecking.
Tail: Mostly white with light flecking.

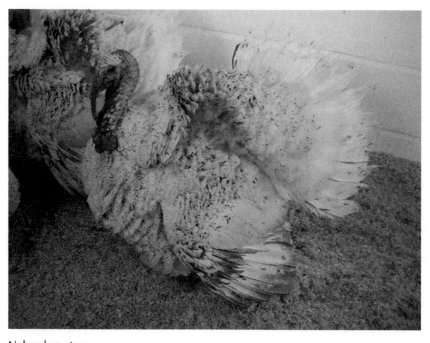

Nebraskan stag

Wings: Secondaries mainly white. Primaries white with flecking. Coverts white with heavy flecking.
Breast: White with flecking.
Body and fluff: Mainly white with some light flecking. Undercolour white in all sections except back.
Legs and feet: Lower thighs white. Shanks and toes salmon.
Toenails: Horn.

Female

Similar to male with less flecking.

Standard weights

Mature stag	13.6–18.14 kg (30–40 lb)	Young stag	11.33–15.87 kg (23–35 lb)
Mature hen	8.16–11.79 kg (18–26 lb)	Young hen	6.35–9.97 kg (14–22 lb)

Defects

Heavy flecking that mask the white. Any other colouring.

Day-old poults

Creamy white with a dark grey/tan spot on back of head.

NORFOLK BLACK

Origin: England
Classification: Light

The Black turkey is believed to have been brought to England via Spain in the 1500s. Many farmers in East Anglia and especially Norfolk liked and kept this bird, hence its name. The Norfolk Black has developed over the centuries through selective breeding and is now recognised as English in origin. It was taken back to America in the 1600s, where it was cross bred with the Eastern Wild and from those matings came the Slate, Narragansett and Bronze.

Male

Head: Fairly long, broad and carunculated. Red, changing to bluish-white. Short black feathers on head and face not a fault.
Eyes: Dark to black.
Beak: Black.
Throat – wattle: Large and pendant.
Plumage: Dense black.
Neck: Of medium length curving slightly backward with an alert carriage.
Legs and feet: Black legs and feet. (Change to pink with age.) Legs short to medium length and well set apart. Thighs full and thick.
Toenails: Black.

Female

Similar to the male.

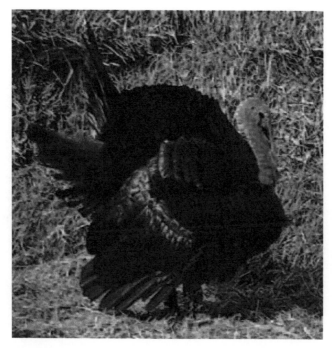

Norfolk Black stag

Standard weights

Mature stag	11.35 kg (25 lb)	Young stag	8.15–10 kg (18–22 lb)
Mature hen	5.90–6.80 kg (13–15 lb)	Young hen	5–5.9 kg (11–13 lb)

Defects

Any bronze colouring (minor fault to be discouraged). Any colour other than black.

Disqualifications

Double breasted.

Day-old poults

The majority of the body is black but the head and face will be a creamy white, along with the breast and the abdomen. There is no distinct pattern to this and poults can have a lesser or greater amount of creamy white down colouration. The pale colour will disappear with age and as feathers begin to grow these should be totally black. The poult's beak will be a pale pink with varying amounts of black on it, especially at the tip. The shanks, feet and toes will be black with some flesh colouring as well.

SLATE

Origin: America
Classification: Light

The Slate turkey is believed to have evolved from crossing Norfolk Blacks, introduced to America, with the Eastern Wild. The breed was admitted to the American Standard of Perfection in 1874. During the turn and early part of the twentieth century, the Slate and Blue turkeys were very popular at the London shows.

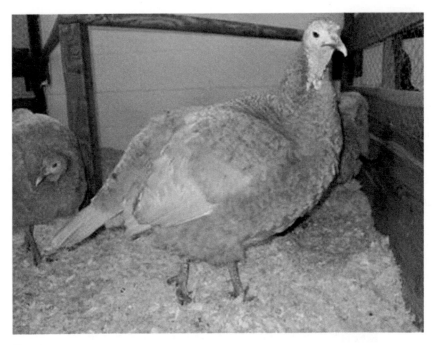

Slate hen

Male

Head: Red, changeable to bluish-white.
Eyes: Dark brown.
Beak: Horn.
Throat – wattle: Red, changeable to bluish-white.
Plumage: Slate blue throughout with black/dark grey flecking.
Legs and feet: Pink in adults; deep pink in young.
Toenails: Horn.

Female

Similar to the male.

Standard weights

Mature stag	10.4–13.6 kg (23–30 lb)	Young stag	7.25–10.4 kg (16–23 lb)
Mature hen	5.4–8.1 kg (12–18 lb)	Young hen	3.6–6.3 kg (8–14 ls)

Defects

Too little flecking. Any entirely black feathers. Dotting rather than flecking. Any other coloured feather.

Day-old poults

The head, neck and back are a yellowish-white with a definite tinge of blue. The throat is a pale yellowish-white to light yellow, going to a yellowish-white underneath the body.

WHITE

Origin: America
Classification: Light

The White turkey has been found throughout the history of the turkey, since the Aztec period. It is believed to be a sport of other breeds, where the white gene has appeared dominant. The White Holland turkey was admitted to the American Standard of Perfection in 1874 and the Beltsville Small White was admitted in 1951. The British White, Austrian White and White Holland have all been bred in the UK. Different strains have been developed for the commercial sector.

Male

Head: Bright rich red, but changeable in the male to cornflower blue and white.
Eyes: Iris dark hazel; pupil blue-black.
Beak: White to pale horn.
Throat – wattle: Red, changeable to pink.
Plumage: White throughout.
Toenails: Horn.

Female

Same as male.

Standard weights

Mature stag   10–12.7 kg (22–28 lb)   Young stag   7.25–10.4 kg (16–23 lb)
Mature hen   5.4–8.1 kg (12–18 lb)   Young hen   3.6–6.3 kg (8–14 lb)

Defects

Any other colour.

Disqualifications

Double breasted.

Day-old poults

Pure white.

OTHER VARIETIES

There are similar variations of the black and white Pied turkey and it is possible to see the Ronquiere from Belgium (which also comes in other colours) and the American Royal Palm, occasionally exhibited in the UK.

The Cornish Palm (a variety of Bronze) and the Crimson Dawn or Black-winged Bronze are both only rarely seen.

Waterfowl

GEESE

The first poultry show of 1845 classified Common Geese, Asiatic or Knob Geese and 'Any other variety'. The first *Book of Standards* described the Toulouse and Embden. Peculiarly enough, these two breeds monopolised our Standards up to recent times, being the chief ones exhibited regularly at shows. At times, other breeds have been exhibited and now the Standards have been extended. The Greylag is said to be the ancestor of all our domestic geese, and the common goose of this country was undoubtedly the English Grey, although a white variety existed, and the Grey Back (Saddleback) may have come from a breed cross.

The sexing of geese may be done via the vent up to four weeks old and after six months old.

The following are classified as wild geese: Canada, Egyptian and all species of British or foreign wild geese.

Goose points

Section	Breed	Carriage	Head and neck	Body	Legs and feet	Condition	Colour	Size
Heavy	African	15	20	20	5	10	10	20
Heavy	American Buff	10	15	20	5	10	25	15
Heavy	Embden	12	22	20	6	10	10	20
Heavy	Skåne	10	15	15	5	10	20	25
Heavy	Toulouse	15	20	20	5	10	10	20
Medium	Brecon Buff	10	15	25	5	10	25	10
Medium	Buff Back	10	10	20	5	10	35	10
Medium	Grey Back	10	10	20	5	10	35	10
Medium	Pomeranian	10	10	20	5	10	35	10
Medium	West of England	10	15	20	5	10	20	20
Light	Chinese	20	30	10	5	10	15	10
Light	Czech	15	20	20	5	10	10	20
Light	Pilgrim	10	15	15	5	10	35	10
Light	Roman	15	20	25	5	10	10	15
Light	Sebastopol	15	10	10	5	40	10	10
Light	Shetland	10	20	15	5	10	25	15
Light	Steinbacher	20	25	10	5	10	20	10

Defects and deformities in waterfowl (for which birds should be passed)

Geese: Undershot mandible, angel or dropped wing, dropped tongue.

British Poultry Standards, Seventh Edition. Edited by J. Ian H. Allonby and Philippe B. Wilson.
© 2019 Poultry Club of Great Britain. Published 2019 by John Wiley & Sons Ltd.

AFRICAN

Classification: Heavy
Origin: China

The African is among the largest and heaviest of the domestic breeds of geese. Both the African and Chinese have evolved from the wild swan goose (*Anser cygnoides*), an Asiatic species, and are distinguished from the Western breeds of geese in having a prominent 'knob' rising up from the base of the beak and having smooth, velvet (pile)-like feathering on their necks. The African also has a soft dewlap which hangs below its beak. This breed has been present in the UK since the late seventeenth century and, although standardised in the USA in 1874, it did not appear in the British Poultry Standards until 1982.

The name African is misleading as the swan goose is an Asiatic species.

Overall type (shape): Male and female

Carriage: Reasonably upright; body at held at 30–40° above the horizontal. Head is held high and the height may often exceed 90 cm (35 in.). Tail carried high above the line of the back, especially in males.
Head: Broad, deep and large. The distinctive knob is large, as broad as the head, protruding slightly forward from the front of the head on the upper mandible (knob should be larger in ganders). Eyes large. Beak rather large, stout at base. A large, smooth, crescent-shaped dewlap extends from below beak to neck below throat.

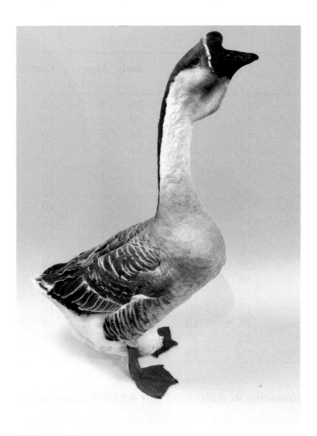

African male

Neck: Long, thick, almost maintaining same thickness along whole length. Slightly arched.
Body: Large, long and almost the same thickness from front to back. Back broad, moderately long and flat. Breast smooth and rounded. Underline smooth and free from keel. If paunch is not smoothly rounded, there should be small, even dual lobes. Stern round, full, free from bagginess.
Wings: Large, strong and folded smoothly against sides.
Tail: Slightly elevated.
Legs and feet: Lower thighs short, stout. Shanks of medium length.
Plumage: Tight and sleek on the body. The neck feathers are soft and smooth, pile like (not furrowed as in breeds developed from the Greylag).

Colour

The brown or grey: Male and female
Head and neck: Beak and knob black. Eyes dark brown. Lower part of head and front of neck a light fawn, which fades to cream in the front of the middle of the neck. A dark brown stripe extends from the crown down the entire length of the back of the neck. Many mature birds display a fine line of white feathers surrounding the beak where it meets the head.
Body: Back ashy brown. Breast light ashy brown shading gradually to light fawn under the body. Sides of body and wing coverts ashy brown, each feather edged with a lighter shade. Patterning on feathers becoming more distinct on the upper side of thigh coverts. Under-body fawn, gradually shading to white on stern.
Tail: Ashy brown heavily edged with almost white shade. Tail coverts white.
Wings: Primaries and secondaries dark slate or brown. Primary coverts light slate or brown. Other large coverts light ashy brown, edged with lighter shade. Scapulars ashy brown with light edging.
Legs and webs: Dark orange or brownish orange. Toenails dark.

The buff: Male and female
Beak and knob: Pinkish brown.
Legs and webs: A dull light orange.
Plumage: Buff with a creamy fawn on the lighter parts. Feather pattern as in the brown.

The white: Male and female
Eyes: Blue.
Beak and knob: Orange.
Legs and webs: Orange-yellow.
Plumage: Pure white.

Weights

Gander   10.0–12.7 kg   (22–28 lb)
Goose   8.2–10.9 kg   (18–24 lb)

Scale of points

Carriage	15
Head and throat	15
Neck	5
Body	20
Legs and feet	5
Condition	10
Colour	10
Size	20
	100

Disqualifications

Undershot mandible (lower beak longer than the upper). Excessive white feathers in coloured plumage except where described.

Faults

Inadequate development or absence of dewlap or knob. Jagged edge to the dewlap. Refined head and neck indicating Chinese input. Lack of reach. Short body. Keel on breast or underside. Baggy paunch. Low tail carriage. Orange in beak or knob of the brown/grey and buff varieties. Twisted neck stripe.

Minor faults (to be discouraged)

Dewlap with folds. Dewlap running excessively into base of beak.

AMERICAN BUFF

Classification: Heavy
Origin: America

The American Buff was developed in North America from common farm geese and is descended from the wild Greylag goose, which inhabits Europe and North Asia. Its history is obscure and there are several theories on how it may have developed. It was standardised in the USA in 1947 and in the UK in 1982. It differs from the other solid buff-coloured geese, i.e. the British Brecon Buff and the German Celler goose, in being larger and having an orange beak and feet.

Overall type (shape): Male and female

Carriage: Rather upright.
Head: Broad and strong. Eyes large and full. Beak of medium length, stout.
Neck: Rather upright and strong in appearance.
Body: Moderately long, broad, plump. Back medium length, broad and smooth. Breast, broad, deep and full. Paunch dual lobed.
Tail: Medium in length, with broad, stiff feathers.
Wings: Medium in size and smoothly folded close to the body.
Legs and feet: Lower thighs medium length, well fleshed. Shanks stout, straight moderately long.

Colour

In both sexes
Head: A soft matt buff. Eyes dark hazel with orange outer eye ring (cilium). Beak orange.
Neck: Soft matt buff shading to a lighter buff as it joins the breast.
Breast: Pale buff.
Body: Back darker buff. Rest of body light buff shading lighter to almost white on abdomen and paunch. Flanks lighter buff, becoming darker. Thighs light buff.
Wings: Primaries matt buff. Secondaries a darker buff with a narrow edging of very greyish buff. Wing coverts soft matt buff with a narrow edging of very light greyish buff.
Plumage: A rich and consistent shade of buff throughout with markings and pattern similar to the Toulouse and the Brecon Buff.
Legs and webs: Orange.

Weights

Gander   10.0–12.7 kg   (22–28 lb)
Goose   9.1–11.8 kg   (20–26 lb)

Scale of points

Carriage   10
Head and throat   10
Neck   5
Body   20
Legs and feet   5
Condition   10
Colour   25
Size   <u>15</u>
                   100

Disqualifications

In both sexes: White in wings.

Faults

In both sexes: White primary or secondary feathers. Distinct dewlap. White feathers under chin. Uneven lobes, back or front. Keel on breast. White line around base of beak in young birds.

Minor faults (to be discouraged)

In both sexes: Narrow white line around base of beak in older birds.

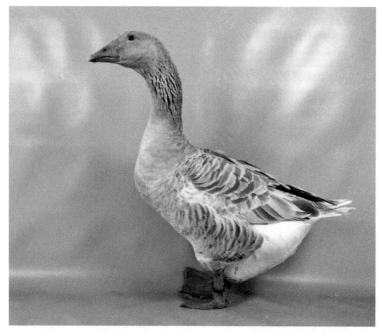

American Buff

BRECON BUFF

Classification: Medium
Origin: Great Britain

As the name suggests, this breed has its origins in the hills of Breconshire, Wales. The overall buff colour, unique among British geese, attracted Rhys Williams, who is credited with collecting and developing this breed in the late 1920s and working with them until they were breeding true. The Standard was initially published in *Feathered World* in 1934 and then in the 1954 *British Poultry Standards*. It is a hardy, active breed.

Overall type (shape): Male and female

Carriage: Fairly upright and alert.
Head: Rounded and neat, with no sign of coarseness. Eyes high set. Beak stout and strong.
Neck: Medium length, fairly stout with no sign of a gullet on throat.
Body: Broad, well rounded and compact. Breast rounded and full. Dual-lobed paunch.
Tail: Medium length, carried almost level.
Wings: Strong and held neatly to the body.
Legs and feet: Legs fairly short, strong shanks.
Plumage: Hard and tight.

Colour

In both sexes

Eyes: Dark brown. Pink outer eye ring (cilium).
Bill: Pink.
Legs and webs: Pink.
Plumage: A deep shade of buff throughout with markings and pattern similar to the Toulouse.

Weights

Gander   7.3–9.1 kg   (16–20 lb)
Goose   6.3–8.2 kg   (14–18 lb)

Scale of points

Carriage	10
Head and throat	10
Neck	5
Body	25
Legs and feet	5
Condition	10
Colour	25
Size	10
	100

Disqualifications

In both sexes: Orange beak, legs or feet. White in wings.

Faults

In both sexes: White feathers under the chin. Blue or light brown eyes. Uneven lobes, back or front.

Minor faults (to be discouraged)

In both sexes: Narrow white line around base of bill in young birds only.

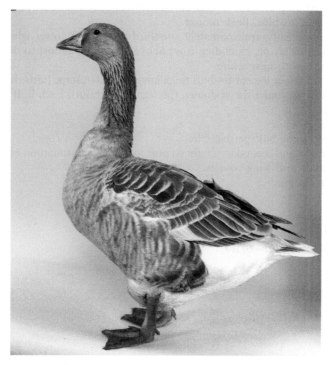

Brecon Buff

BUFF BACK (SADDLEBACK)

Classification: Medium
Origin: Europe

This is an attractive goose with a white background overlaid with buff markings on head, part of neck, a saddleback and thigh coverts. Geese of this kind have long been known as 'Saddlebacks' The Saddleback race, in both grey and buff forms, has been bred entirely for utility throughout Europe for many centuries. Formerly regarded as belonging to the race of Pomeranian geese, it has been distinguished from these in having a dual-lobed paunch and orange beak and feet. It is uncertain how the buff back colour was developed, although there are several theories which have not been proven. This breed was standardised in the UK in 1982.

Overall type (shape): Male and female

Carriage: Almost horizontal.
Head: Fairly broad. Beak of medium length, almost straight and stout. Eyes large.
Neck: Medium length, moderately stout and carried upright with little or no indication of an arch.
Body: Moderately long, plump, deep and meaty, with no evidence of a keel. Deep dual-lobed paunch.
Tail: Closely folded and carried almost level.
Wings: Rather long, with tips crossing over the tail coverts.
Legs and feet: Lower thighs medium length and plump. Shanks moderately long and sturdy.
Plumage: Hard and tight.

Colour

In both sexes

Head: Buff. Solid buff preferred. A small amount of white around base of beak permissible but not desirable. Eyes blue. Beak orange.

Neck: Upper section buff (approximately one-third preferable), lower white.

Back: Buff in a heart shape, extending from above scapulars, almost to the base of tail, each feather edged with near white.

Breast and flanks: White except for buff thigh coverts, and in some birds the buff extends in a broad band right under the abdomen (preferably without). Each buff feather edged with near white.

Paunch and stern: White.

Tail: White, with some buff permissible.

Wings: White flight and secondary feathers: buff forming a continuation of heart-shaped saddle on scapulars and wing coverts.

Legs and webs: Orange.

Weights

Gander   8.2–10.0 kg   (18–22 lb)
Goose   7.3–9.1 kg   (16–20 lb)

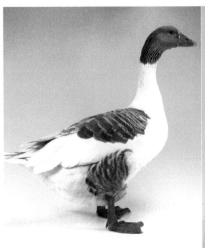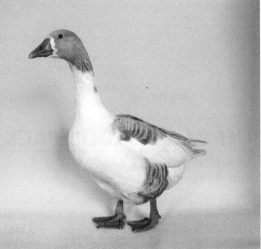

Buff Back pair

Scale of points

Carriage	10
Head and throat	5
Neck	5
Body	20
Legs and feet	5
Condition	10
Colour and markings	35
Size	10
	100

Faults

In both sexes: Uneven markings. White interspersed in coloured plumage. Very uneven division between the colour on the neck. Single lobe or uneven lobes in the paunch.

CHINESE

Classification: Light
Origin: China

The Chinese is an elegant, fine, small goose, active and good at foraging. Although it shares the same wild ancestor (the swan goose) as the African, which can be seen in the similarity of colour and marking, in shape and size the two breeds are very different. Chinese have been present in Britain since at least the early eighteenth century. As mentioned in the UK Standards of 1923 the breed is now standardised in both brown or grey and white varieties. The most distinctive feature is a prominent knob rising from the base of the beak.

They are highly vocal by nature and have a reputation for being good 'watch dogs' – they are famous for guarding some whisky distilleries in Scotland. The Chinese goose is also the most prolific layer of all geese.

Overall type (shape): Male and female

Carriage: Upright with head held high and tail erect.
Head: Medium size. Beak stout at base, medium for size. Knob large, rounded and prominent (smaller in goose than in gander). Eyes bold.
Neck: Long and slender, carried upright, but with graceful arch (longer in gander than in goose).
Body: Compact and plump. Back reasonably short, broad, flat and sloping to give the characteristic upright carriage. Breast well rounded and plump, carried high. Stern well rounded, paunch nicely rounded, without dual lobes.
Tail: Tightly folded and carried erect.
Wings: Large, strong and carried high up.
Legs and feet: Legs medium in length, strong shanks. Feet well spread, straight toes.
Plumage: Tight, firm and sleek.

Colour

The brown or grey: Male and female
Head and neck: Lower part of face and throat light fawn. Front of neck shading from light fawn to cream in mid-section, gradually shading back to light fawn where it joins breast. A dark brown stripe extends from the base of the knob, over the top of the head down the entire length of neck to body. A darkish shaded area extends along the line of the jaw. In older birds there may be a narrow band of white around the base of the beak. Beak and knob black. Eyes dark brown.
Body: Breast light fawn. Back ash brown. Sides of body to thigh coverts a shade of ash brown gradually becoming darker. Each feather edged in a lighter shade, more distinctly on coverts. Underbody gradually fades from fawn to white on stern.
Tail: Ash brown edged with near white. Tail coverts white.
Wings: Primaries and secondaries dark slate or brown. Primary coverts a lighter slate or brown. Remaining coverts light ash brown, edged with lighter shade.
Legs and webs: Dull orange or dark orange-pink feet often with dark markings. Toenails dark.

The white: Male and female

Eyes: Blue.
Beak and knob: Orange.
Legs and webs: Orange.
Plumage: Pure white.

Weights

Gander   4.5–5.4 kg   (10–12 lb)
Goose   3.6–4.5 kg   (8–10 lb)

Scale of points

Carriage   20
Head and throat   20
Neck   10
Body   10
Legs and feet   5
Condition   10
Colour   15
Size   <u>10</u>
                   <u>100</u>

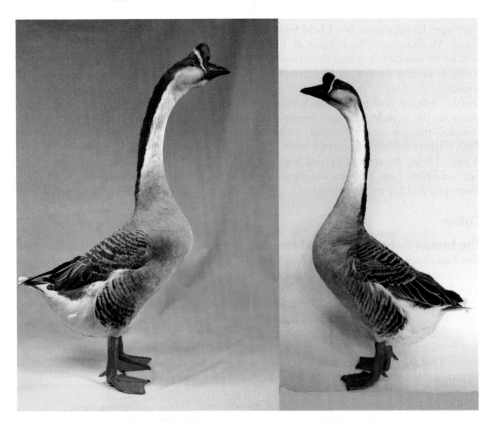

Chinese male (left) and female (right)

Disqualifications

Absence of knob. Any sign of a gullet/dewlap. Kinked neck. Excessive white in coloured plumage except as specified in brown or grey variety. Coloured plumage in the white variety.

Faults

Coarseness or excessive weight. Baggy underbody.

Minor faults (to be discouraged)

Orange marks on knob of older birds of brown or grey variety (this may be caused by damage or by frost).

CZECH

Classification: Light
Origin: Czech Republic

Old, long-established breed of goose from Bohemia, where it was a small table goose that thrived in the damp meadows. It laid plenty of eggs, starting early in the season, and produced a good crop of goslings. The breed was well known in the former East Germany and it was re-imported there in 1959, from whence it passed to West Germany and later to the UK in the 1990s. It was first included in the *British Poultry Standards* in 2008.

Overall type (shape): Male and female

Small goose, broad, full and finely boned body. When viewed side-on the body gives an oval impression. Legs set well apart, giving the impression of a very small goose. Active and alert.

Carriage: Slightly upright, goose more horizontal.
Head: Small, short, well rounded, broad. Well-pronounced cheeks. Well-rounded crown running smoothly into the neck. Throat showing no gullet. Beak short and straight, stout, orange-red with pale pink bean. Neck slightly arched. Strong. About half the length of the body, shorter and stouter in the female.
Body: Medium to long, broad, giving an oval impression from the side. Viewed from the top it is broad, tapering gradually into an egg-shaped form. Slightly upright on the front. The goose is visibly smaller and shorter than the gander. Back moderately long, slightly rounded, gently sloping towards the rear, broad in shoulders tapering slightly towards the rear. Breast very broad, full and well muscled. Undercarriage well rounded and free from bagginess. A small, single lobe situated in the middle of the abdomen is permitted in older females.
Tail: Horizontal, forming a straight line with the back and ending in a point.
Wings: Long, but not to reach beyond the tail, carried high and tight to the body.
Legs and feet: Thighs short, thickset, well muscled; lower thighs hardly visible. Shanks short to medium length, set very well apart, colour orange-red.
Plumage: Tight, sleek and hard.

Colour

In both sexes
Eyes: Blue with narrow orange-coloured eye ring (cilium).

Bill: Orange-red with pale pink bean.
Legs and webs: Orange-red.
Plumage: White.

Weights

Gander   5.0–5.5 kg   (11–12 lb)
Goose   4.0–4.5 kg   (8.5–10 lb)

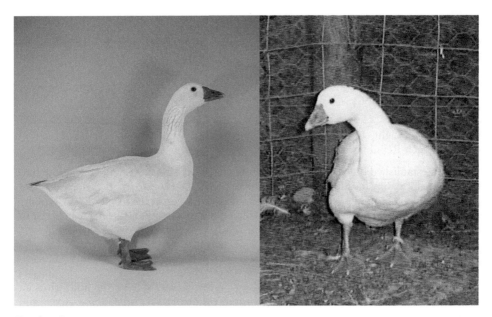

Czech pair

Scale of points

Carriage	15
Head and throat	10
Neck	10
Body	20
Legs and feet	5
Condition	10
Colour	10
Size	20
	100

Faults

In both sexes: Puny overall. Head too short, too long or too narrow. Body mass too bulky or too slight. Top line of body and abdomen running parallel. Too big-boned. Shoulders too narrow. Breast too flat and narrow. Legs too closely set. Lobes in young ganders. Oversized lobe in older females. Odd-coloured patches in the bill, plumage or legs.

EMBDEN

Classification: Heavy
Origin: North Europe

Along with the Toulouse, the Embden has been the longest standardised breed in the UK, both breeds being accepted for Standard in 1865. The Embden was also known as the Bremen and as a breed has been known for several centuries. It is a large, heavy, imposing bird, but gentle in nature. British breeders set about developing the breed and with careful selection increased its size and weight, with a good meat ratio. British Embdens have a slightly different appearance from the continental Embdens in that they are a solid bird with a good strong neck. Continental Embdens tend to have a longer, thinner neck, and this characteristic should be avoided if possible.

Overall type (shape): Male and female

Carriage: Upright and confident.
Head: Strong, bold. Stout beak. Eyes bold and alert.
Neck: Long, well proportioned, without gullet.
Body: Broad, thick and well rounded. Back long and straight. Breast round and full. Shoulders and stern broad. Paunch deep and dual lobed.
Tail: Tail close and carried well out.
Wings: Large and strong.
Legs and feet: Legs of medium length. Shanks large and strong.
Plumage: Hard and tight.

Colour

In both sexes

Eyes: Light blue.
Beak: Orange.
Legs and webs: Bright orange.
Plumage: Pure white.

Weights

Gander   12.7–15.4 kg   (28–34 lb)
Goose   10.9–12.7 kg   (24–28 lb)

Scale of points

Carriage	12
Head and throat	12
Neck	10
Body	20
Legs and feet	6
Condition	10
Colour	10
Size	20
	100

Faults

Undersize. Plumage other than white. Uneven lobes. Indication of a keel. Dewlap. Long thin neck.

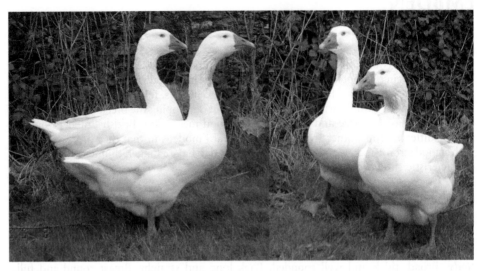

Embden

FRANCONIAN

Classification: Light
Origin: Germany

This is an old breed that developed along the flood plains of the winding Rivers Main and Fränkische Saale. This area was part of the former Duchy of Franconia, in southern Germany. Various coloured (blue, buff and pied) small geese living in this region were selected and bred by farmers, resulting in a small, hardy, active goose capable of raising good numbers of fast growing goslings. They required little feed in harsh winters and were good for meat and feathers.

At the beginning of the twenty-first century, good examples of the breed were collected by Ernst Messinger and Martin Wirsching, who began selective breeding to refine the breed. They produced birds of impressive quality that they took to top shows. They began distributing young stock to other breeders and the breed quickly gained popularity, and was bred and exhibited widely throughout Germany. The blue colour was accepted into the German Poultry Standards in 2008. Small numbers were imported into the UK from this time. It is included in the *British Poultry Standards* for the first time in 2018.

Overall type (shape): Male and Female

Small, fairly stocky, active goose with well-rounded, broad body.

Carriage: Horizontal or slightly sloping.
Head: Relatively short with well-rounded crown, throat with no sign of gullet. Beak short, but not too stout.
Neck: Medium length, strong, nearly straight or slightly curved.
Body: Medium length, broad, well rounded. Chest broad, fully rounded, carried at a slight angle. Undercarriage well defined, neat and smooth, or with a small single lobe, which may be more pronounced in older females. Female slightly smaller and more compact then male.
Tail: Forming a straight line with the back, relatively short and well closed.
Wings: Well set, but not to reach beyond tail. Not or only slightly crossing.

Legs: Thighs well developed, muscular, barely visible. Shanks short to medium length.
Plumage: Tight, dense, close fitting.

Colour

In both sexes
Eyes: Gold-brown with orange-coloured eye ring.
Beak: Orange with pale flesh-coloured bean.
Legs: Orange with horn-coloured nails.
Plumage: Pure medium blue as ground colour on plumage, lower front neck and breast.
Blue shading gradually into white on abdomen and stern. Lower breast, back and wing
feathers have a narrow white lacing. Tail blue with white edging.

Weights

Gander   5–6 kg   (11–13 lb)
Goose   4–5 kg   (9–11 lb)

Scale of points

Carriage   10
Head and throat   10
Neck   5
Body   15
Legs and feet   5
Condition   10
Colour   25
Size   20
                 100

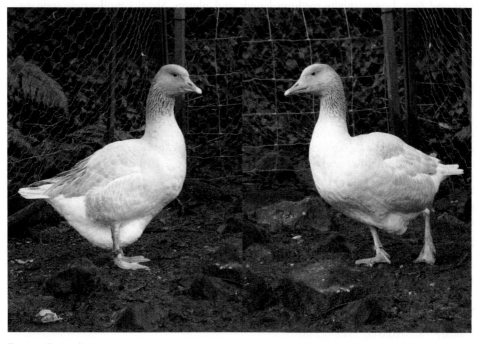

Franconian pair

Minor faults to be discouraged

Oversized, but also specimens which are too small. Dual lobe. Lacking in specified plumage colour, and type.

GREY BACK

Classification: Medium
Origin: Europe

This breed of goose is of the same type and pattern as the Buff Back except that the buff colouring is replaced by grey. Grey and white 'pied' geese occur in many parts of Northern Europe including the UK, where by 1906 these geese had long been known, and esteemed, as Saddlebacks. It has always been a popular colour pattern. This breed should not be confused with the Pomeranian, as, although in appearance they may look similar, the Grey Back is dual lobed with orange beak and feet. It was first included in the *British Poultry Standards* in 1982.

Overall type (shape): Male and female

Carriage: Almost horizontal.
Head: Fairly broad. Beak medium length, almost straight and stout. Eyes large.
Neck: Medium length, moderately stout and carried upright with little or no indication of an arch.
Body: Moderately long, plump, deep and meaty, with no evidence of a keel. Dual-lobed paunch.
Tail: Closely folded and carried almost level.
Wings: Rather long, with tips crossing over the tail coverts.
Leg and feet: Lower thighs medium length and plump. Shanks moderately long and sturdy.
Plumage: Hard and tight.

Colour

In both sexes
Head: Grey. Solid grey preferred. A small amount of white around base of beak permissible. Eyes blue. Beak orange.
Neck: Upper section grey (approximately one-third preferable), lower white.
Back: Grey in a heart shape, extending from above the scapulars, almost to base of tail: each feather with lighter greyish white edging.
Breast and flanks: White, except for grey thigh coverts; in some birds the grey extends in a broad band right under the abdomen (preferably without). Each grey feather with a lighter greyish white edging.
Paunch and stern: White.
Tail: White with some grey.
Wings: White apart from the grey forming a heart-shaped saddle on scapulars and wing coverts.
Legs and webs: Orange.

Weights

Gander   8.2–10.0 kg   (18–22 lb)
Goose   7.3–9.1 kg   (16–20 lb)

Scale of points

Carriage	10
Head and throat	5
Neck	5
Body	20
Legs and feet	5
Condition	10
Colour and markings	35
Size	10
	100

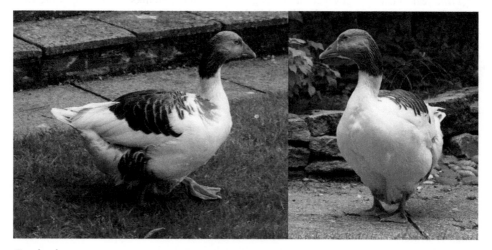

Greyback

Faults

In both sexes: Uneven markings or white interspersed in the coloured plumage. Very unequal distribution of colour on neck. Single lobe or uneven lobes in paunch.

PILGRIM

Classification: Light
Origin: Europe and UK

This is known as an autosexing breed because the males and females are a different colour: the gander is white and the goose grey. Autosexing geese in these colours have been found in the USA, the UK, France, parts of Northern Europe and Australia. Their exact origins are unclear but they may well have been taken to the eastern states of the USA by early settlers from Europe. Oscar Grow, an expert on waterfowl in the USA, claims to have developed the breed in Iowa; when he relocated to Missouri in the Great Depression of the 1930s he named the breed Pilgrim in memory of this move. Alternative evidence suggests they originate from northern Europe and were distributed throughout Europe by human migration and settlement. The breed was first standardised in the USA in 1939 but, despite being common as farmyard geese in the UK, were not standardised in the UK until 1982.

The Pilgrim has a reputation for being an easy to keep, personable bird, with good parenting qualities and a fast growth rate.

Overall type (shape): Male and female

Carriage: Above the horizontal, but not upright.
Head: Medium in size, oval, trim. Beak medium in length, straight, stout and smoothly attached. Eyes moderately large.
Neck: Medium in length, moderately stout, slightly arched.
Body: Moderately long, plump and meaty. Back moderately broad, uniform in width, flat and straight. Breast smooth and without keel. Adult abdomen deep with well-balanced dual lobes, free from bagginess.
Tail: Medium in length, closely folded. Carried almost level.
Wings: Strong, well developed, carried neatly to body.
Legs and feet: Lower thighs medium in length, well fleshed. Shanks moderately short and stout. Toes strong, straight and well webbed.
Plumage: Hard and tight.

Colour

Gander

Plumage: White, some inconspicuous grey permitted in back, wings and tail.
Eyes: Blue-grey.

Goose

Head: Light grey, the forepart may be broken with white, which becomes more extensive with age. Some Pilgrim females have the white extending around the eyes forming 'spectacles'.
Neck: Light grey, upper portion may be mixed with white in older birds.
Back: Light ash grey, laced with lighter grey.
Breast: Very light ash grey, gradually getting lighter as it goes under abdomen, to stern, which is white.
Flanks: Soft ash grey, each feather edged with a lighter shade.
Tail: Ash grey, heavily edged with a lighter grey approaching white.
Wings: Primaries medium grey, coverts light grey. Secondaries medium grey. Remaining coverts light ash grey edged with light grey.
Eyes: Hazel.

In both sexes

Beak: Orange.
Legs and webs: Orange.

Weights

Gander   6.3–8.2 kg   (14–18 lb)
Goose   5.4–7.3 kg   (12–16 lb)

Scale of points

Carriage	10
Head and throat	10
Neck	5
Body	15
Legs and feet	5
Condition	10
Colour	35
Size	10
	100

Faults

In the goose: White blaze on breast. Complete absence of white on head, or all white head. White flights.

In the gander: Solid grey features in plumage. Excessive grey dispersed throughout tail and wings. Any grey, if present, should be inconspicuous.

In both sexes: Flesh- or pink-coloured beak, legs or feet. Single lobe or unbalanced paunch. Undersize.

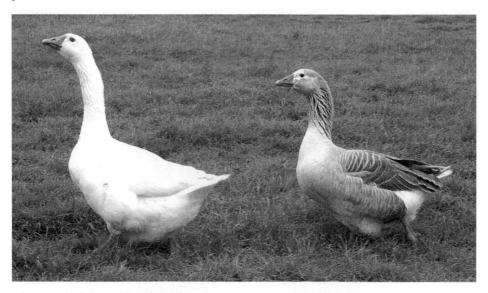

Pilgrim male (left) and female (right)

POMERANIAN

Classification: Medium
Origin: Europe

The Pomeranian gets its name from the former Province of Pomerania, which lay on the southern coast of the Baltic Sea between the estuaries of the Oder and Vistula rivers. This region is now shared between Germany and Poland. The Pomeranian comes in three colour varieties: the grey saddleback, the grey and the white. In the UK the grey saddleback is the most common and the standardised colour. The Pomeranian was first standardised in the 1997 *British Poultry Standards*.

Overall type (shape): Male and female

Carriage: Nearly horizontal.

Head: Fairly broad, crown somewhat flat. Beak medium length, stout and almost straight. Eyes large and prominent.

Neck: Medium in length, stout and carried upright.

Body: Moderately long, plump, deep and meaty. Back long and slightly convex. Breast plump, broad and prominent, no keel. Paunch single lobed, moderately deep and broad.

Tail: Short, closely folded, carried nearly level.

Wings: Long with tips crossing over tail coverts, carried high, neatly and smoothly folded.

Legs and feet: Lower thighs medium length, plump and nearly covered by ample thigh coverts. Shanks moderately long.

Colour

In both sexes

Head: Solid-coloured dark grey head preferred, but some specimens have white feathers around the base of the beak. White under chin is allowed. Eyes blue or brown. Red eye ring (cilium). Beak pink-red to orange-red.

Neck: Upper part (approximately one-third) dark grey, lower part white, separated cleanly and evenly.

Back: Dark grey, feathers with light edging, from point above scapulars to near the base of tail. This should suggest a heart shape.

Breast and flanks: White except for grey thigh coverts, grey feathers again light edged. In some birds a broad band of grey with light edging extends under abdomen (preferably without).

Paunch and stern: White.

Tail: White, but there may be some grey.

Wings: White, but grey heart shape will be on scapulars and neighbouring wing coverts, according to extent of grey saddle. Grey feathers light edged.

Legs and feet: Orange-red.

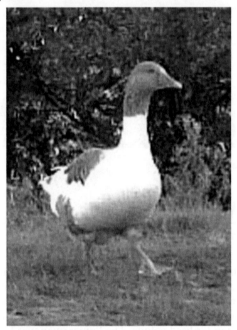

Pomeranian

Weights

Gander   8.2–10.9 kg   (18–24 lb)
Goose   7.3–9.1 kg   (16–20 lb)

Scale of points

Carriage	10
Head and throat	5
Neck	5
Body	20
Legs and feet	5
Condition	10
Colour and markings	35
Size	10
	100

Faults

In both sexes: Dual-lobed paunch. Uneven markings, white interspersed in coloured plumage. Very unequal division between the colours on the neck. Keel on breast.

ROMAN

Classification: Light
Origin: Europe

Supposedly the breed of geese that saved Ancient Rome from a night-time attack by the Gauls: the geese heard the enemy, and the noise the geese made alerted the guards and the Roman citadel was saved.

The Roman is a small, cobby goose which was first introduced into the UK at the beginning of the twentieth century. It was standardised in the 1982 edition of the *British Poultry Standards*. They also occur in a crested form.

Overall type (shape): Male and female

Carriage: Alert and active. Horizontal outline.
Head: Neat and well rounded. Face deep, beak short and not coarse. Eyes bold.
Neck: Upright, medium length and without gullet. Thickness maintained along its length.
Body: Compact and plump, deep and broad and well balanced. Back wide and flat. Breast full and well rounded, somewhat low and without a keel. Stern well rounded, paunch neat and not too pronounced.
Tail: Close, long and carried almost horizontal.
Wings: Long, strong, high up and well tucked up to tail line.
Legs and feet: Legs short, light boned and well apart.
Plumage: Sleek and tight.

Colour

In both sexes

Eyes: Light blue.
Beak: Orange-pink.
Legs and webs: Orange-pink.
Plumage: Pure white.

Weights

Gander   5.4–6.3 kg   (12–14 lb)
Goose   4.5–5.4 kg   (10–12 lb)

Scale of points

Carriage	15
Head and throat	10
Neck	10
Body	25
Legs and feet	5
Condition	10
Colour	10
Size	15
	100

Crested roman

As for Roman on all points, *except* for crest, which takes the form of a tuft of feathers, placed centrally on top of head. The front edge of the tuft should begin just over the back of the eyes. The tuft has been described as a tiny helmet perched on the top of the head.

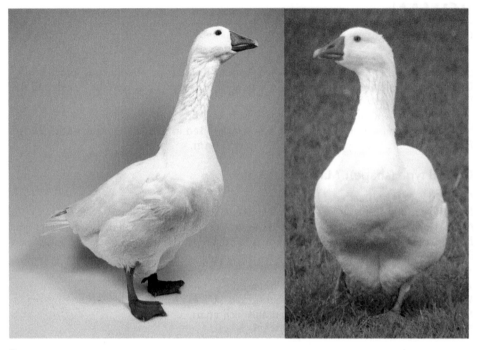

Roman

Faults

Excessive weight, coarseness, oversize or undersize. Ranginess, long thin neck. Plumage other than white. (Traces of light grey may be present on back and rump feathers of yearling females.)

SEBASTOPOL

Classification: Light
Origin: Eastern Europe

The Sebastopol takes its name from the Black Sea port of the same name. They were introduced into the UK by the diplomat Lord Dufferin in 1860, when he was sent to sort out problems in countries surrounding the Black Sea. Sebastopol geese occur widely in these areas and around the Danube and its tributaries.

The Sebastopol is unique and instantly recognisable in that it has curled, soft quilled feathers. There are two forms of the Sebastopol. The smooth breasted has normal feathers on the head, neck, breast and abdomen, with long curled feathers trailing from wings, back and tail. The curly breasted has a more pronounced curl to the feathers, which also cover the breast and abdomen, as well as the back, wings and tail. The curly breasted was standardised in the UK as 'frizzle' in 1982 and the smooth breasted in 1997.

Overall type (shape): male and female

The curly breasted
Carriage: Horizontal.
Head: Neat, rather large and round. Beak of medium length. Eyes large and prominent.
Neck: Medium length, thick and carried upright.
Body: The body appears round because of the full feathering. Back medium length, but looks short, because the long feathers give the body a rounded ball appearance. Breast full and deep, without keel. Paunch neat or dual lobed in older birds, not heavy or sagging.
Tail: Made up of long, well-curled feathers.
Wings: Feathers long, well curled and flexible. They make the bird incapable of flight because they are without stiff shafts.
Legs and feet: Lower thighs short, but stout, each covered with curled feathers. Shanks short and stout.
Plumage: Only feathers of head and upper neck smooth. Feathers on lower neck, breast and remainder of body profusely curly. Feathers of wings and back should be long (the longer, the better), well curled and free from stiff shafts. Birds of good stock and in good condition should display back and wing feathers that almost touch the ground.

The smooth breasted
Carriage: Horizontal.
Head: As curly breasted.
Neck: As curly breasted.
Body: Comparatively short. Back wide, well rounded, sloping gently from shoulders to tail. Breast smooth, full and rounded, without keel. Paunch neat or dual lobed in older birds, not heavy or sagging.
Tail: Short, held closed, carried horizontally or slightly elevated.
Wings: Feathers loosely curled, falling to the ground. The shafts are soft and flexible.
Legs and feet: Thighs short and strong. Shanks short and stout.
Plumage: The feathers of the head, neck, breast, belly and paunch smooth. Feathers of back, saddle, shoulders, wings and thighs are broad, extended in length, profuse, loosely curled and spiralled, falling over wings and rump, often trailing on the ground. The tail feathers are set rather unevenly and slightly 'waved'. The plumage should obscure the legs and feet from view.

Colour

The white (curly or smooth): Male and female
Eyes: Bright blue.
Beak and wings: Orange-pink.
Legs and webs: Orange-pink.
Plumage: Pure white (traces of light grey on back and rump of yearling females allowed).

The buff (curly or smooth): Male and female
Eyes: Brown.
Beak and wings: Orange-pink.
Legs and webs: Orange-pink.
Plumage: Even buff.

Weights

Gander   5.4–6.3 kg   (12–14 lb)
Goose   4.5–5.4 kg   (10–12 lb)

Scale of points

Carriage	15
Head and throat	5
Neck	5
Body	10
Legs and feet	5
Condition and feathering	40
Colour	10
Size	10
	100

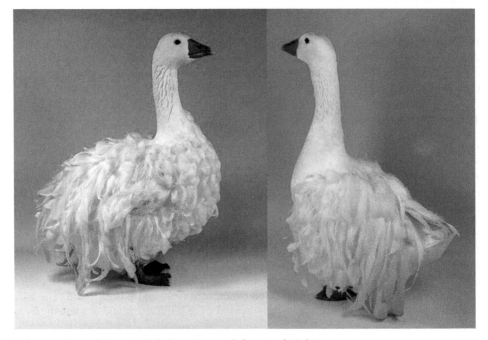

Sebastopol – curly breasted (left) and smooth breasted (right)

Faults

Long thin neck. Flat head. Angel wings. Plumage other than white in the white.

The curly breasted: Silky plumage on the back. Breast curl too low in the breast. Entire lack of curled feathers in the breast.
The smooth breasted: Curled feathers in breast.

SHETLAND

Classification: Light
Origin: Great Britain

This is a small, hardy autosexing breed from Britain's most northerly isles. The breed is a very old breed and was used locally by crofters to reduce the burden of liver fluke that was rife in the wet, marshy land, liver fluke being the enemy of livestock, especially sheep. The geese lay a clutch of eggs before sitting, laying up to 20 when managed well, and they make a meaty carcase. It was first included in the *British Poultry Standards* in 2008.

Overall type (shape): Male and female

Carriage: Only slightly above the horizontal, but not upright.
Head: Neat, not coarse. Eyes moderately large. Bill short, straight and stout.
Neck: Medium length, moderately stout and straight.
Body: Relatively short, giving the impression of a neat, cobby bird. Back broad, slightly convex. Body deep and well balanced. Single lobed.
Tail: Medium in length, closely folded, carried nearly level.
Wings: Long with tips crossing over the tail coverts.
Legs and feet: Thighs medium length, plump and nearly concealed by ample thigh coverts. Shanks moderately long and rather refined, yet sturdy.
Plumage: Hard and tight.

Colour

Gander

Plumage: Pure white throughout. Occasional grey feathers possible on the back of juvenile males.

Goose

Head and neck: The head is predominantly white with some grey, which extends partway down the neck, the white becoming more extensive in older birds. White feathers may be mixed with the grey. Eyes blue. Bill pink.
Back: Small centre back feathers grey.
Breast and flanks: White. Thigh coverts grey, light edged.
Tail: Mainly white with grey in central feathers.
Wings: Primaries, secondaries and tertials normally white, with grey scapulars and coverts forming the saddleback. The amount of grey feathers varies, but should not extend into the neck area. The grey feathers are laced with a paler shade.
Legs and webs: Pink, flesh coloured in immature birds.

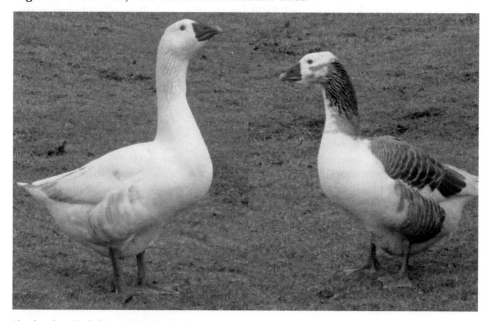

Shetland male (left) and female (right)

Weights

Gander   5.5–6.4 kg   (12–14 lb)
Goose   4.5–5.5 kg   (10–12 lb)

Scale of points

Carriage	10
Head and throat	15
Neck	5
Body	15
Legs and feet	5
Condition	10
Colour	25
Size	<u>15</u>
	100

Faults

Wrong shape or colour of beak. Oversize.

Minor faults (to be discouraged)

In the goose: Over- or undermarking in the grey.

SKÅNE

Classification: Heavy
Origin: Sweden

The Skåne goose or Skånegås (Swedish) is descended from birds (probably Pomeranian types) brought home from Germany by Swedish soldiers in the 1700s. These birds were mixed with other Swedish breeds and the Skåne was the result. Primarily adopted as the farmers' goose, they mature within six months in time for the national 'Goose Day' on 10 November. The Skåne goose has fine meat qualities (skin and meat white), is very easy to fatten and is fast growing and robust. It has a lovely temperament. It lays few eggs (weight 150 g) and is strongly inclined to sit. It was first included in the *British Poultry Standards* in 2008.

Overall type (shape): Male and female

Carriage: Above the horizontal.
Head: Fairly strong, powerful and well shaped. Bill medium thick.
Neck: Medium length, round, upright and quite thick with the upper part bent forward.
Body: Strong, well built and rounded. Back medium length, wide and slightly rounded when viewed from the side; convex line from base of neck to tail. Breast broad, deep and rounded when viewed from the front, with no keel showing. Paunch broad and not too deep, round and single lobed.
Tail: Short and with stiff feathering.
Wings: Big, strong and tight to body. Round sided.
Legs and feet: Thighs fairly short, strong and round. Shanks fairly strong and well set apart; fairly short.
Plumage: Feathering short and tight to the body.

Colour

In both sexes

Head and neck: Head brownish grey with a white ring around the base of the bill. Neck is between a third and a quarter brownish grey with the remainder white – this should be well defined. Eyes small, blue-grey. Bill orange-yellow with flesh-coloured bean.

Body: White with a well-defined and rounded brownish grey feather patch on the back. Similarly there is well-defined brownish grey feathering on the thighs, although this should be a softer hazy colour with the wing as the upper limit. Both back and thigh patches should show light grey edges on the feather.

Tail: White with a dark brownish grey band and a white edge.

Wings: White.

Legs and webs: Pinkish orange.

Weights

Gander   11–14 kg   (24–31 lb)
Goose   9–11 kg   (20–24 lb)

Scale of points

Carriage	10
Head and throat	10
Neck	5
Body	15
Legs and feet	5
Condition	10
Colour	20
Size	25
	100

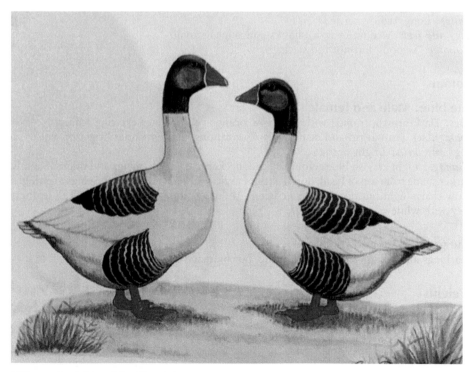

Skåne male (left) and female (right)

Faults

Poor type. Dual lobes (older males and laying females will tend to show more paunch). Poor and irregular colour definition. Grey on lower part of neck.

STEINBACHER

Classification: Light
Origin: Central–East Germany (region of Thuringia)

Often known as a fighting goose, the Steinbacher is probably no more aggressive than any other breed, especially in the breeding season, when all ganders will protect their group. They come from the local geese of Thuringia crossed with Chinese at the end of the nineteenth century, and developed into a distinctive breed described in 'Thüringer Geflügelzüchter', which was standardised in Germany in 1932, but it did not appear in the *British Poultry Standards* until 1997. It has rapidly grown in popularity in the UK due to the blue and lavender colour varieties that are found in this country. In Europe it is available in grey, blue, lavender cream and buff varieties.

Overall type (shape): Male and female

Carriage: Proud stature, fairly upright.
Head: Distinctive shape, with strong, slightly convex beak joining head in a continuous curve to back of head. No sign of knob or dewlap. Eyes large.
Neck: Straight, strong and upright. Medium length.
Body: Slightly stocky. Back strong, wide and slightly sloping downwards to tail. Breast wide and full. Abdomen wide and full, in young birds paunch should be absent, but in older birds a neat, even paunch is allowed.
Tail: Short, pointed and carried level.
Wings: Long, tightly carried.
Legs and feet: Medium length, shanks and thighs strong.
Plumage: Smooth, but not too sleek.

Colour

The blue: Male and female
Eyes: Dark brown, framed with a narrow orange-yellow outer eye ring (cilium).
Beak: Black bean at tip and distinct black serrations, the remainder bright orange.
Legs and webs: Bright orange.
Plumage: Light greyish blue colour to head, neck, breast, back, wings and thighs. Slightly darker shade from top of head, down back of neck. Feathers of shoulders, wings and thighs show sharp, light but not too wide edging. Abdomen and back silver-blue. Tail feathers grey with white edging. Stern white.

The grey: Male and female
Markings and colour pattern as the blue, but plumage colour dark grey.

Weights

Gander 6.0–7.0 kg (13–15 lb)
Goose   5.0–6.0 kg (11–13 lb)

Scale of points

Carriage	20
Head and throat	20
Neck	5
Body	10
Legs and feet	5
Condition	10
Colour	20
Size	10
	100

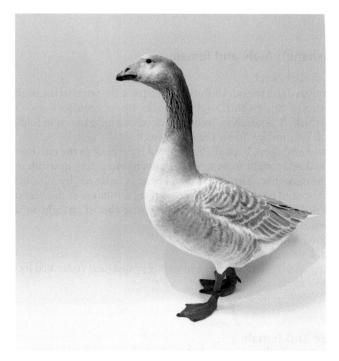

Steinbacher

Faults

In both sexes: Oversize. Body too heavy. Thin neck. Sign of knob or dewlap. Lack of black serrations or black bean on beak. Beak or serration colour other than stated. Feather edging absent. Leg colour other than bright orange. Uneven or lop-sided paunch. Dish-shaped beak. Dark grey (other than in the grey variety) or brown in plumage.

Minor faults (to be discouraged)

In both sexes: Black lines down top of beak.

TOULOUSE

Classification: Heavy
Origin: France

As suggested by its name the Toulouse originated and was developed in the Toulouse region of France. It was bred for meat and was also famous for the production of pâté de foie gras. A large, heavy bird was the result of all this breeding for meat. Because of this the Toulouse became sought after, being brought to the UK in the early 1840s by the then President of the Zoological Society, the 13th Earl of Derby. The Toulouse and Embden were the first breeds of geese to be standardised in the UK in 1865.

The Toulouse was also exported to the USA, and British and American breeders were responsible for further increasing the size of the breed and accentuating some of its features to produce a bird that has a slightly different appearance from the European-bred Toulouse.

Overall type (shape): Male and female

Carriage: Almost horizontal.
Head: Strong, massive and round. Uniform sweep from the point of the beak to the back of the head. Beak strong, fairly short, slightly convex upper beak (culmen). Eyes full.
Neck: Long and thick. A pendulous, well-developed dewlap extends in folds from the base of the lower beak (mandible) down the upper neck.
Body: Long, broad and deep. Back slightly curved from neck to the tail. Breast prominent, deep and full. The keel straight from stern to paunch, increasing in width to the stern and forming a straight underline. The keel on the breast is balanced by muscular supports on either side, which spread along the lower ribs, giving a fullness to the breast. Paunch dual lobed, well rounded, full and even. Stern wide, rising almost straight to the tail. Ample thigh coverts conceal the legs.
Tail: Short, carried high and well spread.
Wings: Large and strong.
Legs and feet: Legs short. Shanks stout and strong boned (legs concealed by thigh coverts).
Plumage: Full and fairly soft.

Colour

The grey: Male and female
Head and neck: Grey, with a slightly darker shade from top of head down back of neck. Eyes dark brown or hazel. Orange outer eye ring (cilium).
Beak: Orange.
Body: Breast and keel a fairly light grey, shading darker to thighs. Back grey. Each feather having a light edging. This edging is more pronounced on thigh coverts. Paunch, stern and tail white, but tail also has a broad band of grey across centre.
Wings: Primaries grey, secondaries darker grey with light edging. Primary coverts light grey; remaining coverts lighter grey with light edging.
Legs and webs: Orange or pink-orange.

The buff
As the grey in all respects, except buff colour plumage instead of grey. Eye, beak, leg and web colour as in the grey.

The white
As the grey in all respects, except pure white plumage instead of grey, blue eyes and orange beak, legs and webs.

Weights

Gander   11.8–13.6 kg   (26–30 lb)
Goose   9.1–10.9 kg   (20–24 lb)

Scale of points

Carriage   15
Head and throat   15
Neck   5
Body   20
Legs and feet   5
Condition   10
Colour   10
Size   20
                   ___
                   100

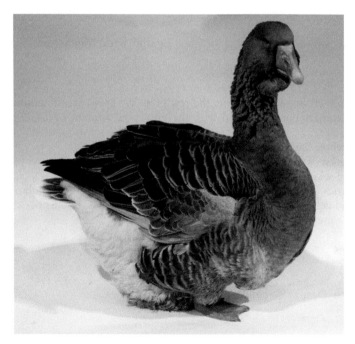

Toulouse

Disqualifications

In both sexes: Dropped, angel or split wings. Dropped tongue.

Faults

In both sexes: Twisted keel. Patches of black or white in plumage. White flights.

Minor faults (to be discouraged)

In both sexes: Narrow white line around base of beak in young birds. Hollows in front of legs.

WEST OF ENGLAND

Classification: Medium
Origin: England

Overall type (shape): Male and female

Carriage: Slightly sloping.
Head: Neat, not coarse. Beak medium sized, straight and stout. Eyes moderately large.
Neck: Medium length, quite stout, with a slight arch.
Body: Moderately long. Body deep. Paunch full, dual lobed. Back broad, slightly convex.
Wings: Long with tips crossing over the tail coverts.
Tail: Medium length, carried horizontally.
Legs and feet: Thighs medium length, plump and nearly concealed by ample thigh coverts, shanks moderately long.
Plumage: Hard and tight.

Colour

Gander

Plumage: Pure white (small traces of grey on the back, thighs and flight feathers permissible).

Goose

Head and neck: Front of head white, the rest grey, the grey extending down the neck, where white feathers may be mixed with the grey. The amount of white on the head increases with age.
Back: Small centre back feathers grey.
Breast and flanks: White, apart from thigh coverts, which are grey laced with light edging.
Tail: Grey and white.
Wings: Primaries, secondaries and tertials normally white, with grey scapulars and coverts forming the saddleback. The amount of grey feathers varies, but should not extend into the neck area. The grey feathers are laced with a paler shade.

In both sexes

Eyes: Blue.
Beak: Orange.
Legs and webs: Orange or pink.

Weights

Gander   7.3–9.1 kg   (16–20 lb)
Goose   6.3–8.2 kg   (14–18 lb)

Scale of points

Carriage	10
Head and throat	5
Neck	5
Body	20
Legs and feet	5
Condition	10
Colour	25
Size	20
	100

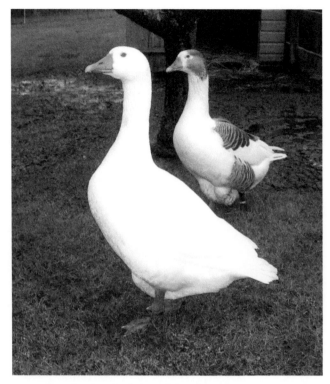

West of England male (left) and female (right)

Crested West of England

As for West of England on all points, *except* for crest, which takes the form of a tuft of feathers, placed centrally on top of the head. The front edge of the tuft should begin just over the back of the eyes.

Faults

In both sexes: Undersize. Pink beak. Uneven lobes to paunch.

Minor faults (to be discouraged)

In the goose: Insufficient grey, especially in the head and neck; overmarking in the grey, extending onto the secondaries and spoiling the back markings.

Ducks

Throughout recent history, it has generally been accepted that all breeds of duck, bar the Muscovy, had their origins in the wild Mallard. This is evident from breeds such as the Rouen, whereas some consider Black East Indians and Cayugas as Mallard sports. The original British white ducks could also have originated as sports from Mallards, being subsequently bred for size and table merits, leading to well-known examples such as the Aylesbury today. Although egg colours are specified for fowl, it has been found, certainly recently, that it is difficult to uniformly specify egg colours in contemporary breeds. A thorough literature search made by Poultry Club of Great Britain Trustee Bill Oldcorn has led to the following table of *suggested egg colours* being formulated, taking information from Edward Brown's *Races of Domestic Poultry*, Lewis Wright's *Book of Poultry* and other historical material. It is assumed that the eggs of geese are indeed uniformly white.

Duck points

Section	Breed	Carriage	Head and neck	Body	Legs and feet	Colour	Size	Condition
Bantam	Black East Indian	10	15	15	5	30	15	10
Bantam	Call	10	18	12	5	30	15	10
Bantam	Crested Miniature	10	35	15	5	10	15	10
Bantam	Silver Appleyard Miniature	10	15	15	5	30	15	10
Bantam	Silver Bantam	10	15	15	5	30	15	10
Heavy	Aylesbury	10	25	20	5	10	20	10
Heavy	Blue Swedish	10	15	15	5	30	15	10
Heavy	Cayuga	10	15	15	5	30	15	10
Heavy	Muscovy	10	20	15	5	20	20	10
Heavy	Pekin	20	20	15	5	10	20	10
Heavy	Rouen	10	15	10	5	35	15	10
Heavy	Rouen Clair	10	15	15	5	30	15	10
Heavy	Saxony	10	15	15	5	30	15	10
Heavy	Silver Appleyard	10	15	15	5	30	15	10
Light	Abacot Ranger	10	15	15	5	35	10	10
Light	Bali	20	30	15	5	10	10	10
Light	Campbell	15	15	15	5	25	15	10

(continued)

British Poultry Standards, Seventh Edition. Edited by J. Ian H. Allonby and Philippe B. Wilson.
© 2019 Poultry Club of Great Britain. Published 2019 by John Wiley & Sons Ltd.

(*Continued*)

Section	Breed	Carriage	Head and neck	Body	Legs and feet	Colour	Size	Condition
Light	Crested	10	40	15	5	10	10	10
Light	Hook Bill	10	30	15	5	20	10	10
Light	Indian Runner	20	20	20	5	15	10	10
Light	Magpie	10	18	12	5	30	15	10
Light	Orpington	10	15	15	5	35	10	10
Light	Welsh Harlequin	10	15	15	5	35	10	10

Defects and deformities in waterfowl (for which birds should be passed)

Ducks: Kinked neck, dished bill, twisted bill, wry tail, roach back, dropped or slipped wing, crest impeding vision, caruncles impeding eyes or nostrils.

Duck breed	Suggested egg colour
Abacot Ranger	White but varies according to strain
Aylesbury	White/greenish white according to strain
Bali	Greenish white but varies according to strain
Black East Indian	Green/grey/white but varies according to strain
Blue Swedish	Pale blue/white
Call	Variable shades according to strain
Campbell	White but varies according to strain
Cayuga	Very dark green/grey (almost black at start of lay)
Crested	Variable shades according to strain
Crested Miniature	Variable shades according to strain
Hook Bill	Variable shades according to strain
Indian Runner	Variable colours according to strain
Magpie	White/greenish white according to strain
Muscovy	Cream fading to white
Orpington	White
Pekin	White
Rouen	Pale green
Rouen Clair	Pale green but varies according to strain
Saxony	White
Silver Appleyard	White
Silver Appleyard Miniature	White/pale green
Silver Bantam	White/pale green
Welsh Harlequin	White but varies according to strain

ABACOT RANGER

Classification: Light
Origin: Great Britain

The Abacot Ranger was one of many breeds developed from (or crossed with) Indian Runners. Starting with 'sports' from khaki Campbells, themselves originally the products of Runner crosses, Mr Oscar Gray of Abacot Duck Ranch, near Colchester, mated their offspring to a white Indian Runner drake. The eventual results were 'light drakes of Khaki carriage and type with dark hoods, and white ducks with blue flight bars and fawn or grey hoods'. This development was begun in 1917 and the Wye College Duck Laying Test of 1922 and 1923 indicates a very successful outcome: the breed came top with 935 eggs in the four bird section.

Originally called the 'Hooded Ranger', this breed almost died out in this country. Imported into Germany via Denmark in 1926, it was 'stabilised' as a colour form by H. Lieker, whence it acquired the name *Liekers Streifere* (Lieker's Ranger or Scout). In 1934 it was eventually standardised under the name of *Streicher-Ente* (Ranger Duck). Later standardised by the British Waterfowl Association (BWA) in 1987, the modern Abacot Ranger owes both its survival and written Standard to the work done in Germany.

Overall type (shape): Male and female

Carriage: Slightly erect, alert and busy.
Head: Well rounded with a slightly raised brow. Bill medium length, rising in a gentle curve to the brow; should not be wedge shaped.
Neck: Medium length, not too thin and only slightly curved, becoming thicker at the base and joining smoothly at the body.
Body: Longish, well rounded but not too full, and without any keel. The almost straight back runs approximately parallel to the underside.
Tail: Only slightly elevated.
Wings: Tight, held close to the body.
Legs and feet: Legs medium length.
Plumage: Tight and glossy.

Colour

Drake

Head and neck: Black with green lustre, terminated above the shoulder by a completely encircling white ring, dividing in a sharp clean line the neck and breast colours. Eyes dark brown. Bill olive green with black bean.

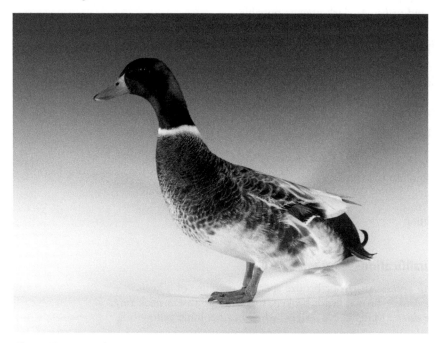

Abacot Ranger male

Back: Upper back feathers white, finely stippled with black and fringed with white. Lower down the back the stippling becomes heavier, each feather preferably fringed with white, until solid black with green lustre on the rump. Black 'sex curls' may also be tipped with white.

Breast, neck base and shoulders: Claret edged with white.
Flanks, underbody and stern: Silvery white to cream (a white ground colour being preferable). A little of the breast colour extending along the upper flank.
Tail: Brownish black, the whole bordered with white. Undertail black, finishing neatly and not running into the stern and flank colour.
Wings: Primaries silvery white with a slightly iridescent dark grey overlay. Secondaries (speculum) bluish green tipped with distinct black then white bars. Greater coverts dark grey with well-defined white rim. Outer scapulars and tertiaries as the breast with wider silver-white edging. Smaller coverts white feathers finely stippled with black (giving the impression of grey), and fringed with white. Underwing creamy white.
Leg and webs: Orange.

Duck

Head and neck: Fawn (a deeper shade in young females) with the brow and crown clearly marked with darker graining. There is a sharp division between the neck and upper white of the breast colour. Eyes dark brown. Bill dark slate tinged with green.
Lower back: Light fawn with darker central streak. Rump fawnish grey with brown tips giving the impression of a triangular pattern.
Upper breast, lower neck, shoulders and flanks: Lightly streaked with light brown on a creamy white ground.
Lower breast, underbody and stern: Creamy white.
Tail: Fawn, edged with cream.
Wings: Primaries and speculum as the drake. Scapulars and tertiaries creamy fawn with brown flecks. Greater coverts dark grey with well-defined white rim. Smaller coverts dark fawn edged with cream. The creamy white ground colour in the bird to prevail. Underwing creamy white.
Legs and webs: As dark grey as possible.

Weights

Drake   2.3–2.5 kg   (5–5.5 lb)
Duck   2.0–2.3 kg   (4.5–5 lb)

Scale of points

Carriage	10
Head, bill and neck	15
Body	15
Legs and feet	5
Colour	35
Size	10
Condition	10
	100

Disqualifications

In both sexes: Absent or bronze specula; presence of a keel.
In the drake: Brown head; broken, too wide or absent neck ring.
In the duck: Mallard eye stripes; white head colour; yellow bill.

Faults

In the drake: Too dark a ground colour; breast colour running too low into body or lacking white edging; blue bill.
In the duck: Absence of graining or streaking; dark ground colour.

Minor faults (to be discouraged)

In the duck: Coarse or black graining on the head.

AYLESBURY

Classification: Heavy
Origin: Great Britain

The Aylesbury derives its name from the town of Aylesbury in Buckinghamshire, where it was bred as a white table duck in the eighteenth century and used in increasingly large numbers to supply the London market. The white plumage was valued for quilt filling and the pale skin contributed an attractive carcass. This light colouration is evident in the pink bill colour that continues to be a key characteristic of the breed.

The Aylesbury was a leading waterfowl exhibit in the first National Poultry Show held at the London Zoological Gardens in June 1845. This was the beginning of *live* poultry exhibitions, and it was the Victorian stress on size that led to the development of the modern Aylesbury with its pronounced keel and long, pink bill. It was standardised in 1865.

Overall type (shape): Male and female

Carriage: Horizontal, the keel parallel to and touching the ground when the bird is standing at rest.
Head: Strong and powerful, with eyes near the top of the skull. Eyes full. Bill long, broad and wedge shaped. When viewed from the side the outline is almost straight from the top of the skull, the head and bill measuring from 15 to 20 cm (6–8 in.).
Neck: Medium length, slightly curved.
Body: Long, broad and keel very deep. Back straight, sloping slightly from shoulders to tail. Breast full and prominent. Keel straight from breast to stern.
Wings: Strong and carried closely to the sides, fairly high but not touching across the saddle.
Tail: Short, only slightly elevated.
Legs and feet: Legs very strong, the bones thick, set to balance a level carriage.
Plumage: Bright and glossy.

Colour

In both sexes
Eyes: Blue.
Bill: Flesh pink.
Legs and webs: Bright orange.
Plumage: White, resembling satin.

Weights

Drake   4.5–5.4 kg   (10–12 lb)
Duck   4.1–5 0 kg   (9–11 lb)

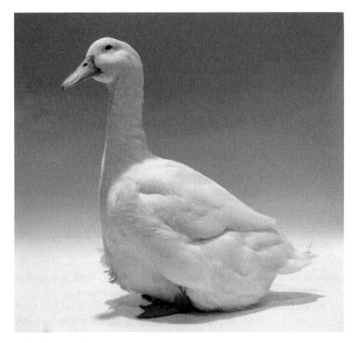

Aylesbury male

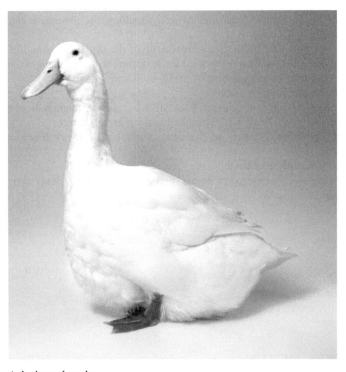

Aylesbury female

Scale of points

Carriage	10
Head, bill and neck	25
Body	20
Legs and feet	5
Colour	10
Size	20
Condition	10
	100

Disqualifications

Plumage other than white. Bill other than flesh pink. Lack of keel.

Faults

In the drake: Any black on the bill.
In both sexes: Primary feathers protruding above the rump. Thin neck.

Minor faults (to be discouraged)

In the duck: Black on the bill.

BALI

Classification: Light
Origin: East Indies

Originally imported from Malaysia in 1925, these ducks take their name from Bali, an island east of Java where they were indigenous. Originally standardised in 1930, the breed has recently been recreated in Britain (in the 1990s) by crossing crested ducks with Indian Runners.

Overall type (shape): Male and female

Carriage: Upright and active (as Indian Runner).
Head: Fine, resembling that of the Indian Runner, but slightly more rounded over the skull, and with a small, single, globular crest on the rear of the head.
Neck: Slim, fairly long, smoothly attached to the shoulders.
Body: Slim and cylindrical with not too much shoulder. Similar to that of the Indian Runner, but with more prominent front, giving the Bali a somewhat heavier appearance.
Wings: Held tight to the body.
Tail: In line with the back.
Legs and feet: Legs strong, set well to the rear of the body to give the upright carriage.
Plumage: Tight and hard.

Colour

The white: Male and female
Plumage: Pure white.

White Bali: Female
Eyes: Blue.
Bill: Orange-yellow.
Legs and webs: Orange.

The coloured
Any colour is permitted but attention should be paid to symmetry of markings.

Weights
Drake   2.3 kg   (5 lb)
Duck   1.8 kg   (4 lb)

Scale of points
Carriage   20
Head, bill and neck   30 (this includes 10 points for the crest)
Body   15
Legs and feet   5
Colour   10
Size   10
Condition   10
                                               100

Disqualifications

In both sexes: Any spinal deformity, in particular twisted or kinked neck. Twisted bill. Wry tail.

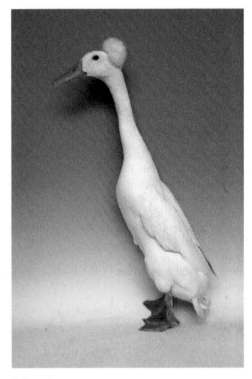

Bali male

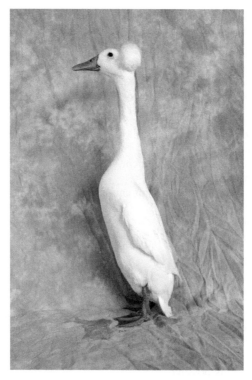

Bali female

Faults

In both sexes: Split, slipped, exaggerated or uneven crest. Crest that interferes with the eyes. Weeping eyes. Domed head. Short body. Not upright in carriage. Thick shoulders or too heavy body reminiscent of the Crested.

Minor faults (to be discouraged)

In both sexes: Wrong bill or leg colour in whites.

BLACK EAST INDIAN

Classification: Bantam
Origin: Uncertain; probably America

First standardised in Britain in 1865, the Black East Indian Duck shares its colour with the North American Cayuga. This bantam duck was alleged to have been imported to Britain by the Earl of Derby in about 1850. However, evidence suggests that it had been already in the possession of the Zoological Society of London (ZSL) since 1831, the same year that the 13th Earl of Derby was elected President of the ZSL. At this time it was known as the 'Buenos Ayres' duck, but there seems to be no evidence that South America or the East Indies were the places of origin. It has been known as 'Labrador', 'Brazilian', 'Buenos Aires' and eventually 'Black East Indie', the first being perhaps the most appropriate geographically.

There is speculation that the black gene may have arrived via a close relative of the northern mallard, the American black duck (*Anas rubripes*). This is the bold assertion of early historians of the Cayuga, and it seems equally applicable to the Black East Indian. The drakes tend to retain their black plumage but the females develop patches of white as they get older. Impure black birds can show elements of brown pencilling, especially under the wings and throat.

Overall type (shape): Male and female

Carriage: Lively and only slightly elevated.
Head: Neat and round, with high skull. Bill medium length and fairly broad. Eyes full.
Neck: Medium length.
Body: Compact. Breast round and prominent.
Tail: Very slightly elevated.
Wings: Strong, closely folded, carried high enough to allow wing tips contact over the back.
Legs and feet: Legs medium length.
Plumage: Smooth, close and glossy.

Colour

In both sexes

Plumage: Black with a beetle-green lustre over as much of the plumage surface as possible.
Underwing: Coverts black with green lustre; main feathers very dark grey.
Eyes: Brown; as dark as possible.
Bill: Black.
Legs and webs: As black as possible.

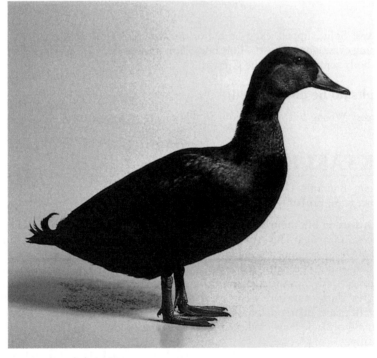

Black East Indian male

Weights

Drake   0.9 kg   (2 lb)
Duck   0.7–0.8 kg (1.5–1.75 lb)

Scale of points

Carriage	10
Head, bill and neck	15
Body	15
Legs and feet	5
Colour	30
Size	15
Condition	10
	100

Disqualifications

In both sexes: Yellow bill; white spot under the bill. Elements of brown pencilling, especially on underwing and throat; brown or conspicuous white in the plumage, including the underwing.

Faults

In both sexes: Purple lustre. Green bill. Oversized. Shallow or narrow boat-shaped body. Pronounced, rounded body as a Call duck. Overlong or flattened bill with exaggerated serrations ('fish billed').
In the duck: Orange in the legs and feet.

Minor faults (to be discouraged)

In both sexes: Grey or olive tip on the bill.

BLUE SWEDISH

Classification: Heavy
Origin: Europe

Blue ducks emerged in northern Europe during the nineteenth century in various breeds. Two of the most popular, the Blue Swedish and the Pomeranian (Pomern), were developed near the Baltic shores of what is now modern Germany and Poland. Both of these breeds have characteristics in common: both have bibs and are blue, but the Blue Swedish has some white primaries. A pair of exhibition Blues will produce a proportion of blue, black and splashed offspring.

Overall type (shape): Male and female

Carriage: From 20° to 25° above the horizontal. Lively and alert.
Head: Oval, bold. Eyes full. Bill medium length, joining the skull in a smooth line.
Neck: Medium length, only slightly curved.
Body: Round, plump, deep; without keel. Breast full. Abdomen free of bulkiness; stern full and rounded. Back flat, straight, about 50% longer than broad.
Tail: Slightly elevated.
Wings: Strong, compact and carried close to the body.
Legs and feet: Thighs well fleshed. Legs medium length; set a little back from centre.

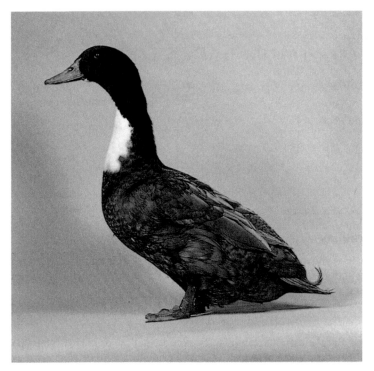

Blue Swedish male

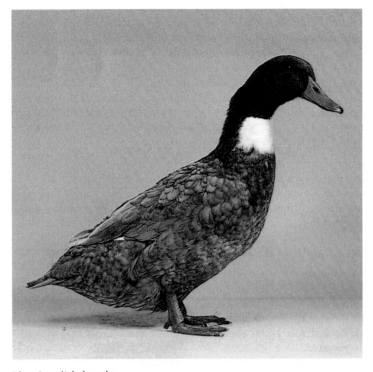

Blue Swedish female

Colour

Head: In the drake, dark blue with greenish lustre. In the duck, dark blue. Eyes brown. Bill in the drake blue preferred to green; in the duck slate blue.

In both sexes: Body plumage a uniform shade of slate blue, strongly laced with a darker shade of this blue throughout except for an unbroken, teardrop-shaped white 'bib' (about 7.5 × 10 cm (3 × 4 in.) in extent in the drake; 5.0 × 7.5 cm (2 × 3 in.) in the duck) upon the lower neck and upper breast. Wings same as body colour, except that the two outer primaries in each should be white. Speculum as inconspicuous as possible. Underwing blue-grey.

Legs and webs: Orange-black in drake, blue-brown in the duck. Irregular paler markings are permitted.

Weights

Drake   3.6 kg   (8 lb)
Duck   3.2 kg   (7 lb)

Scale of points

Carriage	10
Head, bill and neck	15
Body	15
Legs and feet	5
Colour	30
Size	15
Condition	10
	100

Disqualifications

In both sexes: Russet tinge in plumage. Complete lack of bib.

Faults

In both sexes: Lack of size. Visible keel. White bib extending onto belly. Indication of iridescent speculum. Thin neck. Wings meeting over back. More than four white primaries.
In the duck: Paler underbody.

Minor faults (to be discouraged)

In both sexes: Incorrect number of white primaries. Black and green flecks in plumage. White bib extending to lower mandible.

CALL

Classification: Bantam
Origin: Uncertain; probably The Netherlands

While known as Call Ducks nowadays they have been referred to as Decoys or Coys in the past. Francis Willughby, who toured The Netherlands, Germany, Switzerland and Italy between 1663 and 1666, observed how wildfowlers in The Netherlands fitted ponds with channels and nets prior to stocking them with Coy Ducks to entice and entrap wildfowl. He noticed that some Coy Ducks were free winged, but others were pinioned. A painting by Melchior d'Hondecoeter (1636–1695), featuring what appears to be well-grown Call ducklings in the foreground, seems to back this evidence that they existed in The Netherlands in the seventeenth century.

Trapping wildfowl went on in Britain also, with wildfowlers deploying tame or semi-tame ducks to entice their wild relatives. Reverend Edmund Saul Dixon MA revealed in his book *Ornamental and Domestic Poultry*, written in 1848, that a much smaller race of white ducks had been imported from The Netherlands and that their chief merit, indicated by the title Call Duck, consisted in their incessant loquacity. He went on to state that the management of decoys was as well understood in Norfolk as anywhere and that the trained Decoy Ducks there resembled the wild Mallard. While these wild coloured traitors aroused no suspicion the imported conspicuous Dutchmen excited fatal attention and curiosity. The white Call Ducks had a yellow-orange bill unlike the Aylesbury's, which was flesh coloured. Harrison Weir's *Our Poultry*, published in 1902, in quoting from Johnson's Dictionary: 'To decoy, v.a. (from *Koey*, Dutch, a cage), to entrap, to draw into', aptly described why these diminutive ducks were employed.

When the first *Standard of Excellence in Exhibition Poultry* was compiled in 1865 two colour varieties of Calls (known as Decoy at that time) were standardised – the white and the grey. (The latter becoming known as the 'brown' before being termed 'Mallard' at the present time.)

By the mid-1880s, Mandarins and Carolinas had become more popular with exhibitors and Calls were relegated to just the odd exhibit or two being shown in Ornamental duck or drake classes. This state of affairs lasted for over a century until their popularity really took off and more than 300 Call Ducks could be seen at larger shows. This popularity has continued and the Club Show, in current times, can attract in excess of 500 entries. From 1971 onwards, additional colour varieties have been standardised.

Overall type (shape and carriage): Male and female

Carriage: Horizontal, without tipping forward or being too upright.
Type: Body small and compact, short, broad and deep.
Head: Neat and round, with high crown. Full cheeks. Bill short, maximum length 3.1 cm ($1\frac{1}{4}$ in.), and broad, set squarely into the face. Eyes full, round and alert.
Neck: Short and thick.
Legs and feet: Legs short, set midway along the body. Feet straight and webbed.

Self varieties

Black

Plumage of both sexes: Uniform black all over, except head and neck may have some iridescent green sheen.
In both sexes: Bill black; green or grey tip acceptable with age. Eyes dark brown. Legs preferably black, but some orange pigment accepted.
Faults in both sexes: Coloured feathers anywhere other than the required black or iridescent green. Bill, eye and leg colour other than stated.
Minor faults in both sexes: Any evidence of purple or brown sheen or lacing. Grey markings on bill of young birds.

Chocolate

Plumage of both sexes: Uniform dark chocolate, except for the drake's head, which is lustrous dark chocolate.
In both sexes: Bill dark brown with dark bean. Eyes brown. Legs chocolate with darker shading on feet.

Faults in both sexes: Coloured feathers anywhere other than the required chocolate or lustrous dark chocolate. Uneven ground colour (mealiness). Bill, eye and leg colour other than stated.

Minor faults in both sexes: Rust-stippled feathers in drakes or rust-laced feathers in ducks.

White

Plumage of both sexes: Pure white all over.

In both sexes: Bill bright orange-yellow. Eyes blue.

Major faults in both sexes: Any black on bill.

Faults in both sexes: Flesh-coloured bill in adults. Coloured feathers other than the required white. Sappy yellow in plumage. Leg and eye colour other than that stated.

Mallard varieties

Mallard

Drake

Head and neck: Iridescent green with white collar to front and sides of neck. Bill olive green with dark bean.

Breast: Rich claret; clearly defined with no white fringing.

Flanks and underbody: Light grey, stippled with dark grey, with narrow white strip across abdomen and up towards back as far as the tail, forming boundary between underbody and undertail.

Back: Grey, shading to black towards rump.

Rump and undertail cushion: Rump black with green iridescence. Undertail cushion lustrous black.

Tail: Mainly white with dark grey stippling in centre under black sex curls.

Wings: Primaries grey. Scapulars grey, with bronze tinge to outer edge. Tertiaries grey, shading to rich claret on outer edges next to speculum.

Legs: Orange.

Duck

Head and neck: Golden brown with dark brown graining on crown, down back of neck and on eye stripes. Plain, lighter brown throat. Bill dark orange with brown saddle and dark bean.

Breast, flanks, underbody, back and rump: Golden brown pencilled with dark brown.

Undertail cushion: Creamier than underbody but with more pronounced dark brown pencilling.

Tail: Mainly light golden brown irregularly marked with dark brown especially towards centre.

Wings: Primaries brownish slate. Scapulars golden brown pencilled with dark brown. Tertiaries dark brown finely laced with off-white.

Legs: Orange with darker webs.

In both sexes

Wing: Speculum iridescent blue, edged with black then white. Wing bar white then black.

Eyes: Brown.

Major faults

In both sexes: White primaries.

In the drake: Absence of white collar. Spreading of breast colour onto shoulder or underbody.

In the duck: No eye stripes. White neck ring. White throat and/or eye markings.

Faults

In both sexes: Insufficient speculum. Lack of the iridescence required. Incorrect speculum colour. Bill, eye and leg colour other than stated. Spreading of darker central tail stippling markings or peppering to outer white areas of drake's tail or to outer light golden brown areas of duck's tail.
In the drake: White ring completely encircling neck. White fringing on breast in the adult drake. White markings on head, under chin on throat, rump or black part of undertail. Lack of, or incorrect, iridescence on head, rump or undertail. White fringing on black of wing bar.
In the duck: Ground colour too dark. Excessive dark brown pencilling on back feathers (i.e. mossy backed). Lack of any pencilling on back feathers. Light golden brown fringing on white of wing bar. White fringing on black of wing bar.

Minor faults

In the drake: Undefined edges to breast colour. White fringing on breast of drakelets. White strip across abdomen overextending, i.e. onto back or absent.
In the duck: Insufficient eye-stripe markings. Lack of/excess graining on crown and/or neck. Indistinct pencilling on scapulars. Off-white or muddy-looking white of wing bar.

Dusky mallard
Drake

Head and neck: Iridescent green, with no white neck ring or collar. Bill olive green with dark bean.
Breast, flanks and underbody: Light grey, finely stippled with dark grey up to neckline.
Back: Dark grey-brown, shading to black towards rump.
Rump and undertail cushion: Rump black with green iridescence and undertail cushion lustrous black. (*Note*: There is no narrow white strip across abdomen and up towards back as far as the tail, forming boundary between underbody and undertail.)
Tail: Grey-brown, darker towards centre under black sex curls.
Wings: Primaries grey-brown. Underwing coverts pearly blue-grey. Scapulars dark grey, with brown tinge on outer edge. Tertiaries grey-brown.

Duck

Head and neck: Dark golden brown heavily and evenly flecked with very dark brown. Dark flecks on crown show a little iridescence. No eye stripes. Bill dark orange with dark saddle and bean.
Breast, flanks, underbody, rump, undertail cushion and scapulars: Dark golden brown pencilled with dark brown.
Back: Dark golden brown broadly pencilled with dark brown.
Tail: Dark golden brown irregularly marked with dark brown.
Wings: Primaries dull chocolate brown. Scapulars dark golden brown pencilled with dark brown. Tertiaries and lesser wing coverts dull chocolate brown finely laced with off-white.

In both sexes

Wings: Speculum sooty grey with no iridescence and a fine off-white line on leading edge of each feather. Wing bar whiteish grey.
Eyes: Brown.
Legs: Dull orange.

Major faults

In both sexes: White primaries. Iridescent speculum. White feathers on head, under chin or on breast. Evidence of white neck ring or collar.

In the drake: Signs of a claret or white bib. White markings on black part of undertail. Evidence of white strip under abdomen.

In the duck: Any evidence of eye stripes.

Faults

In both sexes: Underwing coverts any colour other than pearly blue-grey, e.g. white. Insufficient speculum. Incorrect speculum colour. Bill, eye and leg colour other than that stated. Spreading of darker central tail stippling markings or peppering to outer grey-brown areas of drake's tail or to dark golden brown areas of duck's tail.

In the drake: Lack of, or incorrect, iridescence on head, rump or undertail.

In the duck: Loss of ground colour and pencilling. Excessive dark brown pencilling on back feathers (i.e. mossy backed). Pencilling too fine, or lacking on back feathers. Insufficient, or lack of, pencilling on underbody feathers.

Minor faults

In the duck: Indistinct pencilling on scapulars.

Chocolate mallard
Drake

Head and neck: Lustrous dark chocolate with white collar to front and sides of neck. Bill dull orange with dark bean.

Breast: Claret; clearly defined with no white fringing.

Flanks and underbody: Blond, stippled with dark chocolate, with narrow white stripe across abdomen and up towards back, forming boundary between underbody and undertail.

Back: Chocolate, shading to dark chocolate towards rump.

Rump and undertail cushion: Lustrous dark chocolate.

Tail: Mainly blond with chocolate stippling in centre under dark chocolate sex curls.

Wings: Primaries light chocolate on outside web of flights with the inner edged with blond. Scapulars blond stippled with dark chocolate. Tertiaries blond, shading to chocolate on outer edges next to speculum.

Duck

Head and neck: Deep buff with dark chocolate graining on crown, down back of neck and on eye stripes. Plain, blond-coloured throat. Bill dull orange with dark chocolate saddle and bean.

Breast, flanks, underbody, back and rump: Deep buff pencilled with chocolate.

Undertail cushion: Lighter buff than underbody but with more pronounced chocolate pencilling.

Tail: Mainly blond irregularly marked with chocolate, especially towards centre.

Wings: Primaries light chocolate on outside web of flights with the inner edged with blond. Scapulars deep buff pencilled with chocolate. Tertiaries light chocolate finely laced with off-white.

In both sexes

Wings: Speculum iridescent dark chocolate, edged with dark chocolate then white. Wing bar white then dark chocolate.

Eyes: Brown.

Legs: Dull orange.

Major faults

In both sexes: White primaries.

In the drake: Absence of white collar. Spreading of breast colour onto shoulder or underbody.

In the duck: No eye stripes. White neck ring. White throat and/or eye markings.

Faults

In both sexes: Insufficient speculum and/or iridescence required. Incorrect speculum colour. Bill, eye and leg colour other than that stated. Spreading of darker central tail stippling, markings or peppering to outer blond-coloured areas of tail.

In the drake: White ring completely encircling neck. White fringing on breast in the adult drake. White markings on head, under chin, on throat, rump or dark chocolate part of undertail. Lack of, or incorrect, iridescence on head, rump or undertail. Spreading of breast colour onto underbody. White fringing on dark chocolate of wing bar.

In the duck: Ground colour too dark. Excessive dark brown pencilling on back feathers (i.e. mossy backed). Lack of any pencilling on back feathers. Buff fringing on white of wing bar. White fringing on dark chocolate of wing bar.

Minor faults

In the drake: Undefined edges to breast colour. White fringing on breast of drakelets. White strip across abdomen overextending, i.e. onto back.

In the duck: Insufficient eye-stripe markings. Lack of/excess graining on crown and/or neck. Indistinct pencilling on scapulars. Off-white or muddy-looking white of wing bar.

Khaki (dusky chocolate mallard)
Drake

Head and neck: Lustrous dark chocolate, with no white neck ring or collar.
Breast, flanks and underbody: Blond, stippled with dark chocolate up to neck line.
Back: Warm khaki shading to lustrous dark chocolate towards rump.
Rump and undertail cushion: Lustrous dark chocolate.
Tail: Blond, darker towards centre under dark chocolate sex curls.
Wings: Scapulars blond, stippled with dark chocolate. Tertiaries blond shading to chocolate brown on outer edges next to speculum. Underwing coverts blond.

Duck

Head and neck: Khaki heavily and evenly flecked with chocolate brown.
Breast: Warm khaki lightly pencilled with grey-brown.
Flanks and underbody: Khaki lightly flecked with grey-brown.
Back, rump and undertail cushion: Warm khaki broadly pencilled with chocolate brown.
Tail: Light khaki irregularly marked with light brown, darker towards centre.
Wings: Scapulars warm khaki broadly pencilled with blue-grey. Tertiaries light khaki finely laced with off-white.

In both sexes

Wings: Primaries warm khaki. Speculum dull chocolate edged with dark chocolate brown then off-white. Wing bar off-white then dark chocolate brown.
Eyes: Brown.
Legs: Dark orange.
Bill: Slate blue preferred.

Major faults

In both sexes: White primaries. Iridescent speculum. White feathers on head, under chin or on breast. Evidence of white neck ring or collar.
In the drake: Signs of a claret bib. White markings on black part of undertail.
In the duck: Any evidence of eye stripes.

Faults

In both sexes: Underwing coverts other than blond, e.g. white. Insufficient speculum. Incorrect speculum colour. Bill, eye and leg colour other than stated. Spreading of darker central tail stippling, markings or peppering to outer blond areas of drake's tail and light khaki areas of duck's tail.

In the drake: Lack of, or incorrect, iridescence on head, rump or undertail.

In the duck: Loss of ground colour and pencilling. Excessive chocolate brown pencilling on back feathers (i.e. mossy backed). Pencilling too fine, or lacking, on back feathers. Insufficient, or lack of, pencilling on underbody feathers.

Minor faults

In the duck: Indistinct pencilling on scapulars.

Marked mallard varieties

Pied

Coloured feathers as in Mallard, with variations in amount of pied (white) markings allowed, symmetry of markings highly preferable. White areas often more extensive in the duck.

Drake

Head and neck: Iridescent green with white surround at base of bill and white line starting at rear of eyes and encircling back of head. Wide white ring completely encircling the neck. Bill light yellow with greenish tinge and dark bean.

Breast: Rich claret, clearly defined with no white fringing.

Flanks and underbody: Light grey, stippled with dark grey, may include white markings especially behind the legs.

Back: Grey, shading to black towards rump.

Rump and undertail cushion: Rump black with green iridescence and undertail cushion lustrous black.

Tail: Mainly white with darker grey stippling in centre under black sex curls.

Wings: Scapulars grey, with bronze tinge to outer edge. Tertiaries grey, shading to rich claret on outer edges next to speculum but may be white.

Duck

Head and neck: Golden brown with dark brown graining on crown, down back of neck and on eye stripes. White surround at base of bill and white line starting at rear of eyes and encircling back of head. Wide white ring completely encircling neck. Bill yellow with light brown saddle and dark bean.

Breast, back and rump: Golden brown pencilled with dark brown.

Flanks, underbody and undertail cushion: Golden brown pencilled with dark brown, may include white especially behind legs but undertail cushion to have more pronounced dark brown pencilling.

Tail: Mainly light golden brown irregularly marked with dark brown especially towards centre.

Wings: Scapulars golden brown pencilled with dark brown. Tertiaries dark brown finely laced with off-white but may be white.

In both sexes

Wings: Primaries white. Speculum iridescent blue, edged with black then white. Wing bar white then black.

Eyes: Brown.

Legs: Orange.

Major faults

In both sexes: Insufficient white markings. Lack of white primaries.

In the drake: Absence of white neck ring. No eye stripes. Spreading of breast colour onto shoulder or underbody. White fringing on breast in the adult drake.

Faults

In both sexes: Insufficient speculum and/or iridescence required. Incorrect speculum colour. Insufficient white markings. Bill, eye and leg colour other than that stated. Spreading of darker central tail stippling, markings or peppering to outer white areas of drake's tail or to outer light golden brown areas of duck's tail.
In the drake: Lack of, or incorrect, iridescence on head, rump and undertail. White fringing on black of wing bar.
In the duck: Ground colour too dark. Excess dark brown pencilling on back feathers (i.e. mossy backed). Lack of any pencilling on back feathers. Light golden brown fringing on white of wing bar. White fringing on black of wing bar.

Minor faults

In both sexes: White cheeks. Lack of symmetry in markings.
In the drake: Undefined edges to breast colour. White fringing on breast of drakelets.
In the duck: Insufficient eye-stripe markings. Eye markings too pale. Indistinct pencilling on scapulars. Off-white or muddy-looking white of wing bar.

Yellow belly

Drake

Head and neck: Iridescent green with white collar almost encircling neck. Bill olive green with dark bean.
Breast: Upper breast rich claret; lower breast pinkish buff extending upwards from underbody to merge with upper breast.
Flanks: Light grey, stippled with dark grey.
Underbody: Pinkish buff.
Back: Grey shading to black towards rump.
Rump and undertail cushion: Rump black with green iridescence and undertail cushion lustrous black with some pinkish buff streaks.
Tail: Mainly white with dark grey stippling in centre under black sex curls.
Wings: Primaries grey. Scapulars grey with bronze tinge to outer edge. Tertiaries grey shading to claret on outer edges next to speculum.

Duck

Head and neck: Golden brown with dark brown graining on crown, down back of neck and on eye stripes. Plain pinkish buff throat. Bill dark orange with brown saddle and dark bean.
Breast, flanks and undertail cushion: Pinkish buff.
Underbody: Light pinkish buff.
Back: Golden brown pencilled with dark brown.
Rump: Dull dark buff irregularly marked with brown.
Tail: Mainly light yellowish buff with some dark buff to brown pencilling in centre of tail.
Wings: Primaries brownish slate. Scapulars golden brown pencilled with dark brown. Tertiaries dark brown finely laced with off white.

In both sexes

Wings: Speculum iridescent blue edged with black then white. Wing bar white then black.
Eyes: Brown.
Legs: Orange.

Major faults

In both sexes: White primaries.
In the drake: Absence of white collar.

In the duck: Evidence of white neck ring. No eye stripes. Pinkish buff extending onto scapulars.

Faults

In both sexes: Insufficient speculum and/or iridescence required. Incorrect speculum colour. Bill, eye and leg colour other than that stated. Spreading of darker central tail stippling, markings or peppering to outer white areas of drake's tail and yellowish buff areas of duck's tail.
In the drake: White ring completely encircling neck. White markings on head, under chin, on throat or rump. Lack of, or incorrect, iridescence on head, rump or undertail. White fringing on black of wing bar.
In the duck: Excess dark brown pencilling on back (i.e. mossy backed). Lack of any pencilling on back feathers. Light golden brown fringing on white of wing bar. White fringing on black of wing bar.

Minor faults

In the drake: Yellow spreading onto chin.
In the duck: Insufficient eye-stripe markings. Lack of/excess graining on crown, head and/ or neck. Off-white or muddy-looking white of wing bar.

Dilute mallard varieties

(It is considered that these have a dilute 'Mallard' colour pattern, i.e. having a dilution of the pattern and in a paler colour. The blue fawn deriving from the Mallard, and the apricot from the blue fawn.)

Blue fawn
Drake

Head and neck: Lustrous charcoal-blue with white collar to front and sides of neck. Bill olive green with dark bean.
Breast: Claret; clearly defined with no white fringing.
Flanks and underbody: Light grey, stippled with charcoal-blue, with narrow white strip across abdomen and up towards back, forming boundary between underbody and undertail.
Back: Blue-grey, shading to charcoal-blue towards rump.
Rump and undertail cushion: Charcoal-blue.
Tail: Mainly white with blue-grey stippling in centre under charcoal-blue sex curls.
Wings: Scapulars light grey, stippled with charcoal-blue. Tertiaries smoke-grey, shading to claret on outer edges next to speculum.
Legs: Orange.

Duck

Head and neck: Fawn with charcoal-blue graining on crown and on eye stripes. Cheeks light fawn and plain light fawn throat. Bill orange-brown with brown saddle and dark bean.
Breast: Fawn, flecked with blue-grey.
Flanks, underbody and undertail *cushion*: Light fawn, flecked with blue-grey but undertail cushion to be creamier with pronounced blue-grey markings.
Back and rump: Fawn, broadly pencilled with blue-grey.
Tail: Mainly light fawn irregularly marked with blue-grey especially towards centre.
Wings: Scapulars fawn pencilled with blue-grey. Tertiaries blue-grey finely laced with off-white.
Legs: Orange with darker webs.

In both sexes

Wings: Primaries smoke grey. Speculum matt charcoal-blue, edged with light blue-grey then white. Wing bar white then light blue-grey.
Eyes: Brown.

Major faults

In both sexes: White primaries.
In the drake: Absence of white collar. Spreading of breast colour onto shoulder.
In the duck: Evidence of white neck ring. No eye stripes. White throat and/or eye markings. Ground colour other than fawn, e.g. rust. Pencilling other than blue-grey, e.g. brown-grey or lavender.

Faults

In both sexes: Insufficient speculum and/or the lustre required. Incorrect speculum colour. Iridescence on speculum. Bill, eye and leg colour other than stated. Spreading of darker central tail stippling, markings or peppering to outer white areas of drake's tail or to outer light fawn areas of duck's tail.
In the drake: White ring completely encircling neck. White fringing on breast in the adult drake. White markings on head, under chin, on throat, rump or charcoal-blue part of undertail. Lack of lustre on head. Breast colour spreading downwards onto underbody. White fringing on blue-grey of wing bar.
In the duck: Black or Mallard coloured feathers anywhere. Light fawn fringing on white of wing bar. White fringing on blue-grey of wing bar.

Minor faults

In the drake: Undefined edges to breast colour. White fringing on breast of drakelets. White strip across abdomen overextending, i.e. onto back.
In the duck: Insufficient eye-stripe markings. Lack of, or excess, graining on crown and/or neck. Off-white or muddy-looking white of wing bar.

Apricot
Drake

Head and neck: Lustrous silver grey with white collar to front and sides of neck. Bill olive green with dark bean.
Breast: Light claret, clearly defined with no white fringing.
Flanks and underbody: Light grey, stippled with apricot-brown, with narrow white strip across abdomen and up towards back, forming boundary between underbody and undertail.
Back: Light blue-grey, shading to blue-grey towards rump.
Rump and undertail *cushion*: Blue-grey.
Tail: Mainly white with light blue-grey stippling in centre under blue-grey sex curls.
Wings: Scapulars light grey, stippled with apricot-brown. Tertiaries light grey, shading to light claret on outer edges next to speculum.

Duck

Head and neck: Apricot with light blue-grey graining on crown and eye stripes. Bill light apricot-brown with brown saddle and dark bean.
Breast and flanks: Even shade of apricot.
Underbody and undertail *cushion*: Light apricot, but undertail cushion to be creamier with pronounced apricot markings.
Back and rump: Apricot very broadly pencilled with light blue-grey.
Tail: Mainly creamy apricot; darker towards centre.
Wings: Scapulars apricot pencilled with light blue-grey. Tertiaries light blue-grey finely laced with off-white.

In both sexes

Wings: Primaries light blue-grey with apricot tinge. Speculum silver grey overlaid with apricot lustre, edged with light silver grey then white. Wing bar white then light silver grey.

Eyes: Brown.

Legs: Orange.

Major faults

In both sexes: White primaries.

In the drake: Absence of white collar. Head colour other than silver grey. Spreading of breast colour onto shoulder.

In the duck: No eye stripes. White throat and/or eye markings. Brown eye stripes. White neck ring. Ground colour ginger instead of apricot.

Faults

In both sexes: Insufficient speculum and/or the required lustre. Incorrect speculum colour. Iridescence on speculum. Bill, eye and leg colour other than that stated. Spreading of darker central tail stippling, markings or peppering to outer white areas of drake's tail or to creamy apricot areas of duck's tail.

In the drake: White ring completely encircling neck. Lack of lustre on head. White markings on head, under chin, on throat, rump or blue-grey areas of undertail. White fringing on breast in the adult drake. Breast colour spreading downwards onto underbody. White fringing on silver grey of wing bar.

In the duck: Uneven ground colour (mealiness). Light apricot fringing on white of wing bar. White fringing on silver grey of wing bar.

Minor faults

In the drake: Undefined edges to breast colour. White fringing on breast of drakelets. White strip across abdomen overextending, i.e. upwards onto back.

In the duck: Insufficient eye-stripe markings. Lack of, or excess, graining on crown and/or neck. Off-white or muddy-looking white of wing bar.

Silver varieties

(Drakes in all silver varieties have an extension of breast colour onto upper flanks, thereby mirroring the colour pattern of the silver drake, i.e. the 'harlequin' pattern.)

Silver

Drake

Head and neck: Iridescent green with white neck ring completely encircling the neck. Bill olive green with dark bean.

Breast and upper flanks: Claret, each feather fringed with white.

Lower flanks and underbody: White.

Back: White stippled with black, shading to black towards rump.

Rump and undertail cushion: Rump black with green iridescence and undertail cushion lustrous black.

Tail: Mainly white with black stippling in centre under black sex curls, which may be tipped with white.

Wings: Primaries white stippled with black especially on outer edges and tips. Scapulars white stippled with black. Lower scapulars rich claret fringed with white to complement upper flanks. Tertiaries white stippled with black, shading to rich claret on outer edges next to speculum.

Duck

Head and neck: White with dark graining on crown extending to back of head. No more than a blush of cream or light fawn on cheeks is permissible on head, while a hint of dark eye stripe in front and behind the eye is desirable. Bill light orange-brown with brown saddle and dark bean.

Breast, back, rump and undertail cushion: White with some brown and charcoal grey mottling.

Flanks and underbody: White.

Tail: Mainly white but matching drake's tail by having charcoal grey markings in centre of tail.

Wings: Primaries white stippled with dark grey especially on outer edges and tips. Scapulars white with some brown and charcoal grey mottling. Tertiaries white with some brown and charcoal grey mottling shading to dark grey on outer edges towards speculum.

In both sexes

Wings: Speculum iridescent blue, edged with black then white. Wing bar white then black. Black of wing bar to be fringed with white.

Eyes: Brown.

Legs: Orange.

Major faults

In both sexes: Pure white primaries. Lack of speculum. Ground colour other than white. Spreading of darker central tail stippling, markings or peppering to outer white areas of tail (i.e. a fringed tail).

In the drake: Any signs of grey stippling on lower flanks. Lack of claret feathers on upper flanks. Lack of white fringing to claret feathers on breast and upper flanks. Well-defined claret breast colour with no bleeding onto flanks.

In the duck: Apricot or fawn-coloured head and/or neck (i.e. a hood).

Faults

In both sexes: Insufficient speculum and/or the iridescence required. Incorrect speculum colour. Bill, eye and leg colour other than stated.

In the drake: Incomplete white neck ring. White markings on head, under chin, on throat or rump.

In the duck: Insufficient brown and charcoal grey mottling on breast, back and especially rump.

Minor faults

In both sexes: Lack of iridescence on speculum. Incorrect speculum colour.

In the drake: Insufficient extension of claret feathers along upper flanks. Excessive extension of claret feathers onto lower flanks or underbody. Signs of white in black part of undertail.

In the duck: Excess dark graining on crown and/or neck.

Dark silver

Drake

Head and neck: Iridescent green with white collar almost completely encircling the neck. Bill olive green with dark bean.

Breast and upper flanks: Claret, each feather fringed with pale grey with fringing less pronounced than in the silver.

Lower flanks and underbody: Light grey stippled with dark grey shading to white towards tail.

Back: Grey stippled with black, becoming darker towards rump.

Rump and undertail cushion: Rump black with green iridescence and undertail cushion lustrous black.

Tail: Mainly white with black stippling especially in centre under black sex curls, which may be tipped with light grey.

Wings: Primaries grey stippled with dark grey. Scapulars grey stippled with dark grey. Lower scapulars claret fringed with pale grey to complement upper flanks. Tertiaries grey stippled with dark grey, shading to claret on outer edges next to speculum.

Duck

Head and neck: Light fawn with dark grey-brown eye stripes and graining on crown. Neck light fawn with plain, pale cream-fawn throat. Bill orange-brown with brown saddle and dark bean.

Breast, flanks, back, rump and undertail *cushion*: Light fawn with dark grey-brown flecking on each feather but undertail cushion to be creamier with more pronounced dark grey-brown flecking.

Underbody: Cream with fine grey-brown flecking.

Tail: Mainly creamy fawn irregularly marked with dark grey-brown especially in centre of tail.

Wings: Primaries creamy fawn to dark brown. Scapulars light fawn with dark grey-brown flecking on each feather. Tertiaries grey-brown finely laced with off-white.

In both sexes

Wings: Speculum iridescent blue, edged with black then white. Wing bar white then black.

Eyes: Brown.

Legs: Orange.

Major faults

In both sexes: Pure white primaries. Lack of speculum. Spreading of darker central tail stippling, markings or peppering to outer white areas of drake's tail and creamy fawn areas of duck's tail (i.e. a fringed tail).

In the drake: Lack of claret feathers on upper flanks. Lack of pale grey fringing to claret feathers on breast and upper flanks. Well-defined claret breast colour with no bleeding onto flanks.

In the duck: Ground colour too dark, i.e. too close to Mallard. Breast and flank colour too light, i.e. too close to Appleyard markings. Evidence of white neck ring. White throat and/or eye markings.

Faults

In both sexes: Insufficient speculum and/or the iridescence required. Incorrect speculum colour. Bill, eye and leg colour other than stated.

In the drake: Insufficient pale grey fringing to claret feathers on lower breast and upper flanks. Insufficient dark grey stippling on lower flanks. White ring completely encircling neck. White markings on head, under chin, on throat, rump or black areas of undertail.

Minor faults

In the drake: Insufficient extension of claret feathers along upper flanks. Excessive extension of claret feathers onto lower flanks or underbody. A complete neck ring.

In the duck: Insufficient eye-stripe markings.

Apricot silver

Drake

Head and neck: Lustrous silver grey with white ring completely encircling the neck. Bill olive green with dark bean.

Breast and upper flanks: Light claret, each feather fringed with white.
Lower flanks and underbody: White.
Back: White stippled with light blue-grey, shading to light blue-grey towards rump.
Rump and undertail cushion: Light blue-grey.
Tail: White with light blue-grey stippling in centre under light blue-grey sex curls, which may be tipped with white.
Wings: Primaries white stippled with light blue-grey especially on outer edges and tips. Scapulars white stippled with light blue-grey. Lower scapulars light claret fringed with white to complement upper flanks. Tertiaries white stippled with light blue-grey, shading to light claret on outer edges next to speculum.

Duck

Head and neck: Light apricot on a white ground, with some light blue-grey graining on crown but no solid apricot hood. Bill light orange with lighter bean.
Breast, back, *rump and undertail cushion*: White with some light apricot mottling.
Flanks and underbody: White.
Tail: White, which can be irregularly marked with a little light apricot in centre of tail.
Wings: Primaries white. Scapulars white with some apricot mottling. Tertiaries white shading to light apricot then light blue-grey on outer edges towards speculum.

In both sexes

Wings: Speculum silver grey, edged with light silver grey then white. Wing bar white, then light silver grey. Silver grey of wing bar to be fringed with white.
Eyes: Brown.
Legs: Orange.

Major faults

In both sexes: Lack of speculum. Spreading of darker central tail stippling, markings or peppering to outer white areas of tail (i.e. a fringed tail).
In the drake: Head colour other than silver grey. Any signs of grey stippling on lower flanks. Lack of claret feathers on upper flanks. Lack of white fringing to light claret feathers on breast and upper flanks. Well-defined claret breast with no bleeding onto flanks.
In the duck: No apricot colour on head. Solid apricot head and neck making a hood. Any charcoal-blue mottling on breast, back or rump.

Faults

In both sexes: Evidence of iridescence on speculum. Incorrect speculum colour. Bill, eye and leg colour other than stated.
In the drake: Incomplete white neck ring. White markings on head, under chin, on throat or rump.

Minor faults

In both sexes: Ground colour other than white.
In the drake: Insufficient extension of light claret feathers along upper flanks. Excessive extension of light claret feathers onto lower flanks or underbody. Head colour other than silver grey. Lack of lustre on head. Signs of white in blue-grey of undertail.
In the duck: Insufficient apricot mottling on breast, back and especially rump.

Blue silver

Drake

Head and neck: Lustrous charcoal-blue with white neck ring completely encircling neck. Bill olive green with dark bean.
Breast and upper flanks: Claret, each feather fringed with white.

Lower flanks and underbody: White.

Back: White stippled with light charcoal-blue shading to charcoal-blue towards rump.

Rump and undertail cushion: Charcoal-blue.

Tail: White with charcoal-blue stippling in centre under sex curls, which may be tipped with white.

Wings: Primaries white stippled with light charcoal-blue especially on outer edges and tips. Scapulars white stippled with light charcoal-blue. Lower scapulars claret fringed with white to complement upper flanks. Tertiaries white with some blue-grey stippling, shading to claret on outer edges next to speculum.

Duck

Head and neck: White with charcoal-blue graining on crown. A hint of charcoal-blue eye stripe in front and behind the eye is permissible. Bill light orange with brown saddle and dark bean.

Breast, flanks and underbody: White.

Back and rump: White with some light charcoal-blue mottling. Mottling heaviest on rump.

Undertail cushion: White with some light charcoal-blue ticking.

Tail: White, which can be irregularly marked with charcoal-blue in centre of tail.

Wings: Primaries and scapulars white. Tertiaries white shading to charcoal-blue on outer edges towards speculum.

In both sexes

Wings: Speculum matt charcoal-blue edged with blue-grey then white. Wing bar white then blue-grey. Blue-grey of wing bar to be fringed with white.

Eyes: Brown.

Legs: Orange.

Major faults

In both sexes: Ground colour other than white. Spreading of darker central tail stippling, markings or peppering to outer white areas of tail. Complete lack of speculum (i.e. a fringed tail).

In the drake: Any signs of charcoal-blue stippling on lower flanks. Lack of claret feathers on upper flanks. Lack of white fringing to claret feathers on breast and upper flanks. Well-defined breast claret colour with no bleeding onto flanks.

In the duck: Solid blue head and neck making a hood. Any apricot on head or apricot mottling on breast, back or rump.

Faults

In both sexes: Evidence of iridescence on speculum. Incorrect speculum colour. Bill, eye and leg colour other than stated.

In the drake: Incomplete white neck ring. White markings on head, under chin, on throat or rump.

Minor faults

In the drake: Lack of lustre on head. Insufficient extension of claret feathers along upper flanks. Excessive extension of claret feathers onto lower flanks or underbody. Signs of white in charcoal-blue of undertail.

In the duck: Excessive dark graining on crown and/or neck. Insufficient charcoal-blue mottling on back and especially rump.

Chocolate silver

Drake

Head and neck: Lustrous dark chocolate with white neck ring completely encircling neck. Bill orange with dark bean.

Breast and upper *flanks*: Claret, each feather fringed with white.
Lower flanks and underbody: White.
Back: White stippled with chocolate, shading to dark chocolate with lustre towards rump.
Rump and undertail cushion: Dark chocolate.
Tail: Mainly white with chocolate stippling in centre under dark chocolate sex curls, which may be tipped with white.
Wings: Primaries white stippled with light chocolate especially on outer edges and tips. Scapulars white stippled with light chocolate. Lower scapulars claret fringed with white to complement upper flanks. Tertiaries white stippled with light chocolate, shading to claret on outer edges next to speculum. Speculum iridescent dark chocolate, edged with chocolate then white. Wing bar white then chocolate. Chocolate of wing bar is fringed with white.

Duck

Head and neck: Light chocolate with some darker chocolate graining on crown with neck shading to white and not forming a solid light chocolate hood. Bill dull orange with darker saddle.
Breast, back, rump and *undertail cushion*: White with some light chocolate mottling.
Flanks and underbody: White.
Tail: White marked with light chocolate markings especially towards centre.
Wings: Primaries white. Scapulars white with some light chocolate mottling. Tertiaries white shading to light chocolate then brighter chocolate on outer edges towards speculum. Speculum slightly iridescent chocolate edged with darker chocolate then white. Wing bar white then light chocolate. Light chocolate of wing bar to be fringed with white.

In both sexes

Eyes: Brown.
Legs: Chocolate-orange with darker shading on feet.

Major faults

In both sexes: Ground colour other than white. Spreading of darker central tail stippling, markings or peppering to outer white areas of tail (i.e. a fringed tail).
In the drake: Any signs of blond stippling on lower flanks. Lack of claret feathers on upper flanks. Lack of white fringing to claret feathers on lower breast and upper flanks. Well-defined claret breast colour with no bleeding onto flanks.
In the duck: Solid chocolate head and neck making a hood.

Faults

In both sexes: Insufficient speculum and/or the iridescence required. Incorrect speculum colour. Bill, eye and leg colour other than stated.
In the drake: Incomplete white neck ring. White markings on head, under chin, on throat or rump.

Minor faults

In the drake: Lack of lustre on head. Insufficient extension of claret feathers along upper flanks. Excessive extension of claret feathers onto lower flanks or underbody. Signs of white in dark chocolate of undertail.
In the duck: Insufficient light chocolate mottling on breast, back and especially rump.

Marked silver varieties

Abacot

Both drakes and ducks to have considerably more colour and a richer shade than traditional silvers. Both sexes are to have evenly fringed tails, as if laced, while silvers have tails that are largely white. (This fringing on the tails of Abacot Calls appears to be approximately half to three-quarters of a centimetre ($\frac{3}{16}-\frac{5}{16}$ in.) in width around the outside edge or perimeter of the tail. It is a collective look rather than a lace on each individual tail feather.) The black or grey stippling on the upper back of the Abacot drake to be heavier than in the silver drake, while the Abacot duck to have a fawn hood as opposed to the silver duck's largely white head with dark graining. The Abacot duck to have far more fawn and brown mottling on her body too.

Drake

Head and neck: Iridescent green, with white ring completely encircling neck. Bill olive green with black bean.

Breast: Rich claret with white fringing but less apparent on upper breast. The white fringing elsewhere not as extensive as in the silver drake (i.e. the Abacot drake shows more claret).

Upper flanks: Rich claret feathers fringed with white to extend boldly along upper flanks.
Lower flanks and underbody: White.

Back: White extensively stippled with black, shading to black towards rump.

Rump and undertail cushion: Rump black with green iridescence and undertail cushion lustrous black.

Tail: Brownish black, evenly fringed with white around the outside edge so that it appears to be laced.

Wings: Primaries white heavily stippled with grey especially on outer edges and tips. Scapulars white stippled with grey. Lower scapulars (shoulders) rich claret fringed with white to complement upper flanks. Tertiaries white stippled with black, shading to claret on outer edges next to speculum.

Duck

Head and neck: Fawn with dark graining on crown with a sharp division between the neck and the white of the upper breast (i.e. females to have a fawn hood). Bill dark slate tinged with green preferred but dull orange-brown with dark brown saddle acceptable.

Breast: White with fawn and brown mottling on upper breast.

Flanks: White with some fawn mottling and darker streaks on upper flanks.

Underbody: White.

Back and rump: White with dark streaks and with fawn and black mottling becoming heavier on rump.

Tail: Fawn, evenly fringed with lighter fawn or off-white around the outside edge of tail so that it appears to be laced.

Undertail cushion: White with some fawn and black mottling.

Wings: Primaries white stippled with dark grey especially on outer edges and tips. Scapulars white with dark streaks and fawn mottling especially on lower scapulars (shoulders). Tertiaries white with some fawn and dark grey mottling shading to grey on outer edges towards speculum.

In both sexes

Wings: Speculum iridescent bluish-green edged with black then white. Wing bar white then black.

Eyes: Brown.

Legs: Orange.

Major faults

In both sexes: Ground colour other than white.

In the drake: Lack of white fringing to claret feathers on breast and upper flanks. Any signs of grey stippling on lower flanks. Lack of brownish black tail evenly fringed with white around outside edge of tail.

In the duck: Lack of fawn hood by being too white in head and neck colour. Any evidence of eye stripes. Lack of fawn tail evenly fringed with lighter fawn or off-white around outside edge of tail.

Faults

In both sexes: Insufficient speculum and/or the iridescence required. Incorrect speculum colour. Bill, eye and leg and eye colour other than stated.
In the drake: Incomplete white neck ring. White markings on head, under chin, on throat, rump or black part of undertail.
In the duck: Lack of required mottling, etc. on upper breast, upper flanks, back and rump.

Minor faults

In the drake: Insufficient extension of claret feathers along upper flanks. Insufficient grey stippling on upper shoulders.
In the duck: Excessive dark graining on crown and/or neck.

Appleyard
Drake

Head and neck: Crown and back of neck iridescent green with white neck ring completely encircling the neck. Base of neck and shoulders below neck ring claret. Face, throat and upper neck creamy white with iridescent green line through the eye and another curved on the cheek. Both lines, not as clearly defined as in the duck, touch behind eye. Bill olive green with dark bean.
Breast and upper flanks: Claret, each feather finely fringed with creamy white. Claret bib to be centrally divided by creamy white as it merges with creamy white of underbody.
Lower flanks and underbody: Some claret feathers finely fringed with light grey extend downwards towards underbody with remainder of lower flanks creamy white stippled with light grey shading to white towards tail. Underbody creamy white.
Back: Grey stippled with black, becoming darker towards rump.
Rump and undertail cushion: Rump black with green iridescence and undertail cushion lustrous black.
Tail: Mainly white with black stippling especially in centre under black sex curls, which may be tipped with light grey.
Wings: Primaries grey stippled with dark grey. Scapulars grey stippled with dark grey. Lower scapulars claret fringed with pale grey to complement upper flanks. Tertiaries grey stippled with dark grey, shading to claret on outer edges next to speculum.

Duck

Head and neck: Crown and back of neck light fawn with dark grey-brown graining; this grained light fawn on the neck should join that of the shoulder without a break. Face, throat and upper neck creamy white. Fawn line through the eye with another curved on the cheek. Both lines to be well defined and to touch behind the eye. Bill orange-brown with brown saddle and dark bean.
Back and rump: Light fawn with dark grey-brown flecking on each feather. Feathers to be finely fringed with creamy white.
Undertail cushion: Creamy white with more pronounced dark grey-brown markings.
Flanks: Upper flanks light fawn with dark grey-brown flecking on each feather. Feathers to be fringed with creamy white.
Breast and underbody: Upper breast creamy white lightly flecked or mottled with dark grey-brown. Mottling becomes heavier on outer sides as breast colour breaks or splits into creamy white on lower breast as it merges with creamy white of lower flanks and underbody.

Tail: Mainly creamy fawn irregularly marked with dark grey-brown especially in centre of tail.

Wings: Primaries mainly creamy fawn to dark brown. Scapulars light fawn with dark grey-brown flecking on each feather; feathers broadly fringed with creamy white. Tertiaries grey-brown finely laced with off-white.

In both sexes

Wings: Speculum iridescent blue, edged with black then white. Wing bar white then black.
Eyes: Brown.
Legs: Orange.

Major faults

In both sexes: Pure white primaries. Lack of speculum. Complete lack of face markings. Spreading of darker central tail stippling, markings or peppering to outer white areas of tail (i.e. a fringed tail).
In the drake: Solid claret bib with no creamy white split on lower breast. Light grey stippling from the lower flanks spreading onto underbody.
In the duck: Lack of a creamy white split on lower breast.

Faults

In both sexes: Insufficient speculum and/or the iridescence required. Incorrect speculum colour. Bill, eye and leg colour other than stated.
In the drake: Lack of pale grey fringing to claret feathers on lower flanks. Incomplete neck ring and excessively wide neck ring.
In the duck: Ground colour too dark. Insufficient face markings. Insufficient creamy white fringing on back feathers. Neck line of light fawn with grey-brown graining at back of neck broken with creamy white. Underbody other than creamy white.

Minor faults

In the drake: Insufficient extension of claret feathers along upper flanks. Excessive extension of claret feathers onto lower flanks or underbody. White markings on black areas of undertail.
In the duck: Completely creamy white undertail.

Apricot Appleyard (butterscotch)
Drake

Head and neck: Crown and back of neck lustrous silver blue-grey with white neck ring completely encircling neck. Base of neck and shoulders below neck ring claret. Face, throat and upper neck creamy white with a blue-grey line through the eye and another curved on the cheek. Both lines, not as clearly defined as in the duck, to touch behind eye. Bill olive green with dark bean.

Breast and upper flanks: Claret, each feather finely fringed with creamy white. Claret bib to be centrally divided by creamy white as it merges with creamy white of underbody.

Lower flanks and underbody: Some claret feathers finely fringed with creamy white extend downwards towards underbody with remainder of lower flanks creamy white shading to white towards tail. Underbody creamy white.

Back: White stippled with light blue-grey, becoming light blue-grey towards rump.

Rump and undertail cushion: Light blue-grey.

Tail: Mainly white with blue-grey stippling especially in centre under blue-grey sex curls, which may be tipped with creamy white.

Wings: Primaries creamy buff. Scapulars bluish buff. Lower scapulars claret fringed with creamy white to complement upper flanks. Tertiaries creamy white, shading to claret on outer edges next to speculum.

Duck

Head and neck: Crown and back of neck butterscotch with darker butterscotch graining. This butterscotch on the neck to join that of the shoulder without a break. Face, throat and upper neck creamy white with a butterscotch line through the eye and another curved on the cheek. Both lines to be well defined and to touch behind the eye. Bill orange-brown with brown saddle and dark bean.

Back and rump: Butterscotch with darker flecking on each feather and feathers to be finely fringed with creamy white on back and rump.

Undertail cushion: Creamy white with more pronounced butterscotch markings.

Flanks: Upper flanks creamy white with pale butterscotch markings fringed with creamy white.

Breast and underbody: Upper breast creamy white lightly flecked or mottled with butterscotch. Mottling becomes heavier on outer sides as breast colour breaks or splits into creamy white on lower breast as it merges with creamy white of lower flanks and underbody.

Tail: Mainly creamy white irregularly marked with butterscotch especially in centre of tail.

Wings: Primaries cream ground colour with light butterscotch. Scapulars light butterscotch with darker flecking on each feather and broadly fringed with creamy white. Tertiaries light butterscotch finely laced with off-white.

In both sexes

Wings: Speculum blue-grey, edged with silver grey then white. Wing bar white then silver grey.

Eyes: Brown.

Legs: Orange.

Major faults

In both sexes: Pure white primaries. Lack of speculum. Complete lack of face markings. Spreading of darker central tail stippling, markings or peppering to outer white areas of tail (i.e. a fringed tail).

In the drake: Solid claret bib with no creamy white split on lower breast.

In the duck: Lack of a creamy white split on lower breast.

Faults

In both sexes: Insufficient speculum and/or the iridescence required. Incorrect speculum colour. Bill, eye and leg colour other than stated.

In the drake: Lack of fringing to claret feathers on lower flanks. Incomplete neck ring and excessively wide neck ring.

In the duck: Ground colour too dark. Insufficient face markings. Insufficient creamy white fringing on back feathers. Neck line of butterscotch with darker graining at back of neck broken with creamy white. Underbody other than creamy white.

Minor faults

In the drake: Insufficient extension of claret feathers along upper flanks. Excessive extension of claret feathers onto lower flanks or underbody. White markings on blue-grey areas of undertail.

In the duck: Completely creamy white undertail.

Marked varieties

Bibbed

Black – Uniform black, except for drake's head and neck, which has some green iridescence.

Blue – Blue laced with darker slate blue except for drake's head, which is lustrous slate blue.
Lavender – Uniform lavender-grey.

Plumage of both sexes

Breast: White bib as even as possible, in a broad tear shape extending from lower neck to upper breast.
Wings: Primaries two or three outer feathers white.
Remainder of body: Black, blue or lavender, as described above.

In both sexes

Eyes: Brown.
Legs: Dusky orange shaded irregularly with greyish black.

Drake

Bill: Olive green with dark bean.

Duck

Bill: Black for black bib; slate blue for blue and lavender.

Major faults

In both sexes: Lack of any white primaries.

Faults

In both sexes: Coloured feathers other than that required in the blacks, blues and lavenders. Too large a bib, including extension onto shoulders. Coloured feathers in bib. Bill, eye and leg colour other than stated.

Minor faults

In both sexes: Incorrect number of white primaries. Too small or too uneven a bib. Undefined edges to white bib. White markings in face. In all colours: rust-stippled feathers in drakes or rust-laced feathers in ducks.

Magpie

Black – Cap and mantle to be uniform black.
Blue – Cap and mantle blue, laced with darker slate blue.
Chocolate – Cap and mantle to be uniform chocolate.

Cap and mantle

Cap to cover the whole of the crown of the head to the top of the eyes. The mantle on the back to be heart shaped. Credit should be given to exhibits displaying both the correct cap and mantle.

Plumage of both sexes

Head and neck: White with black, blue or chocolate cap covering the whole of the crown of the head to the top of the eyes.
Breast, flanks and underbody: White.
Back, scapulars, rump, tail and undertail cushion: Solid black, blue or chocolate to form a heart-shaped mantle of coloured feathers on the back.
Wings: Primaries, speculum, wing bar and tertiaries white.

In both sexes

Eyes: Brown.
Legs: Dusky orange irregularly shaded with greyish black.

Drake

Bill: Olive green with dark bean.

Duck

Bill: Greenish yellow overlaid with either slate blue (in blue) or black (in black) or brown (in chocolate).

Major faults

In both sexes: Lack of any white primaries.

Faults

In both sexes: Lack of correct cap or mantle. Coloured feathers in white areas. Coloured feathers other than required in coloured areas. Bill, eye and leg colour other than stated.

Minor faults

In both sexes: Lack of symmetry in markings.

Weights

Drake   570–680 g   (1¼–1½ lb)
Duck   450–570 g   (1–1¼ lb)

Scale of points

Type and size (general type 10, carriage 10, body size 15, i.e. length, width, depth 5 each)	35
Head, neck and bill (crown – high and round 4; cheeks – full 4; eyes – bold 4; bill – short and broad 4; neck – short and thick 4)	20
Legs and feet	5
Colour (plumage 20; bill 5; legs 3; eyes 2)	30
Condition	10
	100

Disqualifications (type and structure)

In all colour varieties and both sexes
Wry neck or tail. Roach back. Undershot or overshot bill. Cloudy eyed or blind. Obvious sinusitis. Slipped or angel winged.

Major faults (type and structure)

In all colour varieties and both sexes
Dish billed. Fish billed. Down billed. Down faced. Long, slim necks. Oversized/undersized bodies. Unlevel carriage – tipping forward/too upright.

Faults (type and structure)

In all colour varieties and both sexes
Flat crowns. Oval heads. Square heads. Eyes set too high in face. Narrow faced. Uneven cheeks. Long bills. Narrow bills. Narrow, boat-shaped bodies. Long shanks. Shanks too short.

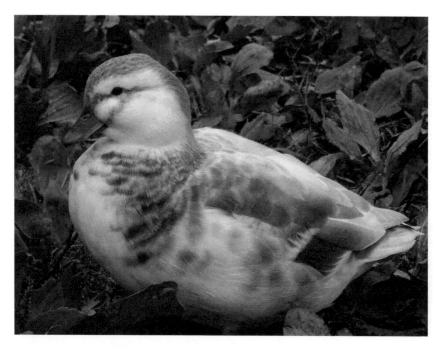

Apricot Appleyard (Butterscotch) Call female

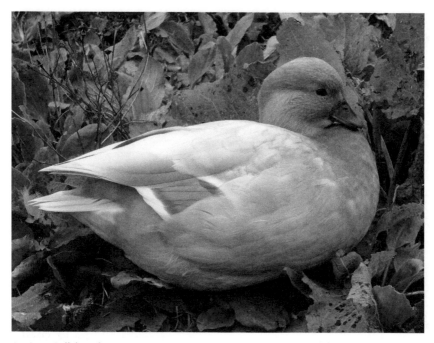

Apricot Call female

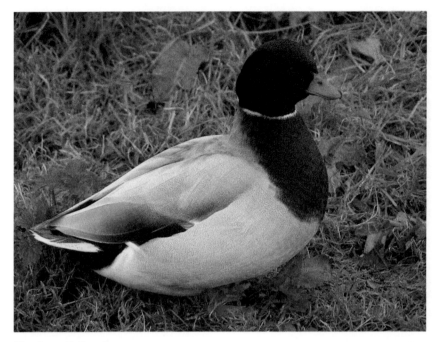

Blue fawn Call male

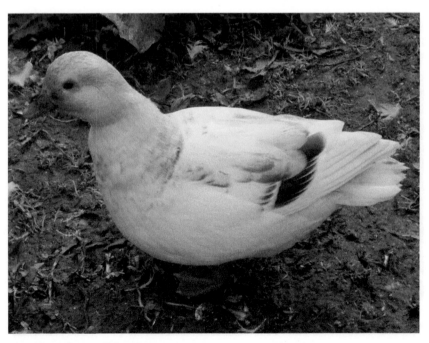

Chocolate silver Call female

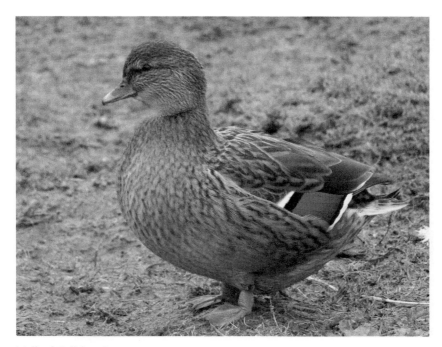

Mallard Call female

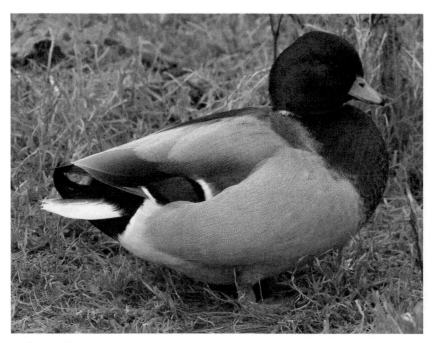

Mallard Call male

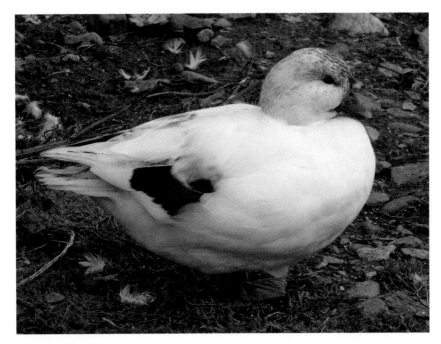

Silver Call female

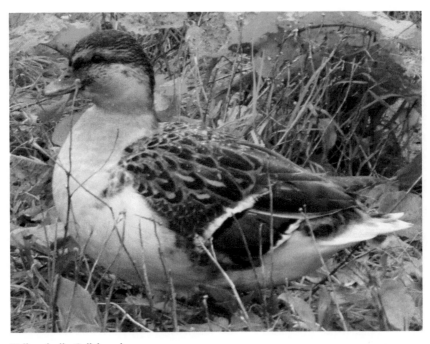

Yellow belly Call female

CAMPBELL

Classification: Light
Origin: Great Britain

One of the first, and certainly the most successful, of the utility breeds designed in the twentieth century from the Indian Runner, the khaki Campbell largely took over as the top egg-laying duck. The colour of farmyard mud, from which it gets the first part of its name, the khaki Campbell proved to be exceedingly agile, very fertile and extremely prolific. It too has spawned many variants: the white Campbell, the dark Campbell, the Welsh Harlequin (a simple mutation of the original khaki), the Abacot Ranger (a cross back to the Runner) and the Whaylesbury hybrid (Harlequin and Aylesbury).

'This breed', writes Captain R.A. Long (1926), 'was produced by mating a Rouen drake with a Fawn and White Runner duck, some Wild Duck blood being added later. Mrs Campbell writes of her ducks that they were meant for utility layers – not show birds – but that since some people wished to show them (and the birds must be bred to a definite type), she drew up a standard of what she would like them best to be in plumage.'

Mrs Campbell's *original* Campbell ducks were not khaki at all. They quite closely resembled Abacot Rangers. It was not until about 1901 when she tried to produce buff-coloured birds, and failed, that the khaki variety emerged.

The white variety was developed by Captain F.S. Pardoe in 1924 and standardised in 1954. It was hailed as having identical utility properties to the khaki but with more attractive selling appearance, at least for the table. The white plumage is the result of a recessive gene that hides other colours. The white Campbell also has a gene that makes the bill appear yellow rather than pink.

The dark Campbell, first standardised also in 1954, was the product of attempts to breed autosexing ducks. Mr H.R.S. Humphreys of Devon is credited with creating this variety in the 3 September 1943 edition of *Poultry World*. The element of sex linkage is caused by a lack of the brown dilution normally in the khaki. Because this is a sex-linked gene, it is possible to cross a khaki drake with a dark Campbell female to produce khaki female ducklings and dark-looking male ones, thus allowing breeders to cull unwanted males in their day-old fluff. Essentially the dark Campbell has the same colour form as the dusky mallard Call. Quite simply it is a khaki without any brown dilution.

Overall type (shape): Male and female

Carriage: Alert, slightly upright, the head carried high. Shoulders higher than the saddle, the back showing a gentle slant. Carriage not too erect (about 35°) but not so low as to cause waddling. Activity and foraging power to be retained without loss of body depth and width.

Head: Refined in jaw and skull; neat boned with smooth face. Eyes full, bold and bright, fairly high in skull and prominent. Bill medium length, depth and width; following a smooth line with the top of the skull.

Neck: Medium length, slender, almost erect.

Body: Deep, wide and compact. Back wide, flat and of medium length. Breast broad and well rounded. Abdomen well developed but not sagging; well-rounded underline from breast to stern.

Tail: Short and small, slightly elevated.

Wings: Tight, held close to the body.

Legs and feet: Legs medium length, set well apart and not too far back.

Plumage: Tight and sleek.

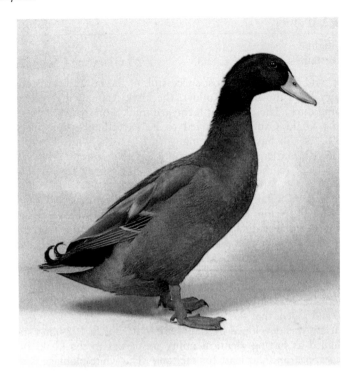

Khaki Campbell male

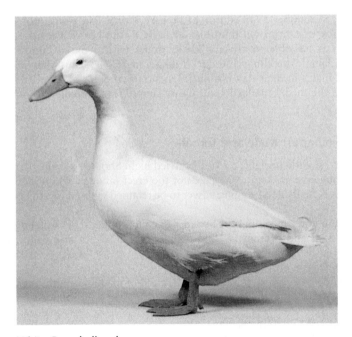

White Campbell male

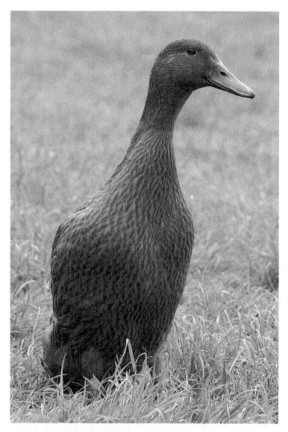

Khaki Campbell female

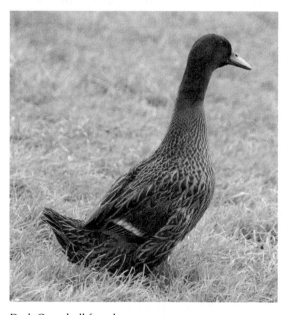

Dark Campbell female

Colour

The dark
Drake
Head and neck: Black with green lustre. Eyes brown. Bill bluish green with black bean.
Shoulders, breast, underbody *and flanks*: Light grey-brown, each feather finely stippled (pencilled) with dark grey-brown, gradually shading to grey at the stern close up to the vent.
Rump: Black with green lustre.

Tail: Dark grey-brown. Tail coverts black with green lustre.
Wings: Primaries dark grey-brown. Speculum dark brown with faint sheen, edged with a thin light grey line. Secondary coverts dark grey with light grey tips. Other coverts dark grey-brown faintly tipped with light brown. Underwing grey.
Legs and webs: Dark orange.

Duck
Head and neck: Dark brown with darker graining on the crown. No eye stripes. Eyes brown. Bill lead colour with black bean.
Back: Brown with darker pencilling.
Shoulders, breast and flank: Brown, each feather distinctly pencilled with darker brown.
Tail: Dark brown.
Wings: Primaries dark brown. Speculum as drake. Smaller coverts tipped with lighter brown. Underwing grey.
Legs and webs: As near body colour as possible.

The khaki
Drake
Head, neck, rump *and secondaries (speculum)*: Green-bronze. Remainder of plumage an even shade of warm khaki shading to lighter khaki towards the lower part of the breast with fine stippled, brown pencilling. Eyes brown. Bill greenish blue, the darker the better.
Underwing: Grey-brown.
Legs and webs: Dark orange.

Duck
The ground colour *is* an even shade of warm khaki.
Head and neck: A slightly darker shade. Eyes brown. Bill dark slate.
Back and scapulars: Pencilled with medium brown.
Breast: Lightly pencilled, on close inspection.
Wings: Khaki; secondaries brown; underwing grey-brown.
Legs and webs: As near the body colour as possible.

The white
In both sexes
Plumage: Pure white throughout.
Bill, legs and webs: Orange.
Eyes: Grey-blue.

Weights

Drake	2.3–2.5 kg	(5–5½ lb)
Duck in laying condition	2.0–2.3 kg	(4½–5 lb)

Scale of points

Carriage	15
Head, bill and neck	15
Body	15
Legs and feet	5
Colour	25
Size	15
Condition	10
	100

Disqualifications

The dark and khaki

In both sexes: White or speckled underwing; white wing feathers; yellow or pink bill.
In the drake: White neck ring; claret bib.
In the duck: Mallard eye stripes; white bib or neck ring.

The white

In both sexes: Flesh-coloured bill. Coloured feathers.

Faults

The khaki

In both sexes: White spot under bill.
In the duck: Complete lack of pencilling on the breast and back; dark pencilling as in the Rouen or dark Campbell.

The white

In both sexes: Dark markings on the bill.

All varieties

In both sexes: Excessive weight or coarseness.

CAYUGA

Classification: Heavy
Origin: America

This breed takes its name from Lake Cayuga in New York State, and is thought to be descended from the wild black duck (*Anas rubripes*). The Cayuga was recorded in North America between 1830 and 1850. It was first standardised in America in 1874 and in Britain in 1901. Its colour is very similar to the smaller Black East Indian: black plumage with brilliant green iridescence. The drakes tend to retain their black plumage but the females develop patches of white as they get older.

Overall type (shape): Male and female

Carriage: Slightly elevated in front; clear of the ground from breast to stern.
Head: Large. Eyes full and bold. Bill wide and moderately long.
Neck: Long and strong with a graceful curve.
Body: Long, broad and deep, without keel; breast prominent.
Tail: Long and closely folded; slightly elevated.

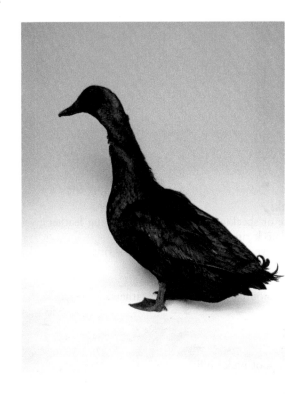

Cayuga male

Wings: Strong, compact and carried close to the body.
Legs and feet: Legs medium length, set a little back from centre.
Plumage: Smooth, close and glossy.

Colour

In both sexes
Plumage: Black with a beetle-green lustre.
Underwing: Coverts black with green lustre; main feathers dark grey.
Eyes: Dark brown.
Bill: Black.
Legs and feet: As black as possible. Some orange permitted in older drakes.

Weights

Drake   3.6 kg   (8 lb)
Duck   3.2 kg   (7 lb)

Scale of points

Carriage	10
Head, bill and neck	15
Body	15
Legs and feet	5
Colour	30
Size	15
Condition	10
	100

Disqualifications

In both sexes: Yellow bill; white spot under the bill. Elements of brown pencilling especially on underwing and throat; brown or white in the plumage, including the underwing.

Faults

In both sexes: Green bill. Purple lustre. Indication of a keel or undercarriage.
In the duck: Orange in the legs and feet.

Minor faults (to be discouraged)

In both sexes: Grey or olive tip on the bill.

CRESTED

Classification: Light
Origin: Uncertain

Darwin described the 'Tufted Duck' (1868) which he obtained from The Netherlands, as well as another sent to him 'from the Malayan archipelago'. The connection is significant. Dutch trading interests in Asia date back at least to 1602, when the Dutch East India Company was formed. Seventeenth century Dutch paintings by artists such as Jan Steen and Melchior d'Hondecoeter feature crested ducks and those with pied markings like the fawn and white Indian Runner. Bali Ducks also emerged from this part of Asia. Since a duck with crested genes would survive with difficulty in the wild, its development and cultivation may be jointly attributed to the inhabitants of the East Indies and the Dutch.

The breed was also described by D.J. Browne in the USA in 1853 and admitted to the American Standard in 1874. Harrison Weir depicted the breed in his work *Our Poultry* in 1902 and the breed was finally admitted to the UK Standard in 1910.

Overall type (shape): Male and female

Carriage: Reasonably upright when active, at approximately 35–40°.
Head: Long and straight, slightly rising to the crown, the centre of which has a well-balanced, even, single globular crest firmly attached to the skull. Eyes bright. Bill long and broad.
Neck: Medium length.
Body: Long, broad and moderately deep. Full, well-rounded breast blending nicely into body.
Tail: In proportion to the bird.
Wings: Strong, carried close to the body.
Legs and feet: Legs medium length.
Plumage: Close and smooth.

The overall picture of the bird, including the crest, is balance throughout.

Colour

The white
In both sexes

Plumage: Pure white.
Eyes: Blue.
Bill: Orange-yellow.
Legs and webs: Orange.

The coloured

Any other colour is permitted but attention should be paid to symmetry of markings.

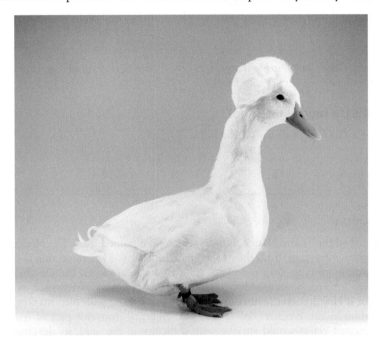

Crested male

Weights

Drake   3.2 kg   (7 lb)
Duck   2.7 kg   (6 lb)

Scale of points

Carriage	10
Head, bill and neck	40
(this includes 30 points for the crest)	
Body	15
Legs and feet	5
Colour	10
Size	10
Condition	10
	100

Disqualifications

In both sexes: Any spinal deformity, in particular twisted or kinked neck, roach back. Twisted bill. Wry tail.

Faults

In both sexes: Split, slipped or uneven crest. Crest that interferes with the eyes. Weeping eyes. Short body.

Minor faults (to be discouraged)

In both sexes: Wrong bill or leg colour in whites.

CRESTED MINIATURE

Classification: Bantam
Origin: Great Britain

This breed is a miniature version of the Crested light duck. It was developed in the British Isles by John Hall and Roy Sutcliffe during the late 1980s and early 1990s, and standardised by the Poultry Club in 1997.

Overall type (shape) and colour: Male and female

As for large Crested.

Weights

Drake   1.125 kg   (2.5 lb)
Duck   0.9 kg   (2 lb)

Scale of points

Carriage   10
Head, bill and neck   35
          (this includes 25 points for the crest)
Body   15
Legs and feet   5
Colour   10
Size   15
Condition   10
                                                  100

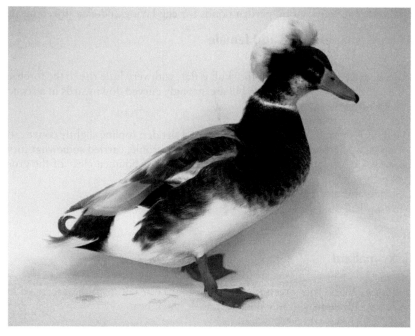

Crested male, miniature

Disqualifications

In both sexes: Any spinal deformity, in particular twisted or kinked neck, roach back and wry tail. Twisted bill.

Faults

In both sexes: Split, slipped or uneven crest. Crest that interferes with the eyes. Weeping eyes. Short body. Oversize.

Minor faults (to be discouraged)

In both sexes: Wrong bill or leg colour in whites.

HOOK BILL

Classification: Light
Origin: Uncertain – possibly from Asia prior to being bred in large numbers at one time in Europe

The Hook Bill is described and illustrated by Francis Willughby (in his *Ornithology*, published in 1678). Harrison Weir (1902) asserts that these birds are of Indian origin. He notes also that he saw them between 1837 and 1840 on the lake at Surrey Zoological Gardens. Weir maintains that the Dutch released their Hook Bills every morning onto the local canals and rivers, a very cost-effective way of feeding them. At dusk the birds flew back to their owners. Fancifully perhaps, he suggests that the bill and white bib made them distinct from the wild targets of the local hunters.

Both Durigen and Broekman (referred to in Schmidt, *Puten, Perlhühner, Gänse, Enten*, 1989) reinforce the Asiatic origin of the bird. Durigen calls it *haken-* or *bogen-schnabel* (hook or bow-bill). The name *Krombekeenden* occurs in the Dutch references and the Germans use the term *Krummschnabel-Enten*. How and when it arrived and later spread in Europe is not reported, although there is evidence (A. Bühle, 1860) that the bird was widely distributed throughout Europe in the mid-nineteenth century, centred particularly in Thuringia, where it was kept on garden ponds for egg-laying and as a prized meat bird.

Overall type (shape): Male and female

Carriage: Almost horizontal.
Head: When viewed from the front, the skull is flat, with very little rise to the forehead. In profile, the upper neck, head and long bill are strongly curved downwards in a semicircle. Eyes set high in the head.
Neck: Vertical, rather long and thin.
Body: Medium length, fairly broad. Back long and slender; topline slightly convex. Breast round when viewed from the front; round and full in profile, carried somewhat forward. Underbody well developed, almost parallel to the back. Abdomen clear of the ground.
Tail: Rather broad, following the line of the back.
Wings: Strong and carried close to the body.
Legs: Medium length.

Colour

The dusky mallard
Drake

Head and neck: Black with green lustre; this colour clear cut from the breast without a white neck ring. Eyes brown. Bill slate grey with black bean.

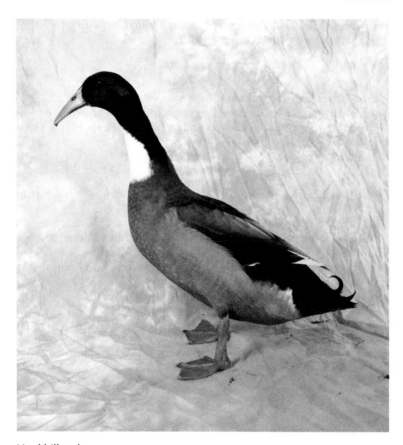

Hookbill male

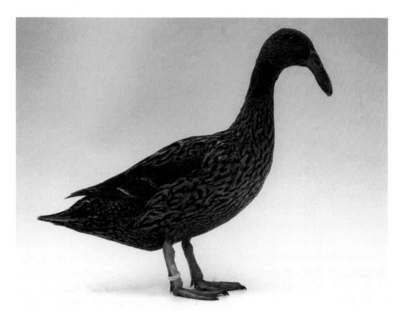

Hookbill female

Back: Upper part ash colour with some green lustre. Rump black with greenish lustre. Tail coverts and sex curls black with some green lustre.
Breast: Steel blue.
Flanks: Dark steel blue with dark grey stippled pencilling.
Stern: Steel blue.
Tail: Dark grey-brown edged with light brown.
Wings: Primaries dark brown-grey. Secondaries (speculum) dull brown or dark slate with very little white bordering. Tertiaries, coverts and scapulars dark slate blue. The scapulars are well pencilled, and tinged with brown. Underwing pearl grey.
Legs: Dark orange.

Duck

Head and neck: Dark brown with darker graining on the crown. No eye stripes. Eyes brown. Bill lead colour with black bean.
Back: Brown with darker pencilling.
Shoulders, breast *and flank*: Brown, each feather pencilled with darker brown.
Tail: Dark brown.
Wings: Primaries dark brown. Speculum as drake. Smaller coverts tipped with lighter brown. Underwing grey.
Legs and webs: Dark orange-brown.

White bibbed dusky mallard

The same colour as the dusky mallard except for a clearly defined, white, teardrop-shaped bib on the lower neck and breast. A small white spot under the chin is permissible. The outer primaries have two to six white feathers.

The white

In both sexes

Plumage: Pure white throughout.
Eyes: Blue.
Bill: Flesh pink.
Legs and webs: Bright orange.

Weights

Drake   2.0–2.25 kg   ($4\frac{1}{2}$–5 lb)
Duck   1.6–2.0 kg   ($3\frac{1}{2}$–$4\frac{1}{2}$ lb)

Scale of points

Carriage	10
Head, bill and neck	30
Body	15
Legs and feet	5
Colour	20
Size	10
Condition	10
	100

Disqualifications

The dusky mallard

In both sexes: White or speckled underwing; blue or green speculum; Mallard eye stripes at any stage of plumage.

In the drake: White neck ring; claret bib.

All varieties
In both sexes: Short or straight bill. Any sign of a keel.

Faults

The dusky mallard and white bibbed dusky mallard
In both sexes: Very distinct light bars on secondary feathers and coverts.

The white bibbed dusky mallard
In both sexes: Missing white flights.
In the drake: Excessive white line through the eye.

All varieties
In both sexes: Oversize.

Minor faults (to be discouraged)

The dusky mallard
In both sexes: Ground colour too pale.

The white bibbed dusky mallard
In both sexes: Uneven or overextended bib. White feathers on either side of the bill.

INDIAN RUNNER

Classification: Light
Origin: East Indies

There are reports of 'Penguin' ducks being imported into Britain as early as 1835. These ducks brought with them brown dilution and also dusky mallard genes, as well as their upright stance and prolific egg-laying capability, as witnessed by Alfred Wallace in Malaya. The term 'India Runner' was largely coined by John Donald in about 1890, when he described similar birds imported also some time in the 1830s. These included all-fawns, whites and pied pattern ducks, the last being the basis of the Poultry Club Standard publication of 1901. The Indian Runner Duck Club's Standard of 1907 described only the fawn-and-white; that of 1913 recognised also the white and the whole fawn.

Black Runners were developed from an early white import that also had a certain amount of black in its plumage. Crossed with a Black East Indian, it allowed the development of both black and chocolate Runners standardised by the Poultry Club in 1930 and the later Cumberland blue Indian Runner, all three of which have extended black genes.

Trout Runners were the next to be standardised. They have mallard (M^+) genes instead of the more common dusky mallard (m^d). When heterozygous for blue dilution (Bl/bl^+), trouts become blue trouts. When homozygous for blue (Bl/Bl) they are apricot trouts (*Blaugelb* in German). A similar use of blue dilution turns the fawn-and-white (pencilled) into the American fawn-and-white.

Silver Runners (*Silber-wildfarbig*) (2008) share the colour genes of the Abacot Ranger and Silver Bantam (dusky mallard, harlequin phase). Apricot and blue duskies (2008) share the colour genes of the fawn Runner, plus the blue dilution gene.

Shape: Male and female

Carriage: Upright, active, nearly perpendicular when at attention, excited or trained for the show pen. When not alarmed, or when on the move, the body may be inclined between 50° and 80° above the horizontal. The proper carriage creates a straight line from the back of the head to the tip of the tail. Total length (fully extended in a straight line, measured from bill tip to middle toe tips): drake 65–80 cm (25–31 in.) and duck 60–70 cm (23–28 in.).

Note: When standing in a show pen the maximum height is closer to an extended measure from crown (above the eye) to tail tip. The following is a rough guide.

Bean to toe, cm (in.)	Crown to tail, cm (in.)
60 (24)	50 (20)
65 (26)	54 (21)
70 (28)	58 (23)
75 (30)	62 (24)
80 (32)	66 (26)
85 (34)	70 (28)

Head: Lean and racy looking with a bill definitely wedge shaped fitting into a skull flat on top, making a clean sweep from the top of the bill to the back of the skull. The eye should be full, alert, bright and so high in the head that the upper part appears almost to project above the line of the skull. The culmen of the bill should be perfectly straight.

Neck: Long, slender, in line with the body. The muscular part should be well marked, rounded and stand out from the windpipe, the extreme hardness of the feather helping to accentuate this. The neck should be neatly fitted to the head. The proportion of neck to body should be 1 : 2.

Body: Long, narrow and cylindrical its entire length, although very slightly flattened at the shoulders, funnelling gradually from body to neck.

Tail: When the bird is alert the tail should extend towards the ground in a straight line from the back.

Wings: Small in relation to the size of the bird; tightly packed to the body and just crossing at the rump.

Legs and webs: Legs set far back to allow upright carriage. Thighs and shanks medium in length.

Plumage: Tight, smooth and hard.

Weights

Drake   1.6–2.3 kg   ($3\frac{1}{2}$–5 lb)
Duck   1.4–2.0 kg   (3–$4\frac{1}{2}$ lb)

Scale of points

Carriage	20
Head, bill and neck	20
Body	20
Legs and feet	5
Condition	10
Colour	15
Size	10
	100

Defects

Disqualifications

In both sexes: Twisted or deformed mandibles. Kinked neck. Low carriage: 'a duck which cannot maintain a natural carriage of *at least* 40° to the horizontal will not be considered a pure Runner, however good its other points may be' (Indian Runner Duck Club of Great Britain – a disqualification since 1913).

White

In both sexes

Plumage: Pure white throughout.
Eyes: Blue.
Bill: Orange-yellow.
Legs: Orange.

Disqualifications

Male: Any black on the bill.
Both: Any coloured feathers.

Major defects

Female: Black bean or line on the bill. Mottled legs.

Minor defects

Female: Black spots on the bill are a common minor fault with age.

Fawn

Male

Head and neck: Dark bronze with metallic lustre, changing to brown claret for the lower neck and upper breast. Eyes brown. Bill pure black to dark olive green mottled with black.
Back: Deep brown, almost black with metallic lustre on the rump.
Breast: Brown claret on the lower neck and upper breast. Lower breast French grey produced by fine stippling of sepia on a lighter ground.
Flanks and underbody: French grey produced by fine stippling of sepia on a lighter ground, extending to the almost black undertail.
Tail: Deep brown, almost black towards the centre.
Wings: Primaries dark brown. Secondaries dark bronze with slight metallic lustre. Coverts fawn, not pencilled or laced. Scapulars red-brown, stippled.
Legs and webs: Black or dark tan mottled with black.

Female

Head and neck: Warm ginger-fawn, a slightly lighter shade than the rest of the body. Each feather is marked with darker red-brown graining. No eye stripes. Eyes brown. Bill black.
Back: Rich and well-marked pencilling on an almost uniform warm ginger-fawn ground with no marked variation of shade.
Breast: The lower part of the neck and neck expansion is a shade warmer than the head and upper neck, each feather pencilled with warm red-brown.
Flanks and underbody: Light fawn, pencilled.
Tail: Light fawn, pencilled.
Wings: Secondaries warm red-brown. Primaries a shade lighter. Scapulars rich ginger-fawn with well-marked red-brown pencilling. Smaller coverts slightly lighter than the scapulars but darkening towards the greater coverts, pencilled.
Legs and webs: Black or dark tan.

Disqualifications

Male: Lack of claret breast colour.
Female: Lack of warm ginger-fawn tone to the plumage and chevron pencilling. Presence of eyebrows or eye stripes.
Both: White body or wing feathers. Blue or green wing bars. Orange or yellow bill. Bright orange feet or legs.

Major defects

Female: Barred feathers on lower flanks.
Both: Light or cream wing coverts or flights. Light tan legs and feet.

Apricot dusky

Male

Head and neck: Pigeon blue with brown tinge, changing to claret for the lower neck and upper breast. Eyes brown. Bill slate green.
Back: Light blue-dun tinged with brown, more grey towards the rump.
Breast: Lower neck, breast and shoulders claret. Lower breast light blue-grey peppered with brown.
Flanks and underbody: Flanks light blue-grey peppered with brown.
Tail: Blue-dun; brown tinge to outer edges.
Wings: Primaries honey-dun. Secondaries darker honey-dun. Coverts light honey-dun edged with brown. Scapulars blue-dun edged with claret.
Legs and webs: Orange-tan.

Female

Head and neck: Uniform apricot-ginger. No eye stripes. Eyes brown. Bill dark slate with dark bean.
Back: Light blue-dun tipped with apricot.
Breast: Uniform apricot-ginger.
Flanks and underbody: Apricot-ginger.
Tail: Outer webs apricot; inner webs blue-dun.
Wings: Secondaries honey-dun. Primaries a shade lighter though darker on the leading edges. Scapulars apricot-ginger. Tertials a shade lighter. Coverts honey-dun edged with apricot.
Legs and webs: Dark tan.

Disqualifications

Male: Lack of claret breast colour.
Female: Presence of eyebrows or eye stripes.
Both: White body or wing feathers.

Major defects

Male: Lack of brown tinge to head. Presence of neck ring.
Female: Very pale ground colour.
Both: Orange or yellow bill. Bright orange feet and legs.

Blue dusky

An intermediate colour form between fawn and apricot dusky. The single blue gene darkens the light blue areas of the apricot to a more charcoal colour; honey-dun becomes blue-dun.

Male: Brown-charcoal head and neck. Dark blue-dun back. Other blue pigment areas darkened. Also darker legs.
Female: Body overall slightly darker ginger than the apricot dusky. Faint blue pencilling on back, body and scapular feathers. Wing feathers blue-dun instead of honey-dun.
Faults: Disqualifications, major and minor defects as apricot dusky.

Mallard

Male

Head and neck: Black with green lustre on the head and upper neck; a distinct white collar almost encircling the neck. Eyes dark brown. Bill green, dark bean.

Back: Dark grey shading to greenish black over the rump.

Breast: Rich claret with no white fringing; margin of claret clearly defined.

Flanks, etc.: Light grey with dark grey stippling. Grey covering as much of the stern as possible.

Tail: Medium dull brown, paler outer feathers; coverts and undertail black.

Wings: Primaries and tertials grey. Speculum blue bordered by black then white. Coverts brownish grey except for greater coverts, which are tipped with white then black. Main scapulars clear steel grey, outer edge bronze tinge. Cream or white underwing.

Legs: Dull orange, darker webs.

Female

Head and neck: Golden brown, each feather with darker brown graining. This graining forms a darker band from the crown down the back of the neck. Eyes brown. Faint eye stripes, i.e. a paler line above the eye, a dark line through the eye and a pale line in front of the eye. Bill dark orange with brown saddle. Plain brown throat.

Back: Brown or chestnut with darker pencilling (chevrons).

Breast and flanks: Brown or chestnut with dark brown pencilling on each feather. Underbody similar.

Tail: Dull dark buff, irregularly marked with brown; darker tail feathers in the centre than the outer edges.

Wings: Primaries brownish slate. Speculum and its borders as drake. Tertials browner than primaries on exposed half. Coverts same colour as back. Scapulars similar to the Rouen. Cream or white underwing.

Legs: Dull orange, darker webs.

Disqualifications

Male: Grey or white in the head colour Absence of neck ring or unbroken neck ring. Claret on flank feathers. Completely white stern.

Female: Presence of white collar. Lack both of eye stripes and of graining on the crown. Light fawn ground colour.

Both: Clear yellow, blue or lead-coloured bill. White primaries. Incomplete, obscure or bronze speculum. Pied markings on the head and neck.

Major defects

Male: White fringing on claret bib feathers.

Female: Unclear pencilling on scapulars and back. Pale throat and eye markings.

Both: White feathers under the bill, under the throat or under the tail. Indistinct speculum and greater covert markings.

Minor defects

Male: Black marks on bill. Lack of dark bronze on scapulars. Lack of black undertail.

Female: Dark ground colour.

Trout

Male

Head and neck: Black with green lustre on the head and upper neck; a distinct white collar almost encircling the neck. Eyes dark brown. Bill golden olive, dark bean.

Back: Silver grey with dark grey stippled pencilling, shading to greenish black over the rump. Lower back fringed with stippled light grey pencilling.

Breast: Lower neck, breast and shoulders claret, with fine white fringing on each feather.

Flanks, etc.: Abdomen, flanks and thighs light grey with mid-grey stippled pencilling, shading to white stern.

Tail: Light stippled grey on outer vane, darker grey-brown on inner vane. Coverts and undertail black.

Wings: Primaries and tertials grey-brown. Speculum iridescent blue bordered with black then white. Coverts silver grey except for greater coverts, which are indistinctly tipped with white then black. Main scapulars silver grey, outer edge faint bronze tinge. Cream or white underwing.

Legs: Orange.

Female

Head and neck: Fawn, each feather with brown graining. This graining forms a darker band from the crown down the back of the upper neck. Eyebrow creamy white; dark line through the eye; pale line in front of the eye down to the bill. Base of the bill and front of the neck creamy fawn. Eyes brown. Bill pinkish orange-brown with spots. Dark bean.

Back: Fawn ground, delicately streaked or pencilled with dark brown. Pencilling best developed on the larger feathers.

Breast and flanks: Fawn ground, delicately streaked or pencilled with dark brown. Pencilling best developed on the larger feathers.

Tail: Buff marked with dark brown; darker feathers in the centre than the outer edges.

Wings: Primaries greyish buff. Speculum and its borders as drake. Tertials showing indications of pencilling. Coverts grey-brown edged with light fawn. Scapulars ideally pencilled with a single V in brown on light fawn. Cream or white underwing.

Legs: Dull orange, somewhat darker than the drake.

Disqualifications

Male: Lack of white stern. Absence of neck ring. Unbroken neck ring.

Female: Any indication of a white collar. Lack both of eye stripes or of graining on the crown. Yellow or lead-coloured bill.

Both: White primaries. Incomplete or obscure speculum. Pied markings on the head and neck. Pigmented underwings.

Major defects

Male: Bill dark or blue-green; grey or white in the head colour; lack of fringing on the claret breast feathers. Claret markings along the flanks.

Female: 'Mossy' or indistinct feather markings on the back.

Both: White feathers under the bill, under the throat or under the tail.

Minor defects

Male: Black marks on bill. Lack of black undertail. Dark bronze dominating the scapulars.

Female: Dark ground colour. Bright orange bill colour. Throat colour extending too far onto the breast.

Both: Indistinct speculum and greater covert markings.

Apricot trout

Male

Head and neck: Head and upper neck pigeon blue. Distinct white ring almost encircling the neck and tapering towards the back and tapering towards the shoulders. Eyes brown. Bill yellow-green; horn-coloured bean.

Back: Oatmeal shading to solid pigeon blue over the rump.

Breast: Lower neck, breast and shoulders claret, with fine off-white fringing on each feather.

Flanks, etc.: Abdomen, flanks and thighs pearl grey, shading to white stern.

Tail: Cream on outer vane of each feather; pearl grey on the inner vane. Undertail pigeon blue.

Wings: Primaries and tertials pearl grey. Speculum pigeon blue tipped with white. Small coverts oatmeal changing to fawn on the greater coverts, which are pigeon blue bordered with white. Main scapulars oatmeal, outer edge claret tinge. Cream or white underwing.

Legs: Orange.

Female

Head and neck: Deep apricot-buff. Eyebrow creamy white; dark line through the eye; creamy white line in front of the eye down to the bill. Base of the bill and front of the neck creamy fawn. Eyes brown. Bill brown-yellow. Pale bean.

Back: Apricot-buff. Lower back and rump pale apricot.

Breast and flanks: Deep apricot-buff.

Tail: Apricot-buff on the outer vane of each feather and light buff on the inner vane.

Wings: Primaries oatmeal. Secondaries (speculum) pigeon blue tipped with white. Smaller coverts light apricot-buff. Greater coverts pigeon blue bordered with white. Main scapulars deep apricot-buff.

Legs: Orange.

Disqualifications

Male: Lack of white stern. Absence of neck ring.

Female: Any indication of a white collar. Lack of eye stripes. Lead-coloured bill.

Both: White primaries. Pied markings on the head and neck. Pigmented underwings.

Major defects

Male: White in the head colour. Bill dark or blue-green; black bean on bill. Lack of fringing on the claret breast feathers.

Female: Claret or excessive white on breast.

Both: White feathers under the bill.

Minor defects

Female: Throat colour extending too far onto the breast.

Blue trout

An intermediate colour form between trout and apricot trout. The single blue dilution gene causes the black pigment of the trout plumage to change to charcoal-blue.

Male: Head, neck, rump and undertail charcoal-blue.

Female: Pencilling on head and body feathers charcoal-blue.

Both: Speculum dark blue-grey instead of iridescent blue.

Faults: Disqualifications, major and minor defects as apricot trout.

Silver

Male

Head and neck: Black with green lustre on the head and upper neck. Distinct white collar completely encircling the neck. Lower neck coloured as for breast. Eyes dark brown. Bill olive green with black bean.

Back: Upper back white feathers finely stippled with black and fringed with white. Lower down the back the stippling becomes heavier, each feather preferably fringed with white, until solid black with green lustre on the rump. Black sex curls, which may be tipped with white.

Breast: Lower neck, breast and shoulders claret fringed with white.

Flanks, etc. : Ground colour silvery whitish cream (white being preferable). A little of the claret breast colour extending along the upper flank.

Tail: Brown-black bordered with white. Undertail black, finishing neatly and not running into the stern and flank colour.

Wings: Primaries silvery white with a slightly iridescent dark grey overlay. Secondaries (speculum) bluish green tipped with distinct black then white bars. Greater coverts dark grey with well-defined white rim. Outer scapulars and tertials as the breast with wider silver-white edging. Smaller coverts white feathers finely stippled with black (giving the impression of grey), and fringed with white. Cream or white underwing.

Legs: Orange.

Female

Head and neck: Head and neck fawn (a deeper shade in young females) with the forehead and crown clearly grained with dark brown. There is a sharp division between the neck and upper white of the breast colour. Eyes dark brown. Bill dark slate green.

Back: White feathers with central dark streak; black and fawn stippling. Lower back light fawn with darker central streak. Rump fawnish grey with brown tips giving the impression of a triangular pattern.

Breast and flanks: Upper breast, lower neck and shoulders lightly streaked with light brown on a creamy white ground. Flanks lightly streaked. Lower breast, underbody and stern creamy white.

Tail: Fawn, edged with cream.

Wings: Primaries and speculum as the drake. Scapulars and tertials creamy fawn with brown flecks. Greater coverts dark grey with well-defined white rim. Smaller coverts dark fawn edged with cream. Underwing cream or white.

Legs: As dark grey as possible.

Disqualifications

Male: Brown head; broken, too wide or absent neck ring.

Female: Mallard eye stripes. White or grey head colour. Yellow bill.

Both: Absent or bronze specula. Solid white or solid brown primary feathers.

Major defects

Male: Too dark ground colour. Breast colour running too low into body or lacking white edging. Blue bill.

Female: Lack of cream or fawn ground colour to the head and upper neck. Lack of any graining on the head. Lack of streaking on the dorsal surface of the body.

Both: Lack of speculum. Ill-defined markings on greater coverts.

Minor defects

Male: Lack of white tips on sex curls; black lines or marks on the bill.

Female: Heavy dark graining on crown and neck.

Fawn and white

Male

Head and neck: The cap and cheek markings are dull bronze-green. The cap is separated from the cheek markings by a projection from the white of the neck extending up to, and in most cases terminating in, a narrow line more or less encircling the eye. The cap should cleanly and smoothly encircle the head. The cheek markings should not extend onto the neck. The bill is divided from the head markings by a narrow prolongation of the neck-white (3–6 mm ($\frac{1}{8} - \frac{1}{4}$ in.) wide) extending from the white underneath the chin. The neck is pure white to where the neck expansion begins, where the meeting is clean cut. Eyes dark brown. Bill light orange-yellow in young birds; green-yellow in adult drakes; black bean.

Back: The base of the neck, scapular feathers, back and rump are similar to the breast colours, darkening to green-bronze on the rump.

Breast, flanks *and underbody*: Uniform soft warm or ginger-fawn, produced by a fine stippling of brown on the cream ground of the individual feathers. The fawn of the thorax should meet the white of the abdomen in a clean line (near the bottom of the breast bone and the top of the thighs). The white extends between the legs to beyond the vent, and also includes the thigh coverts, which obscure most of the coloured thighs.

Tail: Tail feathers cream to medium brown in the central area. Undertail bronze.

Wings: Primaries, secondaries and tertials white; scapulars and some of the smaller coverts fawn, giving approximately a heart shape.

Legs: Deep orange.

Female

Head and neck: The cap and cheek markings are nearly the same shade of fawn as the body colour. The cap is separated from the cheek markings by a projection from the white of the neck extending up to, and in most cases terminating in, a narrow line more or less encircling the eye. The cap should cleanly and smoothly encircle the head. The cheek markings should not extend onto the neck. The bill is divided from the head markings by a narrow prolongation of the neck-white (3–6 mm ($\frac{1}{8} - \frac{1}{4}$ in.) wide) extending from the white underneath the chin. The neck is pure white to where the neck expansion begins, where the meeting is clean cut. Eyes dark brown. Bill light orange-yellow in young birds; spotted green to almost entirely dull cucumber in adult females. Black bean.

Back: The base of the neck, scapular feathers, back and rump are similar to the breast colours.

Breast, flanks and underbody: The coloured plumage is nearly the same shade as the fawn Runner duck; the feathers are pencilled, medium brown on fawn. The fawn of the thorax should meet the white of the abdomen in a clean line (near the bottom of the breast bone and the top of the thighs). The white extends between the legs to beyond the vent, and also includes the thigh coverts, which obscure most of the coloured thighs.

Tail: Fawn to medium brown in the central area.

Wings: Primaries, secondaries and tertials white; scapulars and some of the smaller coverts fawn, giving approximately a heart shape.

Legs: Deep orange.

Disqualifications

Male: Seal grey or seal brown cap, cheek and tail coverts. Any sign of a brown-red bib.
Female: Blue-grey pencilling on coloured body feathers or solid un-pencilled apricot buff feathers.

Major defects

Male: Light-coloured scapulars.
Female: Eye stripes.
Both: Asymmetry of markings. Fawn extending from the back onto the abdomen and thigh coverts ('foul flanked'). Insufficient white plumage.

Minor defects

Male: 'Dribbles' of cap colour onto the white neck. Cheek markings extending onto the neck. Any irregular, blotchy or unclear markings that detract from the symmetry and general cleanness of the colour boundaries. Lack of black bean on bill.

American fawn and white

Male

Head and neck: Pied markings distributed as in the pencilled fawn-and-white (above). Coloured feathers an even light fawn. The cap is grey-fawn. Eyes dark brown. Bill light orange-yellow in young birds; green-yellow in adult drakes. Pale bean.

Back: Pied markings distributed as in the pencilled fawn-and-white (above). Coloured feathers an even light fawn, grey-fawn on the rump.

Breast, flanks *and underbody*: Pied markings distributed as in the pencilled fawn-and-white (above). Coloured feathers an even light fawn.

Tail: Tail feathers cream to light grey-fawn in the central area. Undertail grey-fawn.

Wings: Primaries, secondaries and tertials white; scapulars and some of the smaller coverts light fawn, giving approximately a heart shape.

Legs: Deep orange.

Female

Head and neck: Pied markings distributed as in the pencilled fawn-and-white (above). Coloured feathers an even apricot-fawn. Eyes dark brown. Bill light orange-yellow possibly darkening with age. Pale bean.

Back: Pied markings distributed as in the pencilled fawn-and-white (above). Coloured feathers an even apricot-fawn (without pencilling).

Breast, flanks and underbody: Pied markings distributed as in the pencilled fawn-and-white (above). Coloured feathers an even apricot-fawn (without pencilling).

Tail: Pied markings distributed as in the pencilled fawn-and-white (above). Coloured feathers an even apricot-fawn (without pencilling).

Wings: Primaries, secondaries and tertials white; scapulars and some of the smaller coverts light apricot-fawn, giving approximately a heart shape.

Legs: Deep orange.

Disqualifications

Male: Bronze-green or seal brown cap, cheek and tail coverts.
Female: Medium brown or blue-grey pencilling on coloured body feathers.

Major defects

Both: Asymmetry of markings. Insufficient white plumage. Fawn extending from the back onto the abdomen and thigh coverts ('foul flanked'). Black bean on bill.

Minor defects

Both: 'Dribbles' of cap colour onto the white neck. Cheek markings extending onto the neck. Any irregular, blotchy or unclear markings that detract from the symmetry and general cleanness of the colour boundaries.

Black

In both sexes

Plumage: Black with a beetle-green lustre throughout.
Underwing: Coverts black with green lustre; main feathers very dark grey.
Eyes: Dark brown.
Bill: Black.
Legs: As black as possible. Orange shading permitted in older drakes.

Disqualifications

Female: Any sign of eye stripes.
Both: Conspicuous brown or white in the plumage, including underwing. Yellow bill. Pencilling on the breast.

Major defects

Female: Orange in the legs and feet.
Both: Purple lustre in the plumage. Green bill. White spot under bill. Grey under chin or on the secondaries and coverts.

Minor defects

Both: Grey tip on the bill.

Chocolate

In both sexes

Plumage: A dark, rich, solid chocolate throughout.
Underwing: Underwing pearly brown-grey.
Eyes: Dark brown.
Bill: Black.
Legs: As black as possible. Orange shading permitted in older drakes.

Disqualifications

Female: Any sign of eye stripes.
Both: Yellow bill. Conspicuous white or pencilling in outer plumage, including the underwing.

Major defects

Female: Orange in the legs and feet.
Both: Green bill. White spot under bill.

Minor defects

Both: Grey or olive tip on the bill.

Cumberland blue

In both sexes

Plumage: Rich blue (head and neck darker in the male).
Wings: Rich slate blue with dark lacing on the coverts. Underwing blue-grey.
Eyes: Dark brown.
Bill: Bluish green in the drake; bluish grey in the duck.
Legs: Smoky orange to grey.

Disqualifications

Both: Feathers of any colour other than blue, notably any russet tinge including the underwing.

Major defects

Both: Yellow bill.

Minor defects

Both: Dark flecks in the plumage.

Major defects

In both sexes

Domed head – a rounded skull (rather than flattened) rising beyond the line of the culmen.
Plump head.
Centrally placed eyes – well below the line of the top of the skull.
Dished bill – depression in the line of the culmen.

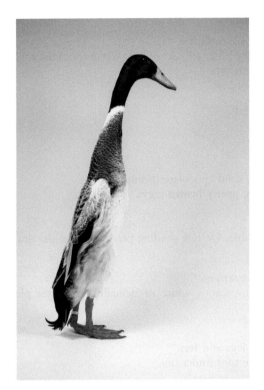

Silver Indian Runner male

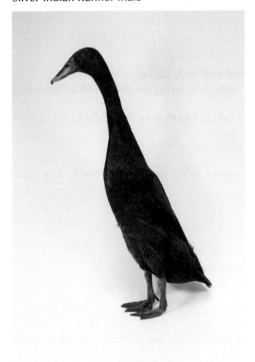

Chocolate Indian Runner female

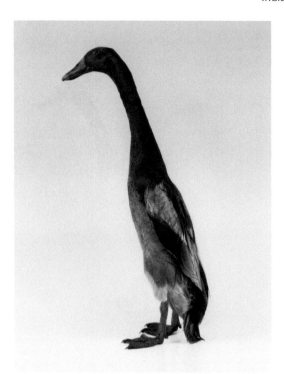

Fawn Indian Runner male

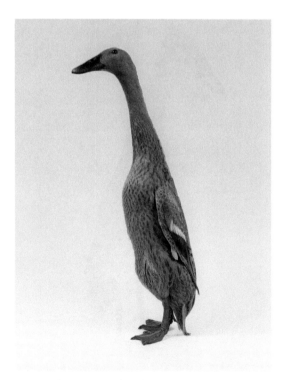

Fawn Indian Runner female

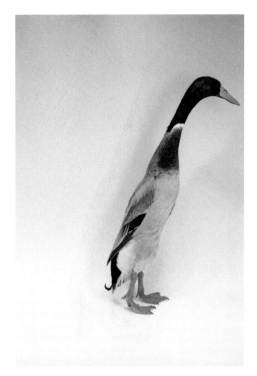

Trout Indian Runner male

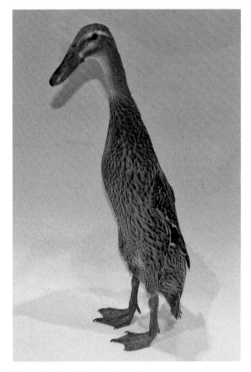

Trout Indian Runner female

Arched neck.

Thick or short neck.

Long neck – beyond one-third of the total length.

Neck expansion that distorts the symmetry of the 'hock bottle' shape.

Prominent shoulders.

Hollow back – angular displacement of the neck to the body, which should be 180° when the bird is standing at attention.

'Gutter' back – a long concavity between the shoulders.

Pointed breast – prominent sternum.

Pigeon breast – prominent chest muscles.

Flat back.

'Cricket bat' – broad, shallow body (flat back and front).

Body squat or short.

Any other major distortion of the narrow, cylindrical shape.

Very short stern – well clear of the ground.

Long stern – touching the ground.

Forward legs – protruding, angular thighs that distort the lines of the body and cause awkward movement or poor carriage.

Turned up tail – when the bird is alert or at attention.

Minor defects

In both sexes: Roman bill. Prominent thighs. Tail between the legs when stressed.

MAGPIE

Classification: Light
Origin: Wales

The Magpie is an unusual duck breed named only according to its original plumage markings of black and white. Developed by Reverend Gower Williams and Mr Oliver Drake in the years following the First World War, the breed was first standardised in the addendum to the 1926 *Poultry Club Standards*. It has a comparable colour form in the later German *Altrheiner Elsterenten* produced by Paul-Erwin Oswald.

Overall type (shape): Male and female

Carriage: Approximately 35° when active. Good length of body, giving a somewhat racy appearance, indicative of strength combined with great activity.

Head: Long and straight. Eyes large and prominent, giving keen and alert appearance. Bill long and broad.

Neck: Long, strong and slightly curved.

Body: Back level and fairly broad. Breast full and rounded.

Tail: Medium length, gently rising from the line of the back, and increasing apparent length of the bird.

Wings: Powerful and carried close to the body.

Legs and feet: Medium length.

Plumage: Close and smooth.

Colour

The black-and-white

In both sexes

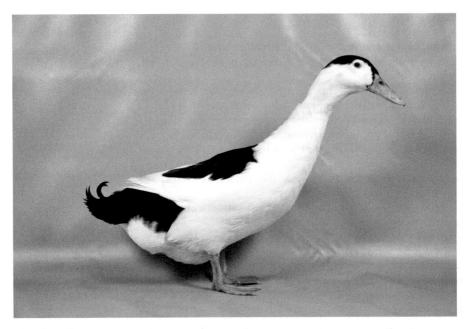

Magpie male

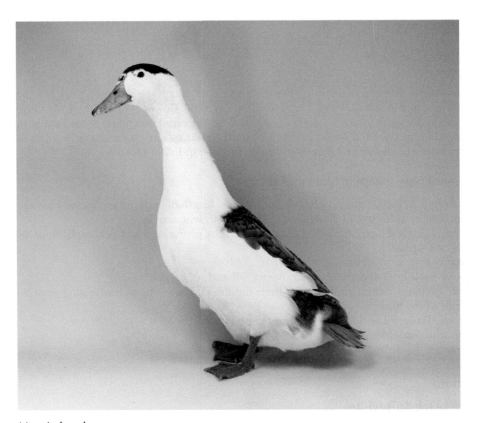

Magpie female

Head and neck: White surmounted by a black cap covering the whole of the crown, down to almost the top of the eyes.

Back: Solid black from shoulders to the tip of the tail.

Breast, flanks, thighs, underbody *and stern*: White.

Tail and undertail: Black.

Wings: White primary and secondary feathers. Scapulars: when the wings are closed there is a heart-shaped mantle of black feathers formed over the back. Underwing white. The outline of the coloured feathers should be sharp, clearly defined and symmetrical.

The blue-and-white

As above, the blue replacing black.

The chocolate-and-white

As above, the chocolate replacing black.

The dun-and-white

As above, the dun replacing black.

In both sexes and all colours

Eyes dark grey or dark brown. Bill in younger birds, yellow; in older birds, drake yellow, spotted with green, and the duck grey-green. Legs and webs: orange; dark mottling permissible.

Weights

Drake   2.5–3.2 kg   (5½–7 lb)
Duck   2.0–2.7 kg   (4½–6 lb)

Scale of points

Carriage	10
Head, bill and neck	18
Body	12
Legs and feet	5
Colour	30
Size	15
Condition	10
	100

Disqualifications

In both sexes: Absence of cap.

Faults

In both sexes: Asymmetry of markings. White feathers in the tail. Markings in the face or thigh. Additional markings other than stated. Cream or pink bill. Excessive weight or coarseness.

MUSCOVY

Classification: Heavy
Origin: America

The wild Muscovy (*Cairina moschata*) is a native of South and Central America, where it was being domesticated long before Columbus arrived in 1492. (White ones were found on

Guadeloupe, by Diego Alvarez Chanca in 1494.) It is allocated to a subgroup of perching ducks known as 'the greater wood ducks', which it shares with the white-winged wood duck and Hartlaub's duck. These are heavy-bodied birds with relatively short legs that give them a horizontal carriage. They have broad wings with bony knobs at the carpal joints and the males show a slight swelling of the forehead during the breeding season. The wild Muscovies are mainly black in plumage with white patches on the wing covert area. These vary, but usually develop with age. This is the basic wild pattern. Other patterns have been developed under domestication, including the magpie pattern and the white-headed magpie pattern. Three other characteristics are readily apparent: Muscovies have an erectile forecrown crest, wart-like 'caruncles' that develop with age, especially in the case of the males, and webbed feet (with strong claws) equally suited to perching as to swimming. The size has increased under domestication. A powerful bird requiring careful handling.

Overall type (shape): Male and female

Carriage: Almost horizontal, low but jaunty.
Head: Large, particularly in the drake. Crowned with a small crest of feathers which are raised in excitement or alarm. Caruncles on the face and over the base of the bill (both crest and caruncles more pronounced in the drake than in the duck). Bill wide, strong, of medium length, and with a slightly curved bean.
Neck: Medium length, strong and almost erect.
Body: Broad, deep, very long and powerful. Breast broad, full, well rounded and carried low. Underbody long and well fleshed, clear of the ground, slightly rounded.
Tail: Long and carried low, giving the body a longer appearance and a slightly curved outline to the back.
Wings: Very strong, long and carried high. Capable of flight.
Legs and feet: Legs strong, wide apart and fairly short. Thighs short, strong and muscular. Feet straight, webbed, with pronounced toenails.
Plumage: Close.

Colour

Colour points to be allocated for *clarity* of the colour in all varieties, and for the *symmetry* of the markings in the magpie pattern and white-headed magpie pattern. In the black, blue, chocolate and lavender, a patch of white (which may develop with age) is permitted on the wing coverts.

The black
Dense black, with metallic lustre.

The blue
Uniform shade of slate blue, strongly laced with a darker shade.

The chocolate
Even shade of chocolate, with metallic lustre.

The lavender
An even shade of pinkish blue-grey.

The white
Pure white throughout.

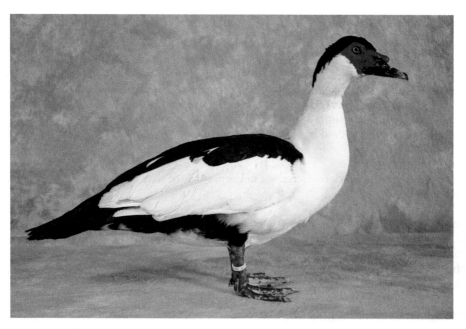

Muscovy male

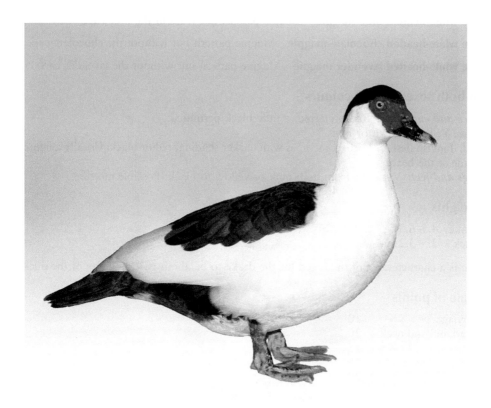

Muscovy female

The magpie pattern

The black magpie

Head and neck white surmounted by a black cap covering the whole of the crown to the nape. Back of the body solid black from shoulders to the tip of the tail. Breast, underbody and stern white. Thigh coverts white, but the outer thighs, tops of the flanks and the undertail are black. White primary and secondary feathers. When the wings are closed there is a heart-shaped mantle of black scapular feathers formed over the back. The outline of the black feathers should be sharp, clearly defined and symmetrical.

The blue magpie

Magpie pattern with black replaced by a uniform shade of slate blue, strongly laced with a darker shade.

The chocolate magpie

Magpie pattern with black replaced by an even shade of chocolate, with metallic lustre.

The lavender magpie

Magpie pattern with black replaced by an even shade of pinkish blue-grey.

The white-headed magpie pattern

The white-headed black magpie   Magpie pattern but without the black cap.

The white-headed blue magpie   Magpie pattern but without the blue cap.

The white-headed chocolate magpie   Magpie pattern but without the chocolate cap.

The white-headed lavender magpie   Magpie pattern but without the lavender cap.

In both sexes and all colours

Face and caruncles: Red preferred, a little black permitted.
Eyes: Yellow, brown or blue.
Bill: Pinkish flesh or horn, sometimes with darker shading, red or black. Usually a lighter shade at the bean.
Legs and feet: Variable, from flesh pink or yellow to black. Possible mottling.

Weights

Drake   4.5–6.3 kg   (10–14 lb)
Duck   2.3–3.2 kg   (5–7 lb)

It is a characteristic of the breed for the drake to be about twice the size of the duck.

Scale of points

Carriage	10
Head, bill and neck	20
Body	15
Legs and feet	5
Colour	20
Size	20
Condition	10
	100

Disqualifications

In both sexes: Caruncles impeding eyes and nostrils.

Faults

In both sexes: Uneven markings in magpie pattern birds. Cap colour extending below the nape; speckled or incomplete cap.

Minor faults (to be discouraged)

In both sexes: Undersize. Lack of caruncling in mature birds.

ORPINGTON

Classification: Light
Origin: Great Britain

The Orpington Ducks were developed by William Cook of Kent, who also bred Orpington chickens in the late nineteenth century. The buff and blue versions are likely to have emerged some time after 1894, and were being advertised for sale in 1898. These ducks were believed to be the result of cross-breeding Indian Runners to Aylesburys, Rouens and Cayugas. The buffs were standardised in 1910, followed by the blue variety in 1926. Black, white and chocolate Orpingtons were also developed but these were not standardised.

The Standard buff Orpington is an attractive but unstable colour form. Standard birds are impure for blue dilution and produce three colour forms, the first of which is the Standard:

Buff: Intermediate head colour in the males (seal brown), a dark grey-brown colour. There is very slight indication of blue on the rump, and the females, like the males, have an overall even buff body colour with little evidence of pencilling.
Blond: Pale buff with a light grey-brown head (in the case of the drake) and possibly more blue on the rump. The females are paler than the buffs and there is even less chance of pencilling.
Brown: Light khaki pencilled plumage on the females; brown heads and rumps on the males; no evidence of blue at all.

Overall type (shape): Male and female

Carriage: Slightly elevated at the shoulders, but avoiding any tendency to the upright carriage of the Pekin or Indian Runner.
Head: Fine and oval in shape. Eyes large and bold. Bill of moderate length.
Neck: Moderate length, upright.
Body: Long and broad, deep, without any sign of a keel. Back perfectly straight. Breast full and round.
Tail: Small, compact and rising slightly from the line of the back.
Wings: Strong and carried closely to the sides.
Legs and feet: Legs of moderate length; strong.
Plumage: Smooth and glossy.

Colour

The buff
Drake

Head and neck: Seal brown (two or three shades darker than the body) with a bright gloss, but complete absence of beetle green. The seal brown terminates in a sharply defined line all the way round the neck. Eyes brown. Bill yellow-ochre with dark bean.

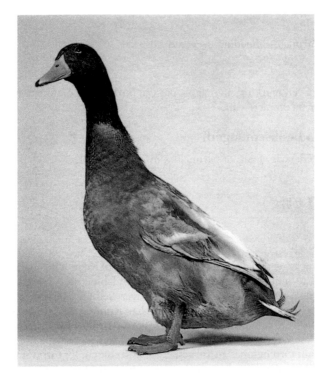

Buff Orpington male

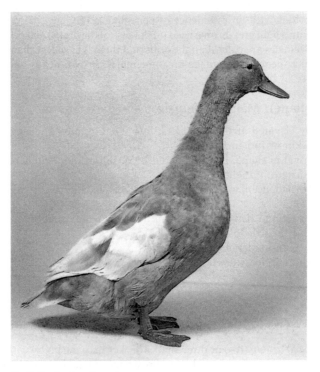

Buff Orpington female

Body: A rich, even shade of deep buff throughout. Rump brown, as free as possible from 'blue'.

Legs and webs: Orange-red.

Duck

Plumage: Body a rich even shade of buff throughout, free from blue, brown or white feathers and any pencilling.

Eyes: Brown.

Bill: Orange-brown with dark bean.

Legs and webs: Orange-red.

Weights

Drake   2.2–3.4 kg   (5–7½ lb)
Duck   2.2–3.2 kg   (5–7 lb)

Scale of points

Carriage	10
Head, bill and neck	15
Body	15
Legs and feet	5
Colour	35
Size	10
Condition	10
	100

Disqualifications

In both sexes: Colour other than stated; evidence of eye stripes at any stage of plumage.
In the drake: Grey, silver or blue head; beetle green on any part.

Faults

In both sexes: Evidence of a keel.
In the drake: White feathers on the neck or under the chin. Brown secondaries. Excessively blue rump. Very green bill. Pencilling.
In the duck: Pencilling. White feathers on the neck or breast. Brown or blue feathers. Green bill.

Minor faults (to be discouraged)

In the drake: Head colour extending onto the breast.
In the duck: Pale primaries, secondaries and wing coverts.

PEKIN

Classification: Heavy
Origin: China

The Pekin was imported from China into Great Britain and America between 1872 and 1874. Crossed with other breeds, it had a large impact on the commercial table bird market. The American strain continues to show a less than upright carriage whilst the British and European Pekins retain the characteristics described below. The British

Standard between 1910 and 1930 insisted on a plumage that was deep cream or 'buff canary', and when this strain 'died out' fresh importations were made from Europe. The present exhibition strain is therefore often referred to as the 'German Pekin', largely to distinguish it from the American. This is a variety that continues to thrive as an exhibition breed and also as basic stock for commercial breeding. In addition, it provided genetic material for several modern breeds, including the Saxony.

Overall type (shape): Male and female

A good description of the general shape of the Pekin is that it resembles a small, wide boat, standing almost on its stern, and the bow leaning slightly forward.

Carriage: Almost upright.
Head: Large, broad and round, with high skull, rising rather abruptly from the base of the bill. Eyes bold, partly shaded by heavy brows and bulky cheeks. Bill short, broad and thick, slightly convex or straight.
Neck: Appears short and thick; with slightly gulleted throat. Erect nape feathers, especially on the drake, can give the impression of a mane.
Body: Medium length, broad, with full shoulders. Breast broad, smooth and full. Broad deep paunch and stern carried just clear of the ground.
Tail: Well spread and carried quite high.
Wings: Short, carried closely to the sides.
Legs and feet: Legs strong and stout, set well back and causing erect carriage.
Plumage: Very abundant and well furnished.

Colour

In both sexes
Eyes: Dark lead-blue.
Bill: Bright orange.
Legs and feet: Bright orange.
Plumage: Deep cream or cream.

Weights

Drake   4.1 kg   (9 lb)
Duck   3.6 kg   (8 lb)

Scale of points

Carriage	20
Head, bill and neck	20
Body	15
Legs and feet	5
Colour	10
Size	20
Condition	10
	100

Disqualifications

In both sexes: Squirrel or wry tail.

Faults

In both sexes: Weeping eyes. Black marks on bill; long or dished bill. Narrow stern; keel on breast. Dropped tail.

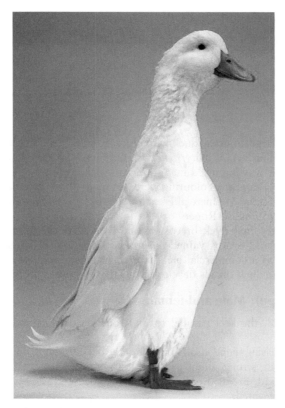

Pekin male

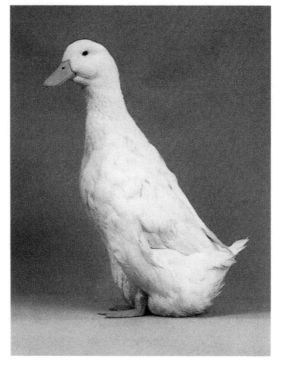

Pekin female

Minor faults (to be discouraged)

In both sexes: White rather than cream plumage.

ROUEN

Classification: Heavy
Origin: France

The Rouen is a very large domestic duck with plumage colour and markings that resemble those of the wild Mallard (*Anas platyrhynchos*). Originally produced in Normandy, from the area of Rouen, it was imported into southern England some time in the eighteenth century. Here its size, shape and colouring were further developed to such an extent that it was distinguished from the commercial French ducks by referring to it as the *Rouen foncé* (dark Rouen) or even 'English Rouen'.

This was one of the first duck breeds standardised in Great Britain (in the original Standards of 1865), and is now valued more for its size and plumage markings in the exhibition pen than as a commercial meat bird. It has also been used as basic stock for breeding many of the duck breeds developed in the twentieth century.

Overall type (shape): Male and female

Carriage: Horizontal, the keel parallel to and touching the ground when the bird is standing at rest.
Head: Massive, skull rising slightly from the base of the bill. Eyes bold. Bill long, wide and flat.
Neck: Medium length, strong, slightly curved but not arched.
Body: Long and broad. Breast broad and deep. Keel deep.
Tail: Very slightly elevated.
Wings: Large and well tucked to the sides.
Legs and feet: Legs of medium length. Shanks stout and well set to balance the body in a straight line.
Plumage: Tight and glossy.

Colour

Drake

Markings throughout the whole plumage should be cleanly cut and well defined in every detail, the colours distinct and not shading into each other.
Head and neck: Black with green lustre to within about 2.5 cm (1 in.) of the shoulders where the ring appears. Ring perfectly white and cleanly cut, dividing the neck and breast colours, but not quite encircling the neck, leaving a small space at the back. Eyes dark hazel. Bill bright green-yellow, with black bean at the tip.
Back and rump: Black with green lustre.
Breast: Rich claret, in the form of a deep, cleanly cut bib dropping vertically in line with the wing butts to beneath the breast.
Flanks and stern: Grey-charcoal stippled pencilling on lighter ground. Undertail black, separated by indistinct, curved line.
Tail: Dark slate-brown. Tail coverts black or dark slate tinged with brown; two or three green-black curled feathers in the centre.
Wings: Primaries and primary coverts dark brown-slate. Secondaries (speculum) iridescent blue tipped with distinct black then white bars. Greater coverts brown-slate tipped with distinct white then black bars. Smaller coverts grey. Scapular feathers similar to, but more brown than, the flank feathers. At the centre of the back and on the edges above the wings, these are rich, dark bronze. Underwing cream or white.
Legs and webs: Orange-red.

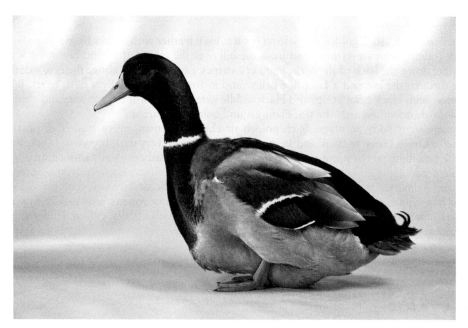

Rouen male

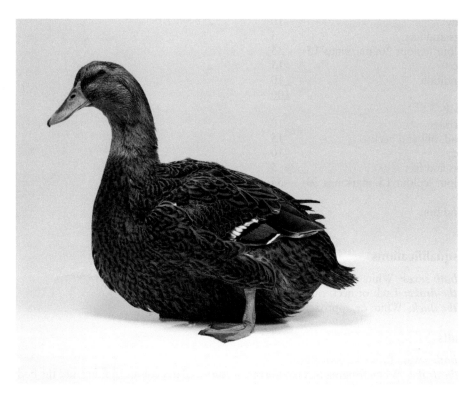

Rouen female

Duck

Head and neck: Rich golden or chestnut brown, each feather with darker brown graining. This graining forms a darker band from the bill over the crown, the band becoming less distinct down the back of the neck. Faint eye stripes, i.e. a faint line above the eye, a dark line through the eye and a faint line below and in front of the eye. Eyes dark hazel. Bill orange, with black bean at tip, and black saddle extending almost to each side and about two-thirds down towards the tip. Plain ground colour on throat.

Remainder of body plumage: Rich golden or chestnut brown, every feather distinctly pencilled from breast to flank and stern, the markings to be very dark brown to black, the black pencilling on the rump having a green lustre. Large feathers ideally show double or triple pencilling.

Wings: Primaries and primary coverts dark brown-slate. Secondaries (speculum) iridescent blue tipped with distinct black then white bars. Greater coverts brown-slate tipped with distinct white then black bars. Smaller coverts edged with a lighter colour. Underwing cream or white.

Legs and webs: Dull orange-brown.

Weights

Drake   4.5–5.4 kg   (10–12 lb)
Duck   4.1–5.0 kg   (9–11 lb)

Scale of points

Drake

Carriage	10
Head, bill and neck	15
Body	10
Legs and feet	5
Colour (colour 20, markings 15)	35
Size	15
Condition	10
	100

Duck

Carriage	10
Head, bill and neck	15
Body	10
Legs and feet	5
Colour (colour 15, markings 20)	35
Size	15
Condition	10
	100

Disqualifications

In both sexes: White primaries. Lack of keel.
In the drake: Lack of neck ring.
In the duck: White or approaching white ring on neck.

Faults

In both sexes: Broken down stern.
In the drake: White fringing on claret breast feathers. Claret colour running into the body colour. Blue-green in the colour of the bill.
In the duck: Indistinct or insufficient pencilling.

Minor faults (to be discouraged)

In both sexes: Indistinct secondary or greater covert bars.
In the drake: Flank feathers with rust. Any white in the stern.
In the duck: Leaden or green bill.

ROUEN CLAIR

Classification: Heavy
Origin: France

The Rouen Clair is a modern development of the traditional Mallard-coloured ducks from the Rouen area of France. It is distinguished from the *Rouen foncé* by the pale (*Isabelle clair*) ground colour of the female, the slightly upright carriage and a number of other characteristics common to the light-phase plumage.

The modern Rouen Clair is largely the result of breeding accomplished by Monsieur Rene Garry between 1910 and 1920. Beginning with birds selected from farms in the area of Picardy, he proceeded to develop bloodlines primarily for size and plumage colour. Further bloodlines, involving Rouen–Mallard crosses, improved the vigour and resulted in a large, light-phase, commercial duck, first standardised in France in 1923 and in Great Britain in 1982.

Overall type (shape): Male and female

Carriage: Rather more upright than the Rouen, 10–20° above the horizontal.
Head: Bold, slight rise to the skull. Eyes bright. Bill medium length, broad.
Neck: Upright and of medium length; not thin.
Body: Very long, with good width, yet more smooth breasted than the Rouen. The important feature of the Rouen Clair is its length (ideally 90 cm (35 in.) from the point of beak to the end of tail with neck extended), which gives it elegance in spite of its heavy body.
Tail: Slightly elevated.
Wings: Neatly folded against the body.
Legs and feet: Legs medium length, set slightly back.
Plumage: Close and smooth.

Colour

Drake

Head and neck: Black with green lustre down to the clear white neck ring, 5–9 mm ($\frac{1}{4}$–$\frac{3}{8}$ in.) wide, which encircles about four-fifths of the neck, leaving a small space at the back. Eyes brown. Bill yellow with greenish tint; black bean.
Back: Pearly grey, darker than the flanks. Rump brilliant greenish black.
Breast: Claret, with white edging at the end of each feather.
Flanks: Pearly grey (grey stippled pencilling on lighter ground).
Underbody: Light grey changing to white.
Stern: White.

Tail: Whitish grey. Undertail black.
Wings: Primaries greyish brown with light edge. Secondaries (speculum) iridescent blue tipped with distinct black then white bars. Greater coverts tipped with distinct white then black bars. Smaller coverts greyish brown. Scapulars grey with bronze edge. Underwing cream or white.
Legs and webs: Orange-yellow.

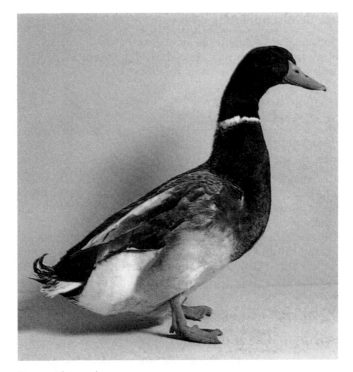

Rouen Clair male

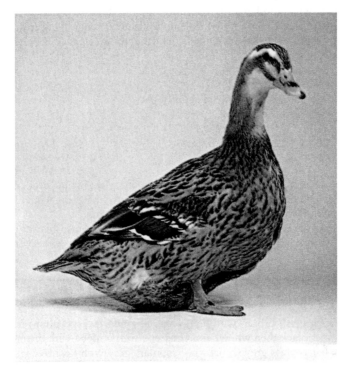

Rouen Clair female.

Duck

Head and neck: Fawn with dark graining on the crown. Eyes brown. Eyebrow of creamy white; dark line through the eye; pale line below and in front of the eye down to the bill. Bill orange-ochre with brown saddle; black bean. Base of the bill and front of neck creamy fawn.

Body: Fawn ground, delicately streaked or pencilled with dark brown. Pencilling best developed as chevrons on the larger feathers.

Tail: Colour as body.

Wings: Primaries greyish brown with light edges. Speculum as drake. Coverts brown edged with cream. Scapulars ideally pencilled with a single V in brown. Underwing cream or white.

Legs and webs: Dull yellow-orange.

Weights

Drake   3.4–4.1 kg   (7½–9 lb)
Duck   2.9–3.4 kg   (6½–7½ lb)

Scale of points

Carriage	10
Head, bill and neck	15
Body	15
Legs and feet	5
Colour	30
Size	15
Condition	10
	100

Disqualifications

In both sexes: White flights.
In the drake: Lack of white stern.
In the duck: Lack of eye stripes; white neck ring.

Faults

In both sexes: Presence of keel; lack of size.
In the drake: Grey in the green of the head. Closed neck ring. Mixture of claret feathers on the flanks. Lack of edging on breast feathers.
In the duck: Throat colour extending too low on the breast.

Minor faults (to be discouraged)

In the drake: Black lines along bill centre.

SAXONY

Classification: Heavy
Origin: Germany

Developed mainly from Rouens, German Pekins and Blue Pommerns around 1930, the Saxony was bred by Albert Franz at Chemnitz. It was first exhibited at Chemnitz-

Alten-dorf at the first Saxony County Show of 1934. However, the breed stock was almost entirely destroyed during the Second World War and in 1952 Franz was forced to begin a revival using small surviving flocks and reintroducing some of the other breeds employed earlier in 1930. The Saxony duck was recognised in East Germany (GDR) in 1957, in West Germany (FRG) the following year and in Great Britain in 1982.

Overall type (shape): Male and female

Carriage: Elevated to approximately 30° when active and alert.
Head: Long, bold, with gentle rise to the forehead. Eyes bright. Bill medium length and broad.
Neck: Medium length, same width from head to breast, not thin.
Body: Large, broad and deep without any suggestion of a keel. Breast full and round.
Tail: Slightly elevated.
Wings: Neatly folded against the body.
Legs and feet: Medium length. Legs set a little back from centre.
Plumage: Close and smooth.

Colour

Drake

Head and neck: Pigeon blue (blue-grey) down to the closed neck ring, which is white and about 5–9 mm ($\frac{1}{4}$–$\frac{3}{8}$ in.) wide. Eyes dark brown. Bill yellow with light green tinge and pale bean.
Back, rump and undertail: Pigeon blue (blue-grey).
Lower neck (below ring), breast and shoulders: Claret with slight silver edging on the shoulders and breast. Lower body oatmeal.
Stern: White.
Wings: Primaries grey. Secondaries (speculum) pigeon blue tipped with distinct dark then light blue bars. Greater coverts tipped with distinct dark then light blue bars. Underwing cream or white.
Tail: Light grey.
Legs and webs: Orange.

Duck

Head and neck: Deep apricot-buff. Eyes brown. Eyebrow of creamy white; dark line through the eye; cream line below and in front of the eye down to the bill. Bill yellow with brownish tinge and pale bean.
Throat: Cream.
Back and rump: Paler buff.
Tail: Buff.
Wings: Primaries oatmeal. Secondaries (speculum) pigeon blue tipped with distinct dark then light blue bars. Greater coverts tipped with distinct light then dark blue bars. Underwing cream or white.
Legs and webs: Orange.

Weights

Drake   3.6 kg   (8 lb)
Duck   3.2 kg   (7 lb)

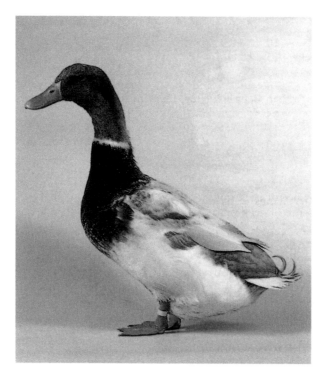

Saxony male

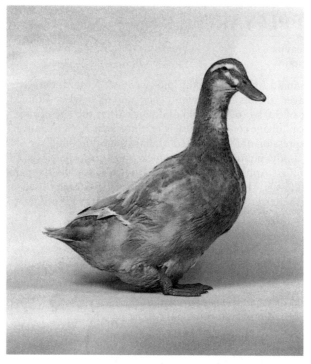

Saxony female

Scale of points

Carriage	10
Head, bill and neck	15
Body	15
Legs and feet	5
Colour	30
Size	15
Condition	10
	100

Disqualifications

In the drake: Absence of neck ring.
In the duck: Presence of neck ring. Absence of eye stripes.

Faults

In both sexes: Keel. Horizontal carriage. Black bean on bill.
In the drake: Broken neck ring. Breast colour running onto the flanks and solid breast colour. Any brown on the head.
In the duck: Claret or excessive white on breast.

Minor faults (to be discouraged)

In both sexes: Upright carriage.

SILVER APPLEYARD

Classification: Heavy
Origin: Great Britain

Originated by Reginald Appleyard in the mid-twentieth century, the Silver Appleyard was developed as a layer of 'lots of big white eggs' and as a white-skinned table bird that attained a weight of 3.0 kg ($6\frac{1}{4}$ lb) (cold and plucked) at the age of nine weeks. For size, carriage and basic plumage colour, it closely resembles the Rouen Clair. Its unique feature, however, is the expression of the restricted Mallard gene that limits the amount of pigment on the face and body plumage of both duck and drake. Little is known about the appearance of the first Appleyards other than from sources like the painting by Wippell commissioned in 1947. The modern Silver Appleyard (standardised in 1982) and its Miniature form (standardised in 1997) are largely the result of breeding by Tom Bartlett of Folly Farm.

Overall type (shape): Male and female

Carriage: Lively, slightly erect, the back sloping gently from shoulder to tail.
Head: Bold, slight rise to the skull. Eyes bright. Bill medium length, broad.
Neck: Upright and of medium length, not thin.
Body: Compact, broad and well rounded. Moderate length.
Tail: Slightly elevated.
Wings: Neatly folded against the body.
Legs and feet: Legs medium length, set slightly back.
Plumage: Close and smooth.

Colour

Drake

Head and neck: Black with green lustre. Faint eyebrow and cheek markings in silver-white.

Bill: Yellow with slight greenish tint, with a dark bean. A white ring (5–9 mm ($\frac{1}{4}$–$\frac{3}{8}$ in.) completely encircles the neck. The throat is silver-white flecked. Base of neck and shoulders below the ring claret.

Back: Claret followed by dark grey mottled back feathers.

Rump: Solid black with green lustre.

Breast: Claret with white undercolour – each feather tipped with a fine, white fringe. The claret bib is broken in the centre and fades to light silver under the body.

Flanks: Grey stippled pencilling on white ground. Claret of breast extends along the upper flank above the thigh coverts, which are pale grey.

Tail: Grey with broad white edging. Undertail black.

Wings: Primaries grey and white, with white edging. Secondaries (speculum) iridescent blue tipped with black then white. Tertiaries grey. Patterned light silver wing coverts match the colour of the breast and underbody. Scapulars grey stipple; outer edge claret. Underwing cream or white.

Duck

Head and neck: Silver-white with crown and back of neck fawn flecked with brown-grey. This fawn on the neck should join that of the shoulder without a break. Deep fawn line through the eye.

Bill: Yellow with a brown saddle and dark bean.

Back and rump: Fawn flecked with brown-grey.

Breast and underbody: Creamy white.

Flanks: Creamy white and fawn, flecked with brown-grey.

Tail: Mottled fawn, darker centre to each feather.

Wings: Primaries creamy white, brown towards the tip. Secondaries (speculum) blue, tipped with black then white. Tertiaries mottled fawn-brown. Coverts white, marked with fawn and grey. Scapulars fawn streaked with grey-brown. Underwing cream or white.

In both sexes

Eyes: Dark hazel.
Legs: Orange.

Weights

Drake   3.6–4.1 kg   (8–9 lb)
Duck   3.2–3.6 kg   (7–8 lb)

Scale of points

Carriage	10
Head, bill and neck	15
Body	15
Legs and feet	5
Colour	30
Size	15
Condition	10
	100

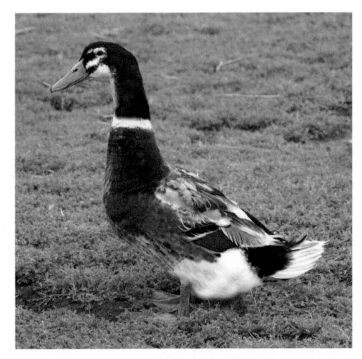

Silver Appleyard male

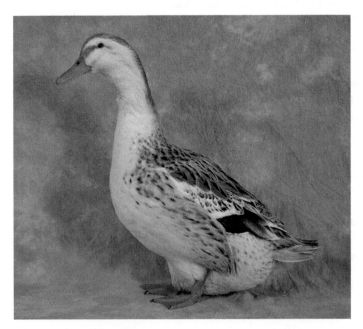

Silver Appleyard female

Disqualifications

In both sexes: Pure white primaries.
In the drake: Solid green head. Dark grey underbody and/or wing coverts. Solid claret bib.
In the duck: Solid brown head.

Faults

In both sexes: Presence of keel. Lack of size. Absence of blue speculum.
In the drake: Open or excessively broad neck ring. Excessive claret along flanks.
In the duck: Lack of eye line. Broken neck line. Excessive colour to underbelly. Completely white wing coverts.

Minor faults (to be discouraged)

In the duck: Completely white undertail.

SILVER APPLEYARD MINIATURE

Classification: Bantam
Origin: Great Britain

Developed in the 1980s and shown at the first BWA Championship Waterfowl Exhibition of 1987 by Tom Bartlett of Folly Farm, this Bantam Duck is a miniature version of the original Silver Appleyard produced by Reginald Appleyard in the mid-twentieth century. The Miniature, first standardised in 1997, is roughly a third of the weight of the original, large breed.

Overall type (shape), colour and scale of points

As for large Silver Appleyard.

Weights

Drake   1.36 kg   (3 lb)
Duck   1.19 kg   (2½ lb)

Disqualifications

In both sexes: Presence of broad band of white extending up the back of the neck. Pure white primaries.
In the drake: Solid claret bib.
In the duck: Solid brown head.

Faults

In both sexes: Oversize. Mallard shape (long bill and racy body). Absence of blue speculum.
In the drake: Open or excessively broad neck ring. Solid grey wing coverts and underbody. Solid claret bib. Lack of silver-white cheek and throat markings.
In the duck: Lack of eye line. Broken neck line. Excessive colour to underbelly.

Minor faults (to be discouraged)

In the duck: Completely white undertail.

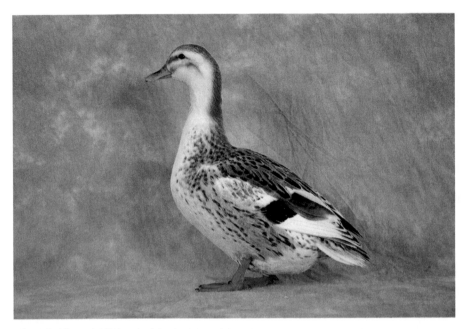

Silver Appleyard Miniature female

SILVER BANTAM

Classification: Bantam
Origin: Great Britain

This bantam breed was formerly known as the Silver Appleyard Bantam. It was produced by Reginald Appleyard from a cross between a small khaki Campbell duck and a white Call drake in the 1940s. The Silver Bantam does not have the same colour genes as the large Silver Appleyard, hence the change of name when the Miniature Appleyard was stand-ardised in 1997. The Bantam is very similar to the Abacot Ranger, which was also developed from khaki Campbells and crossed to a white drake. In this way, the dusky mallard genes were retained and the hidden harlequin-phase genes were revealed.

Overall type (shape): Male and female

Carriage: Slightly erect, head held high, the back sloping gently from shoulder to tail.
Head: Small and neat. Bill medium length.
Neck: Medium length, almost vertical.
Body: Compact, but a more slender shape than the Call Duck. Body clear of the ground for active foraging.
Tail: Medium length and only slightly elevated.
Wings: Held close to the body.
Legs and feet: Legs of medium length.
Plumage: Tight and glossy.

Colour

Drake

Head and neck: Black with green lustre, terminated above the shoulder by a completely encircling white ring, dividing in a sharp clean line the neck and breast colours. Eyes dark brown. Bill yellow-green with black bean.

Back: Upper back white feathers finely stippled with black and fringed with white. Lower down the back the stippling becomes heavier, each feather preferably fringed with white, until solid black with green lustre on the rump. Black sex curls may also be tipped with white.

Breast, neck base and shoulders: Claret edged with white.

Flanks, underbody and stern: Silvery white to cream (a white ground colour being preferable). A little of the breast colour extending along the upper flank.

Tail: Paler outer feathers; central feathers darker, each feather having a dark grey centre and paler off-white edging. Undertail black, finishing neatly and not running into the stern and flank colour.

Wings: Primaries silvery white with a slightly iridescent dark grey overlay. Secondaries (speculum) bluish green tipped with distinct black then white bars. Greater coverts dark grey with well-defined white rim. Smaller coverts French grey with a lighter edging. Scapulars and tertiaries as the breast with wider silver-white edging. Underwing creamy white.

Leg and webs: Orange.

Duck

Head and neck: Fawn (a deeper shade in young females) with the brow and crown clearly marked with darker graining. There is a sharp division between the neck and upper white of the breast colour. Eyes dark brown. Bill yellow to grey-green.

Lower back: White feathers with central dark streak; markings heaviest towards the rump.

Upper breast, lower neck, shoulders and flanks: Lightly streaked with light brown on a creamy white ground.

Lower breast, underbody and stern: Creamy white.

Tail: Feathers white with central dark streak and fawn and black stippling.

Wings: Primaries and speculum as the drake. Greater coverts dark grey with well-defined white rim. Smaller coverts dark fawn edged with cream. Scapulars and tertiaries creamy fawn with brown flecks. Underwing creamy white. The white ground colour in the bird to prevail.

Legs and webs: Orange.

Weights

Drake   0.9 kg   (2 lb)
Duck   0.8 kg   ($1\frac{3}{4}$ lb)

Scale of points

Carriage	10
Head, bill and neck	15
Body	15
Legs and feet	5
Colour	30
Size	15
Condition	10
	100

Disqualifications

In both sexes: Absent speculum. Oversize.

In the drake: Brown head. Broken, too wide or absent neck ring. White under the chin.

In the duck: Mallard eye stripes. White head colour.

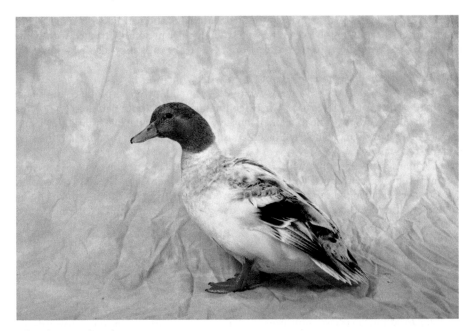

Silver bantam female

Faults

In the drake: Too dark a ground colour; breast colour running too low into body or lacking white edging. Blue bill.
In the duck: Absence of graining or streaking. Dark ground colour.

WELSH HARLEQUIN

Classification: Light
Origin: Great Britain

Originally bred by Group Captain Leslie Bonnet at the end of the Second World War, the breed owes its existence to a chance production of two mutations ('sports') from a flock of khaki Campbells in 1949. These 'Honey Campbells' were renamed 'Welsh Harlequins' when the Bonnet family moved to Wales.

The Harlequins were saved from virtual extinction after the late 1960s by Edward Grayson in Lancashire. He had retained birds from the original Bonnet strain, bred these back to khaki Campbells and eventually stabilised the colour form. This was possible simply because the Harlequin is genetically almost identical to the khaki Campbell. It possesses two recessive genes, which F.M. Lancaster established as harlequin phase. Both khaki Campbell and Welsh Harlequin have dusky mallard genes and sex-linked, brown dilution genes, hence the bronze rather than blue specula. Modern examples of the Welsh Harlequin, however, tend to have bright olive bills, compared with the blue-green of the Campbell and a proportion of the early Harlequins.

Overall type (shape): Male and female

Carriage: Alert and slightly upright, the head carried high with shoulders higher than the saddle, the back showing a gentle slant; the whole carriage not too erect (about 35°) but not so low as to cause waddling. Activity and foraging power to be retained without loss of depth and width of body generally.

Head: Refined in jaw and skull. Eyes full, bold and bright; fairly high in skull and prominent. Bill of medium length, depth and width; following a smooth line with the top of the skull.

Neck: Medium length, slender, almost erect.

Body: Compact, with width well maintained from shoulders to stern.

Tail: Short and small.

Wings: Tight, held close to the body.

Legs and feet: Legs medium length and set well apart; not too far back.

Plumage: Tight and glossy.

Colour

Drake

Head and upper neck: Dark brown with a bronze-green lustre to within about 2.5 cm (1 in.) of the shoulders where a 0.5–1.5 cm ($\frac{1}{4}-\frac{1}{2}$ in.) white ring (finer and more clearly defined at the front than the back) completely encircles the neck. Eyes dark brown. Bill olive green, with black bean.

Back: Upper back feathers white, finely stippled with dark brown and fringed with white. Lower down the back the stippling becomes heavier, each feather preferably fringed with white until solid dark brown on the rump, where there is a slight green lustre.

Breast, neck base and shoulders: Claret, finely fringed with white. This colour washes along the upper flank, finishing at the upper thigh coverts.

Underbody and stern: Creamy white.

Tail: Dark brown bordered with white; undertail bronze.

Wings: Primaries off-white, overlaid with brown. Speculum bronze with green lustre, bordered by a fine line of white. Smaller wing coverts creamy white and finely stippled with dark brown, with white edging. Greater coverts dark brown with white rims. Outer scapulars as the breast colour, edged with creamy white, which gives a dark tortoiseshell effect. Underwing creamy white.

Legs and webs: Orange.

Duck

Head and upper neck: Honey-fawn with brown graining on the crown. Eyes dark brown. Bill dark slate tinged with green.

Main body feathers: Fawn to cream; central shaft of feathers marked with brown. These markings less distinct on breast and underbody.

Rump: Mid-brown with darker brown central streak to each feather.

Tail: Mid-brown.

Wings: Primaries brown edged with white, slightly darker than the drake. Speculum bronze. Well-defined edging on the wing coverts. Scapulars a mixture of fawn, red-brown and cream, producing a rich, tortoiseshell effect. Underwing creamy white.

Note: The general body colour becomes quite diluted when the female is in full egg production.

Legs and webs: Dark brown in mature stock.

Weights

Adult drake 2.3–2.5 kg (5–5$\frac{1}{2}$ lb)
Adult duck   2.0–2.3 kg (4–5$\frac{1}{2}$ lb)

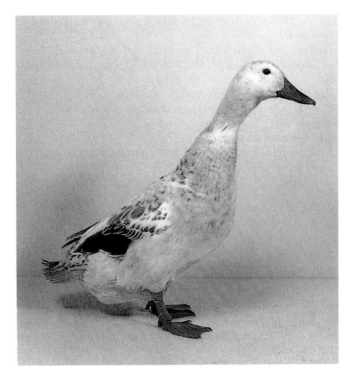

Welsh Harlequin female

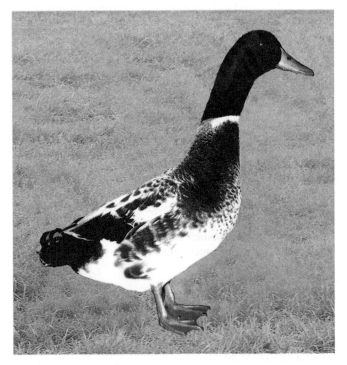

Welsh Harlequin male

Scale of points

Carriage	10
Head, bill and neck	15
Body	15
Legs and feet	5
Colour	35
Size	10
Condition	10
	100

Disqualifications

In both sexes: Blue speculum. Oversize or with a keel.
In the drake: Broken or absent neck ring.
In the duck: Lack of graining on the head.

Faults

In both sexes: Upright carriage. Lack of white edging on the wing coverts.
In the drake: Blue bill.
In the duck: Clearly defined brown hood. Lack of dark feather markings on the rump. Incorrect bill colour.

Minor faults (to be discouraged)

In the duck: Orange legs (legs palest in younger birds; they darken with age).

OTHER BREEDS

The BWA looks after any other breeds of duck not standardised in this edition. Specimens of other breeds appear occasionally, but not so far in sufficient numbers to warrant standardising.

Pomern

A small Blue Swedish without white flights, eastern European in origin.

Shetland

A small and less well-marked version of the Blue Swedish, but black where the Swedish is blue.

Stanbridge white

A medium British breed of white duck, never seen in great numbers but standardised by the Poultry Club a number of years ago.

Standard for utility

Classes may be offered for:

Utility, pure bred for egg production (M/F)
Utility, pure bred for meat production (M/F)
Utility, dual purpose (M/F)
Utility, non-Standard (M/F)
Utility, waterfowl

Note: Any breed to enter utility classes; only birds entered in these classes can win the award for Champion Utility. Non-standard breeds can only compete to win their class, but cannot win Champion Utility. All will be judged for utility using the following points scale:

40 pts	**Capacity**	Size and dimensions of back, breast, abdomen and pelvis appropriate for production. Allow for sex differences and the requirements for egg laying and meat production
40 pts	**Capability**	Good health and fitness as measured by the firmness and quantity of flesh, bloom of feather, state of comb and in layers, width between pin (pelvic) bones. The age of the bird will be taken into account
10 pts	**Breed characteristics**	For commercial hybrids: evenness of feather colour/pattern
10 pts	**Show preparation**	Clean feathers, feet and legs; trimmed toenails and beak, a small amount of olive oil can be applied to comb, wattles and legs

Defects (for which birds should be penalised)

Crooked breast bone, overweight (fat: pin bones are difficult to feel), evidence of parasite damage. In layers, evidence of feather damage on the back due to the cockerel's excessive mating.

Serious defects (for which the bird should be passed and removed from the show)

Any sign of parasites or disease.

British Poultry Standards, Seventh Edition. Edited by J. Ian H. Allonby and Philippe B. Wilson.
© 2019 Poultry Club of Great Britain. Published 2019 by John Wiley & Sons Ltd.

Standard for eggs

The Poultry Club has authorised the following standard and scale of points for judging eggs.

EXTERNAL

Shape: Showing ample breadth, good dome, with greater length than width, the top to be much roomier than the bottom and more curved. The bottom should not be too pointed, and a circular, or even narrow, shape is undesirable. The ideal shape is described as an elliptical cone. In outline it is an asymmetrical ellipse or 'Cassinian oval' and a cross-section at any point across the egg's girth is a perfect circle. This description is best shown by the large fowl egg. Deviations from this ideal are characteristically shown by other breeds but when judging, this is the ideal to aim for. Pullet eggs are less pointed whereas some breeds of bantams characteristically lay more pointed eggs.

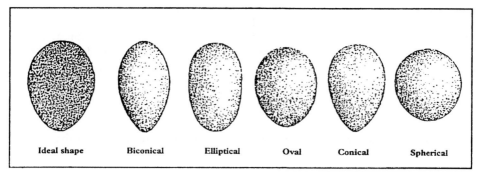

Ideal shape   Biconical   Elliptical   Oval   Conical   Spherical

Shapes of six eggs (description)

Turkeys, ducks and geese are distinct species and each lays eggs of slightly different shape. Hence, they should be shown in their own classes. Turkey eggs are quite short and conical. Duck eggs are slightly elongated, and those of bantam ducks tend to be pointed. Geese lay eggs that are lacking for girth and narrow towards the pointed end.

Size: Mere size is not a deciding point but should be appropriate for the breed and species. A pullet's normal egg when the bird starts to lay is 49.6 g ($1\frac{3}{4}$ oz) and increases quickly to 56.7 g (2 oz), exceeding that after several months of production. There is another increase in the hen egg after the moult. Bantam eggs should not exceed 42.5 g ($1\frac{1}{2}$ oz). Eggs weighing in excess of this should be passed.

Turkey and duck eggs weigh between 70.9 g ($2\frac{1}{2}$ oz) and 92.2 g ($3\frac{1}{4}$ oz). Bantam duck eggs should not exceed 63.8 g ($2\frac{1}{4}$ oz). Goose eggs vary with breed. Light geese lay eggs from 141.8 g (5 oz) and heavy breed goose eggs can weigh up to 198.6 g (7 oz).

Shell texture: Smooth, free from lines or bulges, evenly limed, smooth at each end, without roughness, porous parts or lime pimples.

British Poultry Standards, Seventh Edition. Edited by J. Ian H. Allonby and Philippe B. Wilson.
© 2019 Poultry Club of Great Britain. Published 2019 by John Wiley & Sons Ltd.

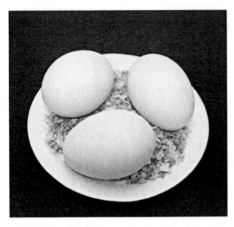

British Waterfowl Association: three waterfowl eggs

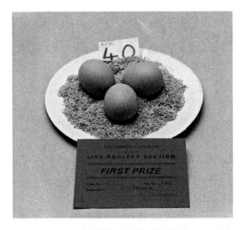

Bantam: three light brown eggs

Colour: White, cream, light brown, brown, mottled or speckled, blue, green, olive and plum. The colour should be even and, in the case of mottled or speckled eggs, regular mottles or speckles are preferred. Mottled or speckled eggs are shown according to their ground colour. Where a Breed Club has stated in its Standard that a particular colour is required, any variations from this should be penalised.

Freshness, bloom and appearance: Shells to be clean, without dull or stale appearance as befits a new-laid egg. Shell surfaces may be shiny or matt, but should be free from blemishes such as stains and nest marks. Eggs may be washed in preparation but not polished.

In duck eggs the position of the air space can be apparent. This is not considered a fault. Muscovy duck eggs often have a wax cuticle which may be removed.

Matching and uniformity: Eggs forming a plate or exhibit to be uniform in shape, shell texture, size, colour and appearance.

INTERNAL

Yolk: Rich, bright golden yellow, free from blood streaks, or 'meat' spots. Well rounded and well raised from the centre of the albumen. One uniform shade. Blastoderm or germ spot not discoloured and there should be no sign of embryo development.

Albumen: This is clear with no signs of blood spots or cloudiness and preferably with no tint of colour. It is of dense substance, particularly around the yolk and the differentiation between this thick albumen and the thin outer should be distinct. Waterfowl albumen must be clear, it is also more viscous and distinct than the hen's albumen; for these reasons waterfowl contents should be exhibited in classes separate from large fowl and bantam.

Chalazae: Each chalaza to resemble a thick cord of white albumen opposite each other and attached to the yolk, keeping it to the centre of the inner albumen. Free of blood and 'meat' spots.

Airspace: Small, about 1.5 cm ($\frac{1}{2}$ in.) diameter (1 cm ($\frac{3}{16}$ in.) bantams), the membrane adhering to the shell. It should be placed at the broad (dome) end, ideally just to one side.

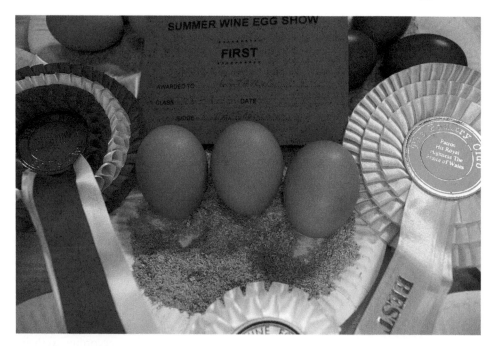

Eggs: three matching

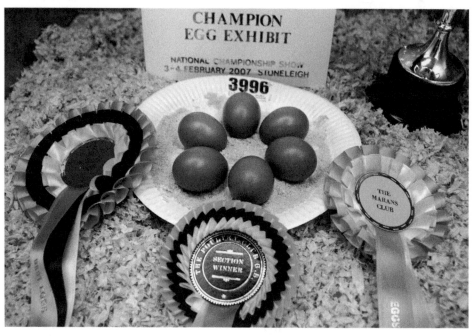

Eggs: six matching

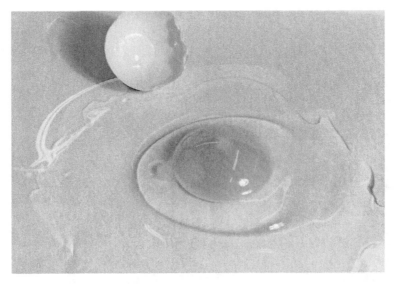

Fresh egg contents: raised yolk, thick albumen and small air sac

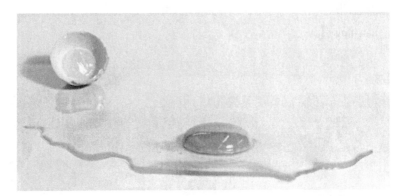

Stale egg contents: flat yolk, thin albumen, large air sac and blood spots.

Freshness: Indicated by small, taut airspace and unwrinkled top surface of yolk, which should be raised and not lacking in height. A stale albumen lacks differentiation and is watery and runny.

Scale of points

External

Shape	25
Size	15
Shell texture	20
Colour	20
Freshness, bloom and appearance	20
	100*

Footnote: May be maximum for each egg, or for a plate of eggs, whatever the number. Add 5 points more for each egg for matching and uniformity.

Internal

Yolk	30
Albumen	30
Chalazae	10
Airspace	10
Freshness	20
	100

Serious defects (for which eggs should be passed)

More than one yolk. Staleness. Polished or overprepared shells. Overweight in bantam eggs, including contents classes. A developing embryo as shown by a 'halo' around the germ spot. Excessive blood streaks and 'meat' spots.

Disqualification

Addition of colouring to shells. Artificial polish or colouring would amount to disqualification and a report to the Poultry Club of Great Britain.

STANDARDS FOR PAINTED, DECORATED AND DISPLAYED EGGS

Shows can provide egg classes for prepared eggs. Variously classified as painted, decorated and displayed.

Painted eggs

These eggs, either blown or hard-boiled, are painted with any of the usual media: oils, watercolours, inks, etc. There must be no other adornment whatsoever, not even beads for eyes or bits of extra shell to provide texture. To set them off nicely, the organisers should provide physical support: about 3 cm ($1\frac{1}{4}$ in.) diameter cardboard rings, 1.25 cm ($\frac{1}{2}$ in.) deep, in which the egg can be placed upright.

Impression/artistic effect	25
Originality/concept/subject matter	25
Quality of painting	25
Use of colour	25
	100

Decorated eggs

Here the egg is often painted, but in addition there is some form of decoration. They range from the very elaborate eggs, whose shells have been cut, revealing painted interiors behind open doors or drawers, to simply decorated eggs. In all cases the egg must be seen and its shape recognisable. Decoration can take the form of beads, cardboard, shells and, of course, colouring.

Impression/artistic effect	20
Originality/concept/subject matter	20
Quality of construction	20
Use of colour	20
Use of materials	20
	100

Displayed eggs

Unlike the other two classes, this is usually for several eggs, usually six, the eggs themselves being unadorned. The exhibit consists of suitably chosen materials (cloth, flowers, bark or cardboard) that serves to highlight the clutch of eggs within the arrangement. It is only in the displayed eggs that credit is given to the eggs used. Ill-matched, poor textured eggs would not enhance the overall effect of the exhibit and be penalised. Arrangements can include bantam, fowl and duck eggs, providing their shape is a match and their shells an even texture. Different colours, too, would not be penalised if such contrast were helpful to the general effect.

Impression/artistic effect	30
Originality/concept/subject matter	25
Use of materials	25
Quality and matching of eggs used	20
	100

Judging is quite subjective, even with the scale of points outlined above. Because of this, these exhibits cannot be awarded Poultry Club Bronze Awards at Poultry Shows, or awards above Bronze tier at Championship Egg Shows.

Glossary

Abdomen   Underpart of body from keel to vent.

A.O.C.   Any other colour.

A.O.V.   Any other variety.

Axial feather   Small feather between wing primaries and secondaries (not waterfowl).

Back   Top of body from base of neck to beginning of tail.

Bands   Stripes straight across a feather (see also 'Cuckoo banding' and 'Pencilling').

Bantam   Miniature fowl, formerly accepted as one-fifth the weight of the large breed it represented, but nowadays one-quarter.

Barring   Alternate stripes of light and dark across a feather, most distinctly seen in the barred Plymouth Rock.

Bay   A reddish brown colour (see also 'Wing bay').

Beak   The two horny mandibles projecting from the front of the face.

Bean   A black spot or mark (generally raised) at the tip of the upper mandible of a duck's bill, seen in Cayugas and other breeds of waterfowl.

Beard   A bunch of feathers under the throat of some fowls, such as the Faverolles, Houdan and some varieties of Poland. A tuft of coarse hair growing from the breast of an adult turkey male, also known as the 'tassel'.

Beetle brows   Heavy overhanging eyebrows, best seen in the Malay.

Bill   A duck's beak.

Blade   Rear part of a single comb.

Blocky   Heavy and square in build.

Booted   Feathers projecting from the shanks and toes, as in the Brahma, Cochin and Booted bantam.

Boule   Hackle starting at sides of throat with a tendency to join behind the neck to form a mane, very thick and convexly arched, reaching to shoulder and saddle and covering the whole back. Seen in some Belgian bantams and Orloffs.

Bow legged   Greater distance between legs at the hocks than at knees and feet.

Brassiness   Yellowish colouring on white plumage, usually on back and wing.

Breast   Front of a fowl's body from point of keel bone to base of the neck. In dead birds, flesh on the keel bone.

Breed   A group of birds answering truly to the type, carriage and characteristics distinctive of the breed name they take. There may be varieties within a breed, distinguished by differences of colour and markings.

Cap   A comb; also the backpart of a fowl's skull; head markings as seen in some ducks.

Cape   Feathers under and at the base of the neck hackle, between the shoulders.

Capon   Strictly speaking a castrated male fowl, but term is also used to describe one treated chemically (now illegal).

Carriage   The bearing, attitude or style of a bird, especially when walking.

Caruncles   Fleshy protuberances on head and wattles of turkeys and Muscovy ducks.

Cere   Coloured skin around eye.

Chicken   A term employed by the Poultry Club to describe a bird of the current season's breeding.

Cinnamon   A dark reddish buff colour.

Cloddy   See 'Blocky'.

Cloudy   Indistinct (see 'Mossy').

Cobby   Short, round or compact in build.

Cock   A male bird after the first moult.

Cockerel   A male bird before his first adult moult.

Cockerel-breeder   A term applied to birds, either male or female, selected to produce good standard bred cockerels.

Collar   A white mark almost encircling the neck of the Rouen drake, also known as the 'ring'.

Comb   Fleshy protuberance on top of a fowl's head, varying considerably in type and size and including cushion (Silkie), horn or V-shaped (La Flèche and Sultan), leaf or shell (Houdan), pea or triple (Brahma), rose (Hamburgh, Wyandotte, etc.), single (Cochin, Leghorn, etc.), cup (Sicilian Buttercup), strawberry or walnut (Malay) and raspberry (Orloff).

British Poultry Standards, Seventh Edition. Edited by J. Ian H. Allonby and Philippe B. Wilson.
© 2019 Poultry Club of Great Britain. Published 2019 by John Wiley & Sons Ltd.

Concave sweep   Hollow curve from shoulders to part way up the tail.

Condition   State of a bird's health, brightness of comb and face and freshness of plumage.

Corky   Light but firm handling characteristic in Old English Game.

Coverts   Covering feathers on tail and wings.

Cow hocks   Weakness at hocks (see 'Knock-kneed').

Crescent   Shaped like the first or last quarter of the moon.

Crest   A crown or tuft of feathers on the head; known also as 'top knot' and in Old English Game as the 'tassel'.

Crow head   Head and beak narrow and shallow, like a crow.

Crown   The area of the head above the eye.

Cuckoo banding   Irregular banding where the two colours are somewhat indistinct and run into each other, as in the cuckoo Leghorn and Marans.

Culmen   The top line of a waterfowl bill when viewed sideways on.

Cup comb   A comb somewhat resembling a teacup with the edges spiked as in the Sicilian Buttercup.

Cushion   A mass of feathers over the back of a female covering the root of her tail, and most prominently developed in the Cochin.

Cushion comb   An almost circular cushion of flesh, with a number of small prominences over it, and having a slight furrow transversely across the middle, as in the Silkie.

Daw eyed   Having pearl-coloured eyes (like a jackdaw).

Deaf-ears   see 'Ear-lobes'.

Dewlap   The gullet (so-called), seen to the best advantage in adult Toulouse geese. Loose pouch of skin on throat under the beak.

Diamond   The wing bay. A term commonly used among Game fanciers.

Dished bill   Depression or hollow in the upper line of the bill of a duck or drake.

Dished lobe   Lobe that is hollow in the centre.

Double comb   see 'Rose comb'.

Double laced   Two lacings of black as on an Indian Game female's feather. First there is the outer black lacing round the edge of the feather and next the inner or 'second' lacing (see 'Lacing').

Down   Initial hairy covering of baby chick, ducklings, etc. Also the fluffy part of the feather below the web and small tufts sometimes seen as faults on toes and legs of clean-legged breeds (see 'Fluff').

Down billed   The waterfowl face is held at a normal angle but the bill has a downward tilt instead of being set squarely into the face, as in a Call Duck.

Down faced   The whole waterfowl head is held permanently at a downward angle from what would be the norm for the breed, e.g. in a Call Duck, with the bill at the correct angle to the face.

Drake   Male duck.

Dual lobed   see 'Lobe'.

Duck   General term for certain species of waterfowl, and also used to describe the female.

Duck footed   Fowls having the rear toe lying close to the floor instead of spread out, thus resembling the foot of a duck.

Dusky   Yellow pigment shaded with black.

Ear-lobes   Folds of skin hanging below the ears, sometimes called 'deaf-ears'. They vary in size, shape and colour, the last named including purple-black, turquoise-blue, cream, red and white.

Eye ring   Ring of coloured skin around the eye in waterfowl.

Face   The skin in front of, behind and around the eyes.

Feather legged   Characteristic of breeds such as the Brahma, Cochin, Faverolles, etc. May be sparsely feathered down to the outer toes, as in the Faverolles, or profusely feathered to the extremity of the middle and outer toes, as in the Brahma. Serious defect in clean-legged breeds.

Fish billed   The bill in waterfowl has convex or flattened sides revealing exaggerated serrations, a defect.

Flat shins   Shanks that are flat fronted instead of rounded.

Flight coverts   Small stiff feathers covering base of the primaries.

Flights   see 'Primaries'.

Fluff   Soft downy feathers around the thighs, chiefly developed in birds of the Cochin type; the downy part of the feather (the undercolour) not seen as a rule until the bird is handled; also the hair-like growth sometimes found on the shanks and feet of clean-legged fowls, and in this case a defect.

Footings   see 'Booted'.

Foxy   Rusty or reddish in colour (see also 'Rust').

Frizzled   Curled; each feather turning backwards so that it points towards the head of the bird.

Furnished   Feathered and adorned as an adult. A cockerel that has grown his full tail, hackles, comb, etc. is said to be 'furnished'.

Gander   The male of geese.

Gay   Excess white in markings of plumage.

Goose   The female of geese.

Grizzled   Grey in the flights of an otherwise black bird.

Ground colour   Main colour of body plumage on which markings are applied.

Gullet   The loose part of the lower mandible; the dewlap of a goose. It appears on fowls, and is seen most distinctly perhaps on old Cochin hens, when it resembles a miniature beard of feathers.

Gypsy face   The skin of the face a dark purple or mulberry colour.

Hackles   The neck feathers of a fowl and the saddle plumage of a male consisting of long, narrow, pointed feathers.

Hangers   Feathers hanging from the posterior part of a male fowl – the lesser sickles and tail coverts known as tail hangers, and the saddle hackle as saddle hangers.

Hard feather   Close tight feathering as found on Game birds.

Head   Comprises skull, comb, face, eyes, beak, ear-lobes and wattles.

Hen   A female after the first adult moult.

Hen feathered   A male bird without sickles or pointed hackles (sometimes called a 'henny').

Hind toe   The fourth or back toe of a fowl.

Hock   Joint of the thigh with the shank, sometimes called the knee or the elbow.

Hollow comb   Depression in comb.

Hollow lobes   Depression in ear-lobes.

Horn comb   A comb said to resemble horns, but generally similar to the letter V, and seen to the best advantage on a matured La Flèche or Sultan male. The comb starts just above the beak, and from it branch two spikes thick at the base and tapered at the end.

In-kneed   see 'Knock-kneed'.

Iris   Coloured portion of eye surrounding the pupil.

Keel   Blade of the breastbone; in ducks the dependent flesh and skin below it. In geese the loose pendant fold of skin suspended from the underpart of the bone.

Keel bone   Breastbone or sternum.

Knob   Protuberance on upper mandible of certain brands of geese.

Knock-kneed   Hocks close together instead of well apart.

Lacing   A stripe or edging all round a feather, differing in colour from that of the ground; single in such breeds as the Andalusian, Wyandotte and Sebright bantams, and double in Indian Game and other females. In the last case the inner lacing not as broad as the outer (see also 'Double laced').

Leader   The single spike terminating the rose type of comb; also known as the 'spike'.

Leaf comb   A comb resembling the shape of a butterfly with its wings nearly wide open, and the body of the insect resting on the front of the fowl's head. It has also been referred to as resembling two scallop shells joined near the base, the join covered with a piece of coral. Seen to the best advantage on a Houdan male.

Leg   The shank or scaly part.

Leg feathers   Feathers projecting from the outer sides of the shanks of such breeds as the Brahma, Cochin, Faverolles, Langshan and Silkie.

Lesser sickles   see 'Sickles'.

Lobe   (see 'Ear-lobes' for fowl) In waterfowl the pouch in between the bird's legs. Dual lobed means two pouches; single lobed one central pouch.

Lopped comb   Falling over to one side of the head.

Lustre   see 'Sheen'.

Main tail feathers   see 'Tail feathers'.

Mandibles   Horny upper and lower parts of beak or bill.

Marking   The barring, lacing, pencilling, spangling, etc. of the plumage.

Mealy   Stippled with a lighter shade, as though dusted with meal, a defect in buff-coloured fowls.

Moons   Round spangles on tips of feathers.

Mossy   Confused or indistinct marking; smudging or peppering. A defect in most breeds.

Mossy backed   Excess pencilling on back or rump feathers in some colour varieties of female Call Ducks, where the darker pencilling on the feather has smudged or peppered to take over as the main colour on the body of the feather. In worst cases just a fine edging or none of the original ground colour remains.

Mottled   Marked with tips or spots of different colour.

Moult   The annual replacement of old feathers with new ones.

Muff   Tufts of feathers on each side of the face and attached to the beard, seen in such breeds as the Faverolles, Houdan and some varieties of Poland; also known as 'whiskers'.

Muffling   The beard and whiskers, i.e. the whole of the face feathering except the crest. In Old English Game the muffed variety has a thick muff or growth of feathers under the throat, differing in formation from that of the breeds named under 'Muff'.

Mulberry   see 'Gypsy face'.

Nankin See breed for colour description.

Open barring Where the bars on a feather are wide apart.

Open lacing Narrow outer lacing, which gives the feather a larger open centre of ground colour.

Outer lacing Lacing around the outer edge of a feather as opposed to 'inner' lacing.

Parti-coloured Breed or variety having feathers of two or more colours, or shades of colour.

Paunch see 'Lobe'.

Pea comb A triple comb, resembling three small single combs joined together at the base and rear, but distinctly divided, the middle of one being the highest; best seen on the head of a well-bred Brahma.

Pearl eyed Eyes pearl coloured. Sometimes referred to as 'daw eyed'.

Pencilled spikes The spikes of a single comb that are very long and narrow; little broader at the base than at the top; generally a defect.

Pencilling Small markings or stripes on a feather, straight across in Hamburgh females (and often known as bands); or concentric in form, following the outline of the feather, as in the Brahma (dark), Cochin (partridge), Dorking (silver grey) and Wyandotte (partridge and silver pencilled) females, and fine stippled markings on females of Old English Game and brown Leghorns.

Peppering The effect of sprinkling a darker colour over one of a lighter shade.

Primaries Flight feathers of the wing, tucked out of sight when the bird is at rest. Ten in number.

Primary coverts See 'Flight coverts'.

Pullet A female fowl before her first adult moult.

Pullet-breeder A term applied to birds, either male or female, selected to produce good standard bred pullets.

Pupil Black centre of eye.

Quill Hollow stem of feather attaching it to the body.

Raspberry comb A comb somewhat resembling a raspberry cut through its axis (lengthwise) and covered with small protuberances.

Reachy Tall and upright carriage and 'lift' as in Modern Game.

Ring see 'Collar'.

Roach back Humped back, a deformity.

Rose comb A broad comb, nearly flat on top, covered with small regular points or 'work', and finishing with a spike or leader. It varies in length, width and carriage according to breed.

Rust A patch of red-brown colour on the wings of females of some breeds, chiefly those of the black-red colour; brown or red marking in black fluff or breast feathers; known also as 'foxiness' in females.

Saddle The posterior part of the back, reaching to the tail of the male, and corresponding to the cushion in a female.

Saddle hackle see 'Hackles'.

Sandiness Giving the appearance of having been sprinkled with sand.

Sappiness A yellow tinge in plumage.

Scapulars Shoulder feathers, which may be elongated in waterfowl.

Secondaries The quill feathers of the wings that are visible when the wings are closed.

Self colour A uniform colour, unmixed with any other.

Serrations 'Sawtooth' sections of a single comb. The filtering apparatus at the side of the waterfowl bill.

Shaft The stem or quill part of the feather.

Shafty Lighter coloured on the stem than on the webbing; a desirable marking in dark Dorking females and Welsummers. Generally a defect in other breeds.

Shank see 'Leg'.

Shank feathering See 'Feather legged'.

Sheen Bright surface gloss on black plumage. In other colours usually described as lustre.

Shell comb see 'Leaf comb'.

Shoulder The upper part of the wing nearest the neck feather. Prominent in Game breeds, where it is often called the shoulder butt (see also 'Wing butt' and 'Scapulars').

Sickles The long curved feathers of a male's tail, usually applied to the top pair only (the others often being called the 'lesser' sickles), but sometimes used for the tail coverts.

Side sprig An extra spike growing out of the side of a single comb, a defect.

Single comb A comb which, when viewed from the front, is narrow, and having spikes in line behind each other. It consists of a blade surmounted by spikes, the lower (solid) portion being the blade, and the spaces between the spikes the serrations. It differs in size, shape and number of serrations according to breeds.

Slipped wing A wing in which the primary flight feathers hang below the secondaries when the wing is closed. This condition is often allied with split wing, in which primaries and secondaries show a very distinct segregation.

Smoky undercolour Defective grey pigment in the undercolour of a bird.

Smut Dark or smutty colour where undesirable, such as in undercolour.

Soft feather Applied to breeds other than the hard feather group of Asian Hardfeather, Indian and Jubilee Game, Old English Game and Modern Game.

Sootiness Grey or smokiness creeping in where it is not wanted, usually in undercolour.

Spangling The marking produced by a spot of colour at the end of each feather differing from that of the ground colour. When applied to a laced breed, such as the Poland, it means broader lacing at the tip of each feather. The spangle of circular form is the more correct, since, when of crescent or horseshoe shape, it favours the laced character.

Spike The rear leader on a rose comb.

Splashed feather A contrasting colour irregularly splashed on a feather.

Split comb The rear blade of a single comb is split or divided.

Split crest Divided crest that falls over on both sides.

Split tail Decided gap in middle of tail at base.

Split wing See 'Slipped wing'.

Sprig See 'Side sprig'.

Spur A projection of horny substance on the shanks of males, and sometimes on females.

Squirrel tail A tail, any part of which projects in front of a perpendicular line over the back; a tail that bends sharply over the back and touches, or almost touches, the head, like that of a squirrel.

Stern In waterfowl, the area between the lower abdomen and the tail.

Strain A family of birds from any breed or variety carefully bred over a number of years.

Strawberry comb A comb somewhat resembling half a strawberry, with the round part of the fruit uppermost; known also as the 'walnut comb'.

Striping The very important markings down the middle of hackle feathers, particularly in males of the partridge variety.

Stub Short, partly grown feather.

Sub-variety see 'Variety'.

Surface colour That portion of the feathers exposed to view.

Sword feathered Having sickles only slightly curved, or scimitar shaped, as in Japanese bantams.

Symmetry Perfection of outline, proportion; harmony of all parts.

Tail coverts see 'Coverts'.

Tail feathers Straight and stiff feathers of the tail only. The top pair are sometimes slightly curved, but they are generally straight or nearly

so. In the male fowl, the main tail feathers are contained inside the sickles and coverts.

Tassel see 'Crest' and 'Beard'.

Tertiaries Feathers attached to the humerus (wing bone closest to the body) and overlying the secondaries. May be elongated in waterfowl.

Thigh That part of the leg above the shank, and covered with feathers.

Thumb-marked comb A single comb possessing indentations in the blade: a defect.

Ticked Plumage tipped with a different colour, usually applied to V-shaped markings as in the Ancona. Also small coloured specks on any part of feathers of different colour from that of the ground colour.

Tipping End of feathers tipped with a different coloured marking.

Top colour See 'Surface colour'.

Top-knot see 'Crest'.

Tri-coloured Of three colours.

Trio A male and two females.

Triple comb see 'Pea comb'.

Twisted comb A faulty shaped pea or single comb.

Twisted feather The shaft and web of the feather are twisted out of shape.

Type Mould, character or shape (see 'Symmetry').

Undercolour Colour seen when a bird is handled – that is, when the feathers are lifted; colour of fluff of feathers.

Uropygium Parson's nose.

Variety A definite branch of a breed known by its distinctive colour or marking – for example, the black is a variety of the Leghorn. Sub-variety, a sub-division of an established variety, differing in shape of comb from the original – for example, the rose-combed black is a sub-variety of the black Leghorn. Thus the breed includes all the varieties and sub-varieties that would conform to the same standard type.

V-shaped comb See 'Horn comb'.

Vulture hocks Stiff projecting quill feathers at the hock joint, growing on the thighs and extending backwards.

Walnut comb see 'Strawberry comb'.

Wattles The fleshy appendages at each side of the base of the beak, more strongly developed in male birds.

Web A flat and thin structure. Web of feather: the flat or plume portion. Web of feet: the flat skin between the toes. Web of wing: the triangular skin seen when the wing is extended.

Well glossed Equivalent to beetle-green sheen.

Whiskers Feathers growing from the sides of the face (see 'Beard' and 'Muff').

Wing bar Any line of dark colour across the middle of the wing, caused by the colour or marking of the feathers known as the lower wing coverts.

Wing bay The triangular part of the folded wing between the wing bar and the point (see 'Diamond').

Wing bow The upper or shoulder part of the wing.

Wing butt or Wing point The end of the primaries; the corners or ends of the wing. The upper ends are more properly called the shoulder butts and are thus termed by Game fanciers. The lower, similarly, are often called the lower butts.

Wing coverts The feathers covering the roots of the secondary quills.

Work The small spikes or working on top of a rose comb.

Wry back A distorted bone structure usually causing a humpbacked condition.

Wry tail A tail carried awry, to the right or left side of the continuation of the backbone, and not straight with the body of the fowl.

Printed and bound by CPI Group (UK) Ltd, Croydon, CR0 4YY

27/10/2024

14580355-0001